The Om Births Approach

How to use your yoga practice to prepare body, mind, and spirit for birth

a book for pregnant yoginis and the people who teach them

Bec Conant

E-RYT 500, RPYT, HBCE, BCCE, SpBCPE

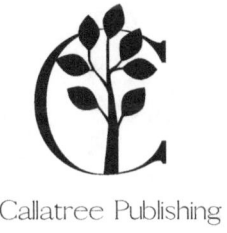

Callatree Publishing

Printed in the United States of America.

ISBN: 979-8-218-14059-5

Cover Photograph: Documenting Life's Moments
Photography: Natalie Nigito Photography
Illustrations: Lauren G. Levine and Bec Conant
Cover and page production: Jenny Putnam

Testimonials for *The Om Births Method*

" I spent three nights in early labor with tons of contractions that came at night and disappeared in the day. I could say I spent three nights in cat/cow. Then Monday, the night before my induction was scheduled, my mind must have subconsciously kicked my system to buck up and birth my baby already. My doula called it a 'precipitous labor' where I literally had my baby 1.5hrs after we reached the hospital.

I can't thank Om Births enough for all the mental and physical tools you gave me through our yoga practice. I must have seen Bec's face and heard her voice telling me to lean into the feeling, dance and be present numerous times that night as it got hard."

Shilpi, Om Births Mom

"I enjoyed Om Births yoga classes so much. Bec made me feel so incredibly empowered as a first time mom with all my crazy body changes. I was in early/active labor for a round 12 hours and pushed for only 50 minutes before he made his debut!!
He was born a healthy 8 lbs 11 oz

I credit so much of it to Bec's INCREDIBLE prenatal yoga classes"

Rebecca, Om Births Mom

"Om Births' classes helped keep me from having a c-section even when I had to be induced 3 weeks early. I still had my son vaginally, which was my birth plan even when all other plans went out the window. Thank you so much!"

Brande, Om Births Mom

Other Published material by Bec Conant and Om Births

Prenatal Yoga with Bec Conant
DVD

Published by Heart of the Moon Media
October 2008

Available on Amazon and through the Om Births platform: www.ombirths.com

A note for pregnant readers

The information contained in this book is for people who have an understanding of yoga who are interested in continuing and using their yoga practice as part of their birth preparation. This book is in no way intended as a substitute for medical advice. If you are pregnant, please consult with your care provider about any practices which you have concern about. Cease practicing and seek medical attention if you have any bleeding during pregnancy or if you have specific medical concerns regarding your pregnancy. Your provider knows your pregnancy better than any book.

A note on pronouns

I grew up and was trained at a time when the default pronouns for expecting people were she/her and mom. I have come to recognize that not all pregnant people identify as female, mom, or use the she/her pronouns—though many also do. In this text I have endeavored to use more gender neutral pronouns and not assume how a pregnant person might choose to identify themselves as they transition into parenthood. That said, there are some places where the terms mom and she/her still remain. I hope readers will bear with this transition in personal identity and forgive places where I may have used a pronoun they did not themselves consider personal.

A seemingly unnecessary disclaimer for yoga teachers

This book by itself will not certify you as a prenatal yoga teacher or provide the prenatal yoga training you need to apply to a certifying body such as Yoga Alliance. There are aspects of teaching prenatal yoga at a certified level which must be transmitted directly from teacher to student. There are also exams, projects, and observations: basically, the down and dirty work of implementing the information laid out in this book. This book is designed to increase your understanding about how to work with a pre- and postnatal population, but a book alone does not constitute a training. For full certification please visit ombirths.com and read more about our Yoga Alliance-certified prenatal teacher training.

Dedication

For all birthing people pre and postnatal and all the people working with them,
and for Sawyer

Table of Contents

Introduction

There is nothing in this universe more primal, more powerful, or more sacred than a mother giving life to her child.

—Unknown

Why are you here?

I start every prenatal teacher training with this question. "Why are you here?"

I borrowed the question from a meditation in Nancy Bardacke's book *Mindful Birthing.* In this meditation, students close their eyes and visualize themselves dropping a stone, symbolizing the question, into a deep well. As the stone sinks, different answers arise from ever deeper parts of their consciousness. After allowing whatever is ready to arise, which may include nothing, we open with the sound of Om.

Often, students come to training weekends with ideas about what it means to work with pregnant women. Often, they come with a great deal of fear. Sometimes, there is a lack of information—or worse, misinformation—about yoga and pregnancy. Students may arrive with highly medicalized images of pregnancy, or they may be enthralled with the earth/mother/goddess aspect of the birth experience. And sometimes it is all of the above. What I have found is that getting these expectations on the table is vital to working with the clarity, precision, and gentleness required to unpack a topic as big as yoga during pregnancy.

I ask you the same question: Why are you here? You may be seeking guidance on how to practice yoga yourself, and you may yourself be pregnant. If that is the case, welcome! This book will absolutely give you tools for structuring and deepening your practice while pregnant. It will also delve into why we might practice in certain ways while pregnant which differ from the classic yogic *asanas* and *pranayamas.* You'll learn ways to practice during pregnancy and how that practice can affect not only your comfort throughout pregnancy but the process of labor and birth itself. Our yoga practice during pregnancy literally has the potential to impact how we welcome our babies into our arms and shape the next generation of humans coming into this world. I am delighted to welcome you into this yoga family!

Or maybe you found this title because you currently teach yoga and are curious about how to apply it to a pregnant population. At the time of this writing, there are over 18,000 yoga studios in the United States producing graduates from their teacher training prgrams, but few of these new teachers emerge knowing how to confidently work with pregnant students.

Why would you want to teach yoga to pregnant people? Whether your reasons are to better serve whomever walks into your room or possibly to delve deeper into the world of pregnancy and birth itself, this book aims to help. My goal is to remove some of the fears, misconceptions, and myths that have developed around prenatal yoga and give you a solid teaching foundation to help you guide pregnant women with confidence and compassion.

My story

My journey here started in 2000, in New York City, where I took my first yoga teacher training. At the time, I had no real interest in pregnancy or women's health. I was a budding modern dancer, and yoga seemed a good way to explore movement and connection to my body, not to mention improve my flexibility.

I finished the five months of course work, observed and assisted the required classes, taught my final exam class, and received my shiny new 200-hour Registered Yoga Teacher certification. Armed with my newfound knowledge and yogic understanding, I began offering small group sessions at a local gym. Shortly thereafter, I was offered the chance to teach an open level class at the studio where I had trained. Thrilled at the chance to join this revered group of yoga faculty, I painstakingly planned out my sequence and cultivated my playlist.

On the day of my first class, fighting both anxiety and excitement, I walked into the room. Before me sat seven students with their mats and props neatly arranged. Five of the students were clearly pregnant—and of those five, three were evidently in their third trimester!

My mind froze. I attempted to "take my seat" (our school's term for stepping in and embodying the space of the teacher) at the front of the room—but everything was buzzing. As I welcomed the students into class and began my centering meditation, my thoughts raced back to the half day at the start of my training when we had covered what to do and not do with pregnant students. I couldn't remember any of it. That information had long since been replaced with details about backbends and how to create a dynamic sequence. With a not-so-small prayer to the universe to give me guidance, we chanted our opening Oms and off we went.

I'm fairly certain I did not give those five pregnant people much of a yoga class that day. The only thought I remember working with was "Um, breathe, and don't hurt the baby!" I should clarify that this story is not meant to disparage the quality of my 200-hour training program. The challenge I faced is endemic to all 200-hour trainings. There simply is not enough time to explore the intricacies and nuances of yoga during the perinatal[1] experience—not when you are also covering the *yamas* and *niyamas*, *pranayama*, *Tadasana*, *Shavasana*, and everything in between. Again, the level of teaching in those trainings is not at issue. The issue is that there is too much content around pregnancy and the postpartum period to cover everything in detail within that setting. And, to be fair, not all students are interested enough to want the full experience.

After that extremely humbling moment, I began casting around for someone who could give me guidance on how to better serve pregnant students who walked into my yoga classes. I happened upon a one-day training entitled "Teaching Yoga to Pregnant Women." "Thank

---

[1] Perinatal: The period from conception until one year following the baby's birth

goodness!" I thought. "Here is the very information I'm seeking!" But while the workshop was filled with interesting tidbits on the birth process and physiology of pregnancy, the general teaching when it came to *asana* was, "Just trust the pregnant woman. She will know what she should and shouldn't be doing…" (You have to imagine that being said with a very breathy, flower-child air to it.) This guidance left me feeling uncertain. Like a vast river with no banks to give it direction, I could feel myself becoming lost in the sea of yoga postures and breathing practices, unsure of which might feel better or worse to a pregnant student.

So I kept searching, happening upon a three-day training taught north of the city. Figuring that the problem had been that a single day was not long enough to give the full scope of yoga during pregnancy, I eagerly enrolled. This training immediately contradicted nearly everything the previous one had suggested. Whereas my previous training had introduced the idea that a pregnant woman could be trusted to know her own body, this training took the opposite approach. I left the weekend with a long list of postures and movements that pregnant women apparently should never attempt. They were not to twist, lie on their backs, or do any breathing practices at all. They certainly could not invert or lie prone—even with props. And above all, they were so hypermobile that any posture with the feet wider than three feet apart was destined to destroy their pelvic integrity. (We will address some of these claims in later chapters.)

Needless to say, I came out of that weekend even more confused. Was the pregnant body a fragile, delicate, high-risk object that should only be moved with the greatest of care? Or could the pregnant woman be trusted to move and bend as she felt was best? I didn't know. As if I wasn't uncomfortable enough, the studios where I was teaching asked if I would offer prenatal classes on their schedules! I needed the work, so I accepted, and I began piecing together these two opposing pictures as I observed my students and their practices during pregnancy.

It is here that I must thank Judith Hanson Lasater for bringing some clarity into the picture at last and providing the bridge (or perhaps yoke?) between the two extremes of the prenatal yoga world. In the midst of what was turning into my own personal trial by fire teaching pregnant women, Judith was teaching in New York and mentioned that she would be leading a weeklong training on teaching "prenatal yoga and yoga during pregnancy" in San Francisco. "Ah!" I thought, "A full week will clearly be enough time to put these two pictures together!" What I didn't realize was that along with being a yoga training, this was also a training to become a birth doula[2] and would include sections taught by a midwife and a doula.

As it turned out, it was the doula training, not the yoga, which provided the missing piece of how to bring the full yoga practice to pregnant mothers. My earlier trainings had either focused purely on safety concerns or waxed too poetic about the goddess quality of motherhood. The doula perspective offered a deep understanding of the physicality and process of labor and birth—but also an inherent trust in the body's ability to birth a baby without

---

[2] Professional support person for a pregnant person during the labor process, sometimes referred to as a birth coach

intervention unless the mother wished for it, at least most of the time. This training got into the structure of the pelvic joints, and how and why to fully support them. It walked through the different stages of labor and birth and addressed why each phase might need different levels of support and mental focus.

The message was clear: the pregnant body is strong. It is not sick or injured, just different in special ways. If you can understand how this body is specifically different from the body of a novice yoga student, then it becomes clear what yoga can be done, where it needs modification, and which practices should be avoided to best support the growing mother/baby dyad. I also began to realize that teaching "prenatal yoga" was something different than "teaching yoga to pregnant people." The latter is a basic yoga practice modified for the pregnant body. The former includes the full experience of the transformation of pregnancy, the preparation for labor, the cultural ideas and judgments around types of birth and ways of parenting, and even the time following the baby's birth, when moms and babies meet one another and move into a new type of yoga together. The yoga practice can be a method to better understand, and maybe embrace, the entire experience of pregnancy, birth, and motherhood. It is from this principle that this book is born.

Birth is more than a physical process. Our cultures also surround us with assumptions, stories, and images of birth. There may be no topic which has greater fear and emotion surrounding it than the birth of a baby. For some of you, this book will be the first time you interact with the effects of modern medicine on the birth experience (both good and bad) or the first time you directly consider the cultural stories we have around birth and motherhood. Yoga teachers addressing the needs of your pregnant students, it is worth examining the prevailing views your students will face during their pregnancies, whether they wish to or not.

A quick history of birth

What comes to mind when you think of childbirth? I also ask this question during my prenatal yoga teacher training. It is an exercise I borrow from my HypnoBirthing® childbirth classes as a way of surfacing deeply held, and usually unquestioned, images and assumptions about the childbirth process. The answers range from comical (screaming "You did this to me!"), to idealistic (transformative life affirmation), to technical (hospitals, needles, blood). Inevitably, two concepts come up every single time: pain and fear.

Birth has serious baggage. Linked with the miraculous emergence of the baby is the long history of controlling the body, controlling women's bodies, and controlling women. If you think these ideas don't come into the room when practicing yoga pregnant, think again. Everyone has a story in their head, whether they know it or not. Some are positive, and I revel when I find students who have come into matrescence[3] excited and standing in their power. But all too often, the images we carry are of intense pain, life-threatening complications, disempowerment, and, in extreme cases, death. Women want to bask in the exciting, celebratory

---

[3] A term coined by Psychologist Aurelie Athan in the 1970s to describe the transition and process during which one becomes a mother, similar to the transition involved in adolescence.

aspects of birth, but as their estimated due date approaches, many women's experiences come to be dominated by fear. They wonder whether their bodies are capable of birthing, how they will survive (not endure—survive) the pain, and what they will do afterwards. Given that women have been birthing babies for thousands of years, it would seem that the birth process works. So where does this fear come from?

There have been numerous books written on the history of birth, but for our purposes we need only skim the surface to find the origins of fear. (A note here: For the moment I'm going to discuss the major cultural events that have influenced current attitudes towards pregnant and birthing women in the US, events that are largely rooted in European history. Those beliefs are not representative of all beliefs in all cultures, and I acknowledge that not all history, or culture, is "Western" or European.).

At the moment, in Western cultures, birth usually occurs in a hospital setting, where a series of protocols and interventions guide the process to bring a sense of order and "safety." But birth was not always medically controlled and managed. Once upon a time, the birth of a child was a community event. It took place in the home where the child being born would grow up, with many wise women to nurture, support, and guide the mother through the course of her labor. In some ways, we are better off with modern medical advances, and in some ways we are not. The intersection of Western medicine and the birth process has brought about many life-saving techniques, but it has also eroded belief in the ability of a woman's body to give birth without intervention, or, for that matter, without a skilled attendant. The power of women as birth-givers has been steadily degraded and replaced by the science of obstetrics. As a culture, we have nearly forgotten that the female body was in fact designed to give birth and is capable of bringing the baby into the world all by itself.

In a time before medical science, birth was something of a mystery. The connection between sex and pregnancy was not fully understood, and communities were smaller and possibly more female-centric. We have archeological accounts of early Mesopotamian societies where women were revered as the creators of life. Statues of pregnant female figures signify the importance of the mother goddess. Paintings from as far back as the Bronze Age depict female fertility rituals focused on women's ability to create and give birth. We can imagine a baby being welcomed with great celebration. We can also imagine women being revered, viewed as mysterious and a little terrifying. They alone seem to hold the power of continuing the survival of the tribe.

What happened? The big shift seems to start just before the

Middle Ages. A series of legal decrees by the Catholic Church dictated that women were to be secluded and isolated during late pregnancy and birth. These decrees were enforced by local governments that were primarily controlled by the church, whose emphasis on original sin and the subjugation of women led to a societal shift towards centralized control and governance. Rather than being a time when a woman was supported and surrounded by a trusting and wise community, birth became a solitary event.

This period also coincided with the witch burnings in western Europe. During this time, any free-thinking or powerful woman was at risk for persecution and execution. Many of these women were midwives. Who would be more powerful than a woman armed with the knowledge of herbalism and the birth process, who could apparently decide which babies lived and which died? The Church said that this power was reserved for God alone. It is well documented that many of the women who were burned at the stake or drowned during this time were highly skilled, older midwives who could help new mothers work with their labors rather than being trapped in them. The result? Rather than having wise, loving, and supportive women around them, mothers were left to birth by themselves, forced to navigate any twists and turns on their own without guidance.

Many more women birthed in fear, and consequently much greater pain and difficulty, because of the lack of basic maternal wisdom. Nobody was there to suggest different positions or advise on how to avoid a mal-positioned baby. Not coincidentally, it is around this time that the King James Bible has the first mention of Eve's curse: being forced to give birth in pain and suffering. Previously, the words for Adam's and Eve's burden had been the same, "labor," just in different places. Birthing women were denied the presence of a doctor since they were not supposed to be aided in their "labor." They were destined to "suffer" anyway, so why have a doctor's assistance? Although the doctors of the time were not the highly skilled surgeons we now think of as obstetricians. Obstetricians were initially the failing students, who, since they couldn't be trusted to do actual surgery, were allowed to attend "that base process of childbirth." Many graduated medical school without ever having even seen a live baby being born.

The big shift towards obstetrical birth probably began with the invention of forceps in 17th century France. The story goes that King Louis XIV wanted to watch his mistress give birth, so to convenience the king, they laid the woman on her back on a table. As we'll discuss, this isn't the best position for a baby to be born, but the doctors then availed themselves of a new instrument known as forceps and were hailed as geniuses for having discovered how to "get the baby out of mom." I'm sure there was a midwife around somewhere, quietly wondering what the poor woman was doing on her back in the first place. But the result was that Western medicine became focused on getting the baby out, a problem that doesn't actually need solving (unless you force someone into a non-physiological position for birthing).

The introduction of forceps also created a cultural shift whereby doctors were finally allowed to attend to birthing women. Previously they had been forbidden, and the task had fallen to midwives who, because of the knowledge lost in the Middle Ages, were less skilled than their predecessors. Remember, they had burned all the good ones at the stake. Even with medical attendance, birth still retained some odd conventions, such as denying anesthesia (chloroform), because women were seen as destined to suffer during labor. There are many gender-based power dynamics present in the perinatal field. For further reading on this topic, see *Birth as an American Rite of Passage* by Robbie Floyd-Davis or *The Surprising History of How We are Born* by Tina Cassidy.

In 1853, Queen Victoria of England demanded chloroform for her birth with Prince Leopold. Being the Queen, she got whatever she wanted; she was head of the Anglican Church by that time, too, so out went any celestial decrees about hearing women scream in labor. Victoria emerged from the anesthesia hailing it as the best thing ever, and she decreed that henceforth, all women in the British Empire were allowed chloroform for their labors. The British Empire at this time circled the globe, and her pronouncement had a dramatic impact. It opened the door for anesthesia during labor, but it also brought on an additional complication.

The dosage of anesthesia was not standardized, and individual reactions were unpredictable. Mothers had to be closely monitored while under its effects. While birth was actually fairly safe in the home, anesthesia was not. Many labors began shifting into hospitals so doctors could keep a closer eye on their patients. The hospital was put forth as the "modern" way to birth the baby, but the shift had more to do with monitoring, regulating the dosage of anesthesia, and administering resuscitation drugs for either mother or baby if necessary. The downside was that hospital maternity wards at the time were appallingly dirty. Infections ran rampant, and many more women began dying of what became known as "childbed fever," a name for any untreated infection following birth. The death rate for women who birthed in hospitals far exceeded that of women who birthed in their own homes.

Much of the credit for changing birth conditions can be attributed to Florence Nightingale. Using her ability to raise money as influence, she insisted that maternity wards adopt sanitation and cleanliness standards and also saw to it that incompetent doctors were removed from the birth scene.

Unfortunately, once the shift towards anesthesia had been made, the pendulum swung very quickly from unsupervised to overprescribed. Instead of anesthesia being a choice for women, it became the standard practice. Over the years, the methods of anesthetizing women during the birth process moved from chloroform, to ether, to scopolamine (a very dark time in especially the American history of birth when women were strapped down to beds and left half-aware, often in disinhibited and psychotic states, from the drug's side effects). For several generations, women gave birth under various types of anesthesia, in semi-conscious or unconscious states, where babies—often heavily drugged—were pulled out via forceps.

This practice of managing birth with anesthesia and mechanical devices continues in many hospitals. Today, most women give birth with anesthesia known as an epidural, or a combined spinal-epidural, which numbs the sensory nerves below the ribs, allowing a woman to remain awake while feeling hardly anything of her labor. In some ways, the epidural exemplifies the mind-body split in our culture: you can be fully present and rational for the birth of your baby—but not feel anything from the chest down. Certainly epidurals can be a useful tool, and in no way am I suggesting that they should not be used when needed. The same goes for the cesarean section (C-section). Thank goodness we have safe surgical birth in this country for when it is truly needed.

But these interventions are not without consequences. Along with the general medical risks, one major downside to the epidural can be that the nerves to the muscles for pushing are numbed, as is the sensory feedback loop which would normally tell a mother to change positions to help her baby better fit through the birth canal. This limits her ability to work with her body and assist in the birth of the baby. Meanwhile, the medical focus is still on the procedures and possible complications that could arise rather than on the body's innate ability to birth. The result is that 1 in 3 babies in the United States is currently born by major abdominal surgery, and the United States has one of the highest maternal and fetal mortality rates in the industrialized world.[4] Even women who wish for an unmedicated birth often give birth in this anxiety-producing hospital setting.

This is one side of the history of birth in the West, but it is not the whole story. Along with this increasing shift towards medicalization there has more recently been a secondary movement away from technology and back to trusting women and their bodies. Begun during the 1960s and 70s, this "natural childbirth" movement is now sweeping the world. Women have begun asking if there might be a more holistic method for birthing and what techniques they might use to avoid taking drugs or being numbed or cut as they give birth. Popular techniques for natural childbirth include Lamaze®, Bradley®, HypnoBirthing®, Birthing from Within, Mindful Birthing, and Spinning Babies®. The birth community is becoming increasingly polarized, with one side looking for better ways to intervene and the other looking for total autonomy outside the hospital setting. One woman wants to give birth in a tidal pool assisted by dolphin midwives; the other wants a scheduled cesarean without ever having to go into labor.

Natural childbirth takes the approach that birth is something which can, and perhaps should be, accomplished without drugs and without numbing sensation. It is a chance for mom to more fully experience what her body is doing, and if she can do that, then she may even be able to assist her body's own natural processes. As natural childbirth becomes more popular, more hospitals are trying to accommodate patients' wishes. But the very model of the hospital is set up to look for complications and to intervene, not to presume that the process of birth works perfectly well in the first place. The birth process can be adversely affected if that internal wisdom is not respected. Many hospitals still function from the presumption that birth is a medical event that should be highly regulated and controlled in case of an emergen-

---

[4] Centers for Disease Control and Prevention. (2021, March 23). Products - health e stats - maternal mortality rates in the United States, 2019. Centers for Disease Control and Prevention. www.cdc.gov/nchs/products/hestats.htm

cy. Many studies now show that those same regulations interfere with a mother's ability to tap into the internal wisdom she has within her own body.[5]

A woman's body is designed to manage the challenges of pregnancy and birth. Female pelvic structure has wider internal dimensions, allowing for movement not present in the male pelvis. Hormones during pregnancy create even greater pelvic mobility to ease the baby's journey into the world. The body adjusts its posture and carriage throughout the pregnancy to accommodate both the growing belly and increase in weight. During birth, the muscles of the uterus work together to alternatively contract and release, resulting in the thinning and eventual opening of the cervix to create an open passage for the baby. At the same time, the baby goes through specific movements which work with its mother's body to bring it into the world. Without any education or intervention, the body will begin a series of uterine contractions all on its own, the cervix will dilate, and the baby will move down and out of the body. Oxytocin, the hormone which ultimately produces the uterine contractions, is secreted in large amounts during the birth process, and this hormone also brings about an intense bonding between mother and baby that continues as the child grows up. In short, the process of birth works, and it works well. But we have gotten away from the wisdom inherent in the pregnant body, instead turning to medical procedures to ensure birth happens in one specific manner, often according to predictable timelines and landmarks.

This is where yoga comes in. The root word of yoga, *yuj* in Sanskrit, literally means "yoke." Yoga is often defined as a union or yoking of things; mind and body, breath and movement, exercise and our greater life, little self and big self. What about yoking inherent trust in the mother's ability, and her body's ability to birth, with safe medical practices done only when actually necessary? If mothers learned to trust the body's wisdom, to feel what the body is guiding them towards, then maybe birth itself could yoke modern technological advances with ancient wisdom to find its own yoga. And just maybe, that would affect the next generation of humans who come onto this planet…

With the entire range of the yoga experience, a pregnant woman could:

- Learn the practical knowledge of how her body works
- Give voice and understanding to her fears
- Gain the capacity to adjust to inner and outer changes with extraordinary flexibility
- Gather techniques to minimize the fear-tension-pain spiral in labor
- Connect to her growing baby
- Relieve many of the common aches and pains of pregnancy
- Restore the body's overall balance, making space for a possibly easier labor and birth
- Learn to listen to, and to trust, the body's instinctual wisdom
- Embrace sensation while staying present in the moment
- Find space to be herself
- Choose and be supported in the birth that is right for her

---

[5] Jansen, L., Gibson, M., Bowles, B. C., & Leach, J. (2013). First do no harm: Interventions during childbirth. *The Journal of Perinatal Education*. www.ncbi.nlm.nih.gov/pmc/articles/PMC3647734/

Prenatal yoga is about giving power back to women and to pregnant people at large. Pregnancy is not an affliction or illness; mom is not injured or weak during birth. In giving the power back to the birthing person, we empower her to make whatever choices she wants from a place of strength. She can know that her body was specifically designed for birth and then choose whatever birth style she wishes, be it "natural" or not.

How to use this book

This book is divided into three sections intended to break down the enormous topic of yoga and pregnancy into more manageable components: Anatomy, Practice, and Birth. Whether you come to this book with a seasoned yoga practice, a budding pregnancy, a background as a yoga teacher, all, or none of the above, there are several ways to use this material. For pregnant people, I hope this book provides insight and understanding about what is happening in your body and how you can recruit your yoga practice to best serve you in preparing for birth. For those interested in physiology, I hope this book will serve as a reference guide and prompt some reflection on how to truly see and support your pregnant students.

The Anatomy section delves into the structure of the body from both a medical and a yogic perspective. I have found that understanding how the structures of the female body and pelvis fit together, along with the interconnection between the bones, muscles, fascia, and organs, can greatly influence which postures and practices we choose to explore. It also informs how we practice certain *asanas*, especially during pregnancy. Some of the alignment and "classic" yoga instructions are not well suited to the pregnant body, nor are they helpful preparation for birth. I've also included guided exercises for self exploration and discovery that are available as recordings through the Om Births website (look for the urls listed alongside the written descriptions). Please feel free to practice at your own comfort level.

From Anatomy, we move into the Practice section. I'll address some of the major myths still being perpetuated in the general yoga community as well as specific postures and practices that can be performed during pregnancy, with specific instructions around practicing while expecting. The postures are separated into "beginning" and "advanced" segments, as certain postures may require more attention and awareness than others. Additionally, the home practice chapter covers daily movements that can be employed to use yoga as a preparation for labor and birth. I believe that yoga during pregnancy can do more than help the body feel better as it changes shape. If done carefully, and with awareness, a prenatal yoga practice has the potential to more fully prepare the body and mind to work with the birth process and may even make that process easier by balancing connective tissue and focusing mental attention.

Finally, we come to the section on Birth. Having discussed the structure of the pregnant body, and the appropriate yoga practices, how does it come together? It would be remiss to not discuss the very event, and following postpartum experience, which every pregnant person will eventually undergo. Understanding the birth process is a crucial link to practicing yoga during pregnancy. We will explore the physiology of the birth process and how it intersects with our yoga practice. We'll also delve into what I call the "4 Cornerstones of

Working with Labor" as a framework for working with the birth experience, no matter what arises, and what it means to fully prepare for birth with yoga rather than to simply practice while pregnant. This section finishes with a taste of yoga appropriate for postpartum and exercises for rediscovering one's center (literally and figuratively) in the midst of the transformation into motherhood.

I hope this book will inspire you to explore pregnancy as well as the intersection between the changing body and the practice of yoga. I firmly believe that if we understand how the body is changing, and how our movements, thoughts, and awareness affect that body, then we can dramatically impact the entire process of birth, motherhood, and beyond.

Anatomy

"As a yoga teacher you have to develop x-ray vision in your students."

— Cyndi Lee

1 — It Starts with the Pelvis

It all started in a pelvis. At least, our personal journey did. After we were that "twinkle in our parent's eyes," the two halves of our DNA ultimately came together in our mother's pelvis. We were conceived there.[6] We were born from there. The pelvis is the center of gravity for the female body and the emotional center for the energy body. It supports the weight of the organs and baby during pregnancy and encases the pathway through which a baby enters the world. Over 30 different muscles intersect with the pelvis, and dozens of ligaments and fascial structures support (or impede) the function of the uterus and the process of birth. Simply put, when it comes to pregnancy, the pelvis is the nucleus from which most other things radiate.

Nearly every yoga training I have taken contained a section about the anatomy and structure of the pelvis. You may have studied the pelvis yourself in some context. You might have seen or held a plastic model of a pelvis or examined one as part of a standing skeleton. You may have reviewed pictures or photographs in anatomy textbooks or colored in bones and joints in an anatomy coloring book. This is certainly what I did in my initial 200-hour and subsequent weekend-long specialized yoga trainings.

But unless you had a unique and well-informed workshop or training program, I am willing to bet a great deal of money that the pelvis you examined, observed, and colored in with your pencils had a fundamental flaw concerning prenatal yoga: IT WAS MALE! Nearly all pelvic models available on the market depict the male pelvis rather than the female. And throughout medical history, the male body has always been taken to be the default, the standard, while the female is considered the deviation. Never mind that it is the introduction of testosterone and the Y chromosome which causes the reproductive tissues to shift from the female structure to the male during gestation. Yes, you read that right. We all start out female, and then shift to be male. It really does all start with the pelvis![7]

Despite the best attempts to represent the female body, nearly all skeletal models, both in yoga trainings and general anatomy trainings, make assumptions based on the male structure for the pelvis. This is true even though most students practicing yoga in the West are female—it's just how things are currently done. As we'll see, there are some decided differences between the male and female pelvic structures, and those differences result in somewhat different responses to certain movements and yoga shapes.

Let's take a moment and review pelvic anatomy, so everyone starts out on the same foot—or maybe hip?

---

[6] Or in the case of IVF, an embryo is implanted in its mother's pelvis—but we still begin here

[7] *The Developing Human*, Moore and Persaud, Saunders; 11th edition (March 15, 2019)

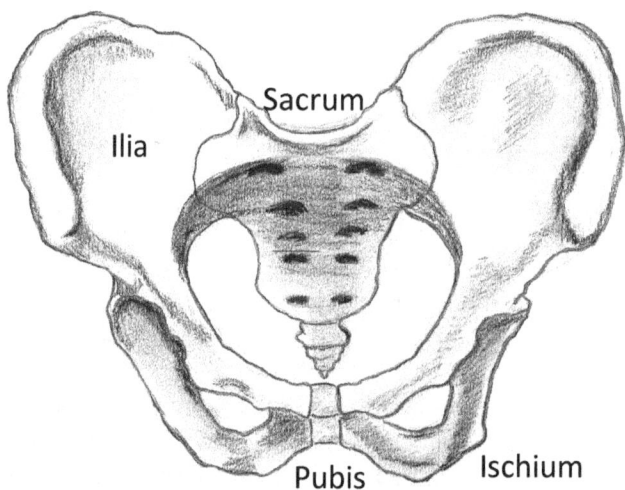

The pelvis is composed of three main bones which form a bowl in the mid-body. The root of the word "pelvis" actually means "bowl" in Latin. This bowl serves as both the cradle and support for our internal organs and the transfer point for weight from the upper body to the lower body and the earth. The two wing bones are divided into three sections: the ilium (plural ilia), which is the curving wing you can feel if you rest your hands on your hips; the ischium, or the lower segment extending into the buttocks where we rest our weight in good sitting posture; and the pubis, or the segment wrapping around and joining in—guess where—the pubic region!

Trick question for my anatomy geeks: Those are the sections of the bone, but what's the actual name for the bone made up of these three components? In my prenatal teacher training I often pose this question to students. After much sputtering and calling out the names of the different parts of the bones, I admit that the technical Latin name for this bone is the os-inominata, or the inominate bone. Translated into English, it means the "no name bone" (os=bone, in=negation or no, nom/nominate=named). We all have a good laugh realizing why no one can ever remember the name for this wide curving structure; there isn't one.

The commonly used name for the curving hip bone is the ilium: the flat, wide section we can feel. The two ilia, one on each side, combine with the sacrum in the back to create the pelvic bowl structure. At the front of the ilia, we can also feel a hard point sticking out. In yoga classes you might hear a teacher refer to these as points as hip points or "headlights," and they are generally used as a reference for where the pelvis is pointing. Anatomically, they're called the anterior superior iliac spine (ASIS) bones (or as I like to call them, the "as is bones," because really we should be leaving them as is). These reference points are useful in assessing where the bowl of the pelvis is pointing and whether it is sitting in a neutral posture.

A note about pelvic alignment: It is common when looking at a pelvic model to think of the bowl being fully upright—as though carrying a full punch bowl of liquid—but this often leads to a common mistake in positioning. The sacrum actually sits as an angle in the back of the pelvis, completing the curvatures of the spinal column above it and creating the final spring of the shock absorbers in the spinal curves. If we focus on tipping the pubic bone upwards (commonly cued as "tucking the tailbone"), we flatten the angle of the sacrum and decrease the springiness of the spinal curves above. As we'll see during pregnancy, this

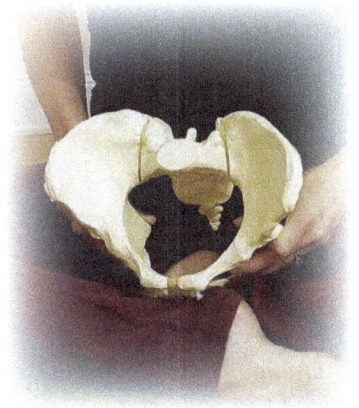

tucking action has a detrimental impact on the body's ability to adjust to its changing shape. Even more concerning, it leads to tension and constriction around the uterus and posterior pelvic floor—the very space into which the baby must descend in order to be born. The bowl does support the weight of the organs, but it does so by sharing that load between the pelvic bones and the legs below, not by dropping it all onto the pelvic floor. Bottom line (no pun intended): when aligning the pelvis, bring the weight to rest on the front of the sitting bones in a seated posture, and stop tucking the tail when standing! I'll come back to more specific instructions for this alignment shortly.

As we talk about the bones, we can recognize the first major differences between the male and female pelvis. These differences also illustrate why certain classic yoga alignments might not be appropriate for a pregnant body.

Look at the images of the two pelvises in Figure 1 In the male pelvis, the ilia are tall and straight, the sacrum is more steeply angled and closer to the sitz bones, the sitz bones themselves are narrower, and the pubic arch is much narrower than in its female counterpart. As a result, the male pelvis is taller and more narrow while the female is wider, more shallow, and flexible. The female pelvic bowl is better able to handle shifts in the internal organs (to accommodate a growing baby, for example). This adaptability comes from greater potential mobility in both the hip socket and the internal pelvic joints.

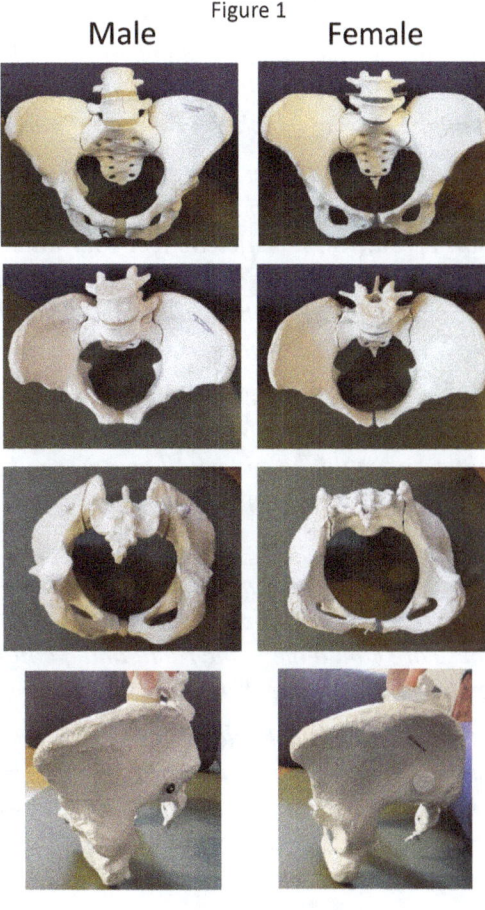

Figure 1

Male   Female

Pelvic landmarks
(recorded instructions available at www.om-births.com/ombirthsbook/pelviclandmarks)

Here's an exercise to explore your own anatomy and pelvic shape. I have found personal exploration to be one of the best methods in fully understanding anatomy. It is one thing to look at pictures and models, another to physically feel your own landmarks and experience how your bones, muscles, and tendons fit together. Follow along if you like. Even better, if you have a willing friend, you might be able to feel a couple of landmarks on another body and discover any differences between the two of you. Obviously if you do this with a friend, get permission before touching, and don't get too personal with someone else's body.

Standing in a comfortable position, take your hands to your waist and feel your way down until you come to two bones curving around the sides (the place we usually place our hands when we rest them on our hips). These are your iliac crests. Make your hands flat and press down on the top of this curve. Feel how the increased weight shifts in your body. If you feel along this bone towards the front you'll find two bony points roughly above your hip creases. These are your ASIS landmarks, the bones we use as references for where the pelvis is pointing.

Now feel around the iliac crest towards the back of your pelvis. The bony ridge will eventually disappear into the ropy muscles of your back, then flatten out into the expanse of the sacrum. Just before the flat of the sacrum, you may be able to find the two bony points of your posterior superior iliac spine (PSIS) on the back. Take note, are they very prominent? Shallow? Is there a clear dimple just inside them? If you can feel the dimple, that is your sacroiliac (SI) joint. If you have experienced SI pain, you may be familiar with this spot, and it might even feel good to give it a light massage.

Now take the hand on your sacrum and turn it so your fingers point towards your feet. Feel how the fingers and palm can cup around the curvature of the sacrum. If you slide the hand down a bit, you'll be able to feel your tailbone at the base of your sacrum, almost between your butt cheeks. In good alignment there will be about a 30 degree angle between the sacrum and the plumb line of gravity, but that may also depend on how your pelvis is resting on your legs. Can you get a sense for how your sacrum is currently aligned?

If you now bring your hands back to the ASIS and slide your hands closer towards the body's midline, you'll move off bone and into the soft tissue of the abdomen. Move the fingers down between the thighs and you'll contact the bony ridge of your pubic symphysis. Take note again, is this area tender? Does one side seem higher or more forward than the other?

If you feel like getting personal with yourself, try reaching beneath and slightly behind the pubic joint. (I would not recommend doing this in a yoga class, folks! And definitely not with your friend!) You'll find a space where you can feel the ridge of the pubic bones (technically these are called the pubic rami) and a couple of your fingers will fit between them. How many? Two? Three? This gives you a sense of how wide your own pubic arch might be.

Still with me? Reach underneath the flesh of your buttocks. Feel for two bony points buried under the muscle and fat padding; those are your ischial tuberosities. We more commonly refer to them as the sitz bones. These are what you would sit on if the pelvis was upright, and the name actually comes from the German "sitzen," meaning "to sit." Now imagine the space between your sitz bones, your pubic bone and your tailbone. This circle is the opening to the lower segment of the pelvis, known as the pelvic outlet, and this section, along with the deeper spaces within the pelvic bowl, is what we are concerned with in the process of childbirth.

There's another problem with most training in pelvic anatomy, especially when it concerns yoga. The plastic models are usually fixed together with bolts and screws, giving the impression that the pelvis is a solid, barely moving bowl structure. While the male pelvis is more structurally rigid than its female counterpart, the pelvis is actually a living, breathing, moving structure that varies from person to person and posture to posture. Learning anatomy from books and models is useful for cognitive understanding, but yoga also offers the chance to learn experientially. Ultimately, we encounter our anatomy as a living, breathing system, not static pieces. All of this needs to be taken into account when thinking of practicing yoga during pregnancy. The pelvis isn't just a bowl. It has joints!

The internal pelvic joints consist of two sacroiliac (SI) joints in the back where the sacrum meets the ilia and the pubic symphysis in the front where the two pubic bones join together. To find the SI joints, we can feel for another bony landmark similar to the ASIS, but in the back. This posterior superior iliac spine (PSIS), can often have a small divot just inside it which marks the SI joint. These joints are gliding joints, meaning they slide along one another rather than folding as our knees or elbows do. As we bend and flex the spine, the sacrum lightly nods and twists at the sacroiliac joints. Far from being a locked joint, the bones are able to glide and rotate slightly with one another. Depending on the positioning and structure of your pelvis, some move more than others.

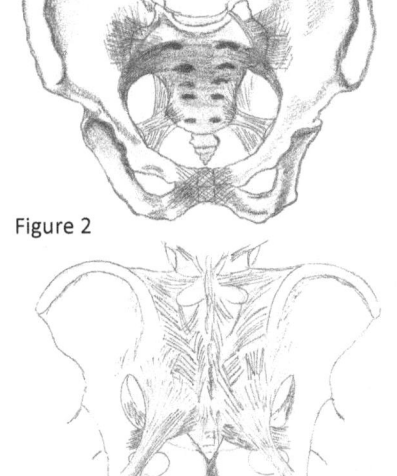

Figure 2

At the lowest end of the sacrum there is also the coccyx, or tailbone, and the sacro-coccygeal joint. The joint between the sacrum and the tailbone is usually more rigid, but it can still flex and extend as the pelvic floor and sacrum move. Osteopaths and chiropractors are well aware of the "breathing" quality of a sacrum that comes with balanced alignment and can actually feel this subtle motion. The curve of the sacrum is far more pronounced in the female pelvis than in the male pelvis, as is the distance between the sacrum and a mid-pelvic bony landmark called the ischial spine. Indeed, if you take a look at the lower section of the classic female pelvis, the interior looks nearly spherical—again, as though something round were supposed to fit into it… Hmmm…

The stabilizing network: pelvic ligaments and fascia

The anatomy of the female pelvis—wider, shallower, more curved—compared to the male allows female pelvic joints to move further and with greater ease. But so much potential mobility raises a challenge: how does the female pelvis stay together? After all, this is where the weight of the upper body transfers into the legs. How can something so flexible also be asked to support so much?

Enter the fabulous network of ligaments and fascia to provide the needed stability. Fascia is an interconnected web of tissue that weaves throughout our bodies. In some ways, it is like plastic wrap, encasing each internal structure but also holding the body together. You can think of it as a second "skin" woven in and throughout the body, thick at some places, thinner at others. Like our skin, fascia responds to pressure, temperature, hydration level, and even emotional state.

All of the body's joints are stabilized by strong lines of fascia called ligaments. Ligaments connect bone to bone (and bone to organ) and provide tensile strength, meaning they do not stretch very much. If the fascia is healthy and well hydrated, the ligaments should provide solid resistance to movement without being rigid or brittle. Look at the picture of pelvic ligaments in Figure 2. The pubic symphysis at the front has an entire sheath of ligaments spanning from one pubic bone to the other to hold the joint together. The SI joints, in the back of the pelvis, likewise have similar ligaments bridging the front side of the sacrum to the Ilia. The SI joint is also reinforced by two big ligaments on the back side of the pelvis: the sacro-spinous ligament, which connects to the ischial spine, and the sacro-tuberous ligament, which connects to the ischial tuberosity.

Why are these two thick ligaments on the back side as well? The reason has to do with the shape and angle of the sacrum and its role in the internal infrastructure of the skeleton.

The keystone of the arch

Have you ever seen an old-fashioned stone bridge or an archway in a medieval cathedral? The center stone, known as the keystone, always has a triangular shape. The shape of the keystone allows the weight above the arch to be redistributed down the sides of the arch without falling to the ground.

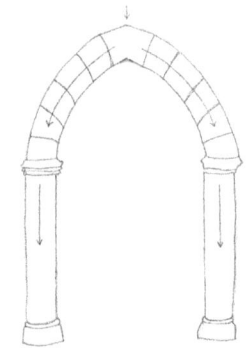

The forces within the body that act on the sacrum naturally create a similar arch structure. The weight of the upper body comes down through the spine, contacts the sacrum, and is distributed down through the pelvis into the femurs. From there weight flows down through the legs and into the ground. The sacrum is the keystone of this organic arch! But wait, there is more to this story.

If the pelvis is aligned so that the spine provides shock absorption (which it is supposed to do), then the sacrum sits at an angle of around 30 degrees, pointed away from the body at the base. If we apply pressure to the top side (as the lumbar spine does) the lever action on the top of the sacrum would cause the base to swing upwards, leading to a collapse of the much-needed arch. To solve this problem, the body has laid down tension lines (the sacro-spinous

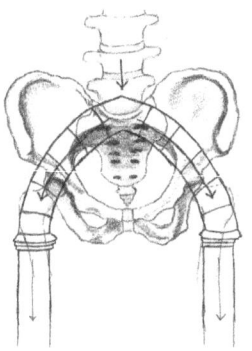

and sacro-tuberous ligaments) that hold the sacrum in its keystone position but still allow it to shift as it needs to for balance. Without these lines, the normal weight of the upper body would cause the sacrum, and the entire pelvis, to become unstable. Why is this important to consider for yoga during pregnancy? Well, for that we have to consider the hormonal changes in effect as the baby grows.

Pelvic movement
(recording at www.ombirths.com/ombirthsbook/pelvicmovement)

This exercise demonstrates that your pelvis is not a static bowl but a moving structure.

Sit with your legs crossed (Sukhasana, or "easy seat"). Feel for your sitz bones, and then squeeze your butt cheeks together. Try to "walk" your sitz bones together and make things as narrow as possible. Now place your thumb on one sitz bone, and then stretch your middle finger across the space between to measure the distance between your ischial tuberosities (It's OK, you can touch your body here—it's your body!). Holding your hand as still as you can, bring your fingers to where you can see them and observe roughly how many inches are between your thumb and middle finger. I have maybe 3.5 or so. Don't judge how wide it is; just get a base measurement.

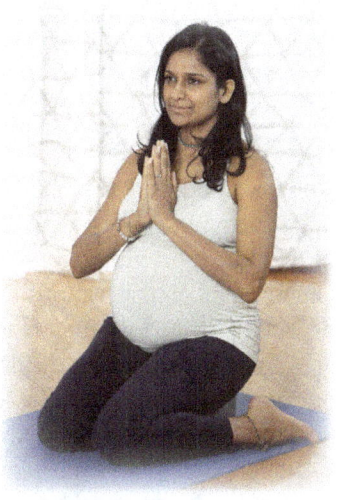

Now shift to sit in Virasana (knees together with the feet apart and the thighs rotated inward). Tilt the pelvis forward and use your hands to spread your butt cheeks, making things feel as wide as possible. Now reach back and take the same measurement, thumb to middle finger across the sitz bones. Was there a difference? Was it significant? For most people, changing the orientation of the pelvis and the femur bones changes the distance between the sitz bones. For some the difference can be an inch or more (I shift to nearly 5 inches across!).

If you have female anatomy, all that movement you felt during the exploration is the result of your pelvic anatomy. If you have male anatomy, your sitz bones probably didn't move nearly as much. If the bones can move this much under normal conditions, what happens during pregnancy when the hormonal balance in the body shifts?

Relaxin: it ain't just in the mind

When the female body becomes pregnant, hormones immediately shift to help maintain the pregnancy and, eventually, prepare the body to give birth. Progesterone and estrogen levels rise during the first trimester, signaling the body first to maintain the uterine lining for implantation and then to support the growing fetus and placenta. Around the end of the first trimester, the placenta will take over production of these hormones. Before then, they are maintained by the corpus luteum, which is formed from the follicle from which the egg emerged. The increase in progesterone and estrogen leads to a softening of connective tissues in the body as well as a slowing of the smooth muscle function in some organs. These changes ensure that the muscles of the uterus don't begin contracting, as they would for menstruation, and unintentionally expel the growing fetus. And they help the uterus maintain the blood-rich lining for the fertilized egg to implant and grow.

The pregnant body also produces a rather aptly named hormone called relaxin. Relaxin, just as it sounds, "relaxes" all connective tissue in the body. This hormone hits a peak in the first trimester as it prepares the uterus for implantation and then stops the body from following its usual cycle of menstruation,[8] literally keeping the uterus relaxed so it doesn't expel the growing baby by shedding the uterine lining. High levels of relaxin continue throughout the pregnancy, maintaining a relaxed uterus as the baby grows. Relaxin softens not only muscles but also fascia and even cartilage, and it acts on the entire body. It literally doesn't know your a** from your elbow. The combination of relaxin, progesterone, and estrogen makes it possible for the pelvic joints to stretch and move further during the birth process, so the baby has more room to descend, rotate, and eventually emerge. What happens when a pregnant person actively stretches their body in different positions, as we do during a yoga practice? Consider how much we just discovered our own pelvic bones can move, and then consider how the body becomes more pliable and flexible during pregnancy. Can you see the potential problem? The hormones don't distinguish between a baby asking to move through and a deep yoga posture that promotes greater range of motion. If our joints can move significantly without pregnancy hormones, how much more can those of a pregnant woman move once progesterone, estrogen, and relaxin get involved?

Keep in mind, too, that the pelvis is the arch structure holding up the spinal column and the upper body. If the keystone of the sacrum is destabilized, it compromises the entire integrity of the body's architecture. As we'll see, protecting this integrity leads to some alignment changes and considerations for the pregnant body when moving through yoga *asanas*, especially if the tendency is to overstretch or lean into ligaments rather than promote stability. While those ligaments (fascial lines meant to hold joints stable for weight bearing) might normally be able to bear the load, they too become more flexible as a result of pregnancy hormones. Consistent overstretching can increase the resting length of a ligament. Once stretched, ligaments take a long time (possibly years) to return to their previous condition, leaving joints in a semi-permanent destabilized state. As a result, we get issues like SI joint pain, which occurs when the joint shifts more than intended, leading to compression of the nerves radiating from the pelvis. Ask any group of female yoga students, and you'll probably find that at least half have dealt with either sciatica or low back pain—the result of the compression of these nerves.

Remember how the pubic symphysis joint is stabilized laterally by a sheath of ligaments run-

---

[8] Plant, R. (2021, June 14). What is relaxin? *Verywell Family.* https://www.verywellfamily.com/what-is-relax-in-5180381

ning from one side to the other? This sheath holds the two halves of the pelvis together at the front of the body, creating the bowl into which the sacrum sits as the keystone. Like the structure of a beautiful crystal, the bones of the pelvis are elegantly organized to provide strength and flexibility. Add in pregnancy hormones, and the whole structure becomes more pliable. If, with this increased flexibility, a yogi puts increased pressure on the pubic symphysis (think: fully turning the pelvis to the side of the yoga mat without adjusting the feet, dropping into a deep lunge without internal support, or constantly tucking the tailbone), the stabilizing connective tissue in this area is overstressed. Too much stress can lead to a separation of the two pubic bones, a painful condition called symphysis pubis dysfunction (SPD). In extreme cases, women who already had loose connective tissue to begin with (like advanced yogis or ballet dancers) may even have difficulty walking. If the pelvis lacks stability to bear weight on one leg, walking becomes impossible because the weight shift from one foot to another creates a shearing (and extremely painful) force through the midline of the pelvis.

And we haven't even touched on the impact that unstable and misaligned pelvic bones can have on the function of the pelvic floor, the internal position of the uterus, and the overall space available for the baby to grow, position, and eventually birth. Movement patterns during pregnancy have the ability to impact far more than just our day to day comfort and flexibility levels. I'll come back to this point in subsequent chapters.

Bottom line: Keep the pelvic bowl intact!!!

The levels of the pelvis

In order to keep this bowl intact, we have to understand the different parts of the bowl which can be affected and how those different levels interact with pregnancy and the birth process. The upper segment of the bowl, known in medical circles as the pelvic inlet, is the circle created by the top of the ischium, pubis, and sacrum. This segment creates the arch system for the body's weight, and it needs to be stable for a person to stand up and move well.

During pregnancy, maintaining this integrity is key to the body being able to shift as the belly and baby grow. But how we maintain the integrity matters too, because the pathway for a baby to be born is neither completely straight nor uniformly shaped. The way you load the pelvis during pregnancy with yoga and everyday movements will impact the internal space created by the muscles and fascia, which the baby will have to navigate through during birth.

There are three levels to the pelvic birth pathway, the inlet, the mid-pelvis, and the outlet. During the birth process, baby must navigate through each of them individually. This means the pelvis must both support and shift during labor, and how much a pregnant person has encouraged the pelvis to do each movement during pregnancy can influence how easily the body navigates labor and delivery. If our movement diet was fully balanced, pregnant women would have no need for prenatal yoga—we would probably have no need for exercise at all— but I'll get back to that.

Baby begins labor by sliding their head into the top circle of the pelvic inlet. Since this circle is usually wider side to side, most babies will begin labor looking right or left rather

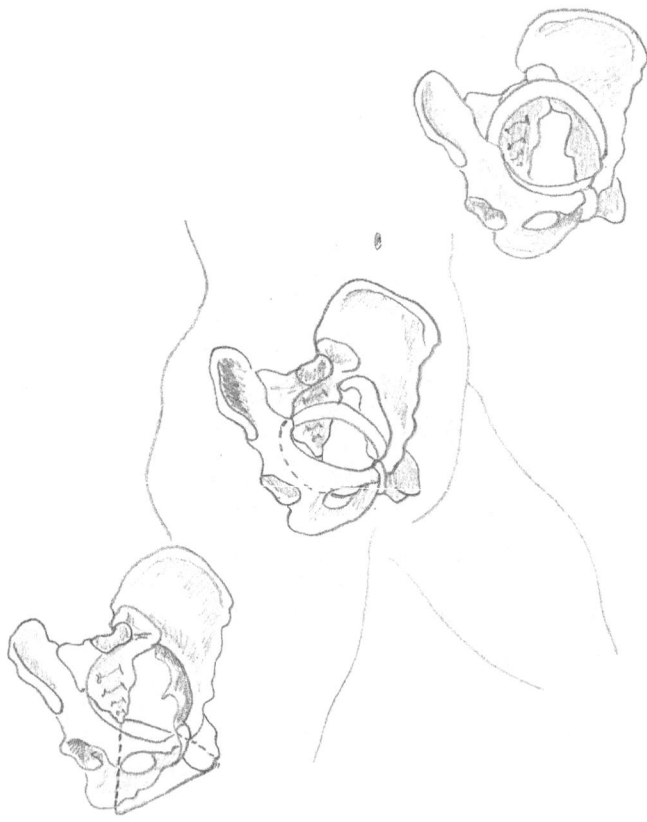

Each of the three levels of the pelvis comes into play as the baby descends and rotates during the birth process.

than straight back. Once in the pelvic inlet, the baby must rotate through a curved path in the mid-pelvis where the ischial spines protrude into the pelvic space and the muscles of the pelvic floor align front to back in the body. The muscles of the pelvic floor guide the head through a gentle rotation to align baby's nose towards mom's spine.

Once through the mid-pelvis, the baby's head must extend under the pubic arch, drawing the head towards the diamond formed by the ischial tuberosities, pubic symphysis/pubic arch, and the coccyx. The movements that open each level of the pelvis can differ. Think about what movements shifted your sitz bones during the pelvic movement exploration. Did the base of the pelvis open with the knees moving apart? Or together?

Depending on factors such as maternal position, the relative tone of the muscles around the pelvis, and whether mom is able to move, mom can make space for the baby and release the area where the baby sits by shifting her position to move the bones and muscles at each section of the pelvis. Daily posture and movements can impact this relative flexibility or stability. A yoga practitioner who spends too much time tucking the tail forward may tighten the fascia in the back of the pelvis, leading to restrictions in the posterior pelvic ligaments, which have to yield for the sacrum to move backwards as the baby descends. Again, simple movements can have big impacts on the body's space for birth. What postural patterns have we been holding in the years leading up to pregnancy? How have we been moving our bones? Have we kept the birthing path, which was there when we were born, open? If we were moving as our ancient grandmothers did, our bodies would probably be in far better tone and balance—and we wouldn't be exercising because we'd just move throughout the day. But most of us don't have this kind of holistic movement diet. And this is where *asana* comes in to start restoring balance.

Key Takeaways

The pelvis is a bowl made of three connected bones (sacrum and the two ilia), plus the tailbone (coccyx) at the base, and supports the weight of the organs and upper body.

There are marked differences between the male and female pelvis, and most yoga postures focus on the male pelvis, which is more stable than the female structure.

Ligaments in the front and back of the pelvis stabilize and support the pelvic joints.

During pregnancy hormonal changes make the pelvic ligaments more pliable and susceptible to overstretching. We need to exercise caution in deep yoga postures.

Balanced alignment in the pelvic bowl involves aligning the bowl so the weight of the upper body transfers through to the legs. This results in the sacrum serving as a keystone in the arch of the pelvis and legs holding up the spine.

When practicing yoga during pregnancy it is important to align the pelvis properly and to protect the internal joints within the pelvic bowl so as not to destabilize the support structure of the body. Key among the alignment cues is to stop tucking the tail, which jams the pelvic joints.

Balancing the pelvic position allows for the muscles and connective tissues to relax, which creates more room for the baby during pregnancy and birth. Angling the front of the pelvis down encourages baby to align best for birth.

2 — The Pregnant Spine

My first yoga teacher, Cyndi Lee, once described Tadasana as "the underpants of every standing posture in yoga." She meant that underneath all the contortions and bends of the standing postures is the foundation of Tadasana. Done well, Tadasana (Mountain pose) sets us up to stand in balance within the field of gravity and can even assist the body in managing changes to the center of gravity during pregnancy. Done incorrectly or without awareness, however, it has the potential to affect every posture that involves standing on the feet. Like a ripple in a pond, shifts made within Tadasana can probably apply to every subsequent standing pose. This posture is often overlooked in yoga practice or done with a stylization that actually misses the intricacies of the pose. So it only makes sense that we start with Tadasana in our exploration of *asana*.

Tadasana: standing up
(recording available at www.ombirths.com/ombirthsbook/tadasana)

Start with the feet at the base. During pregnancy, you want to increase the stability of the foundation because of everything that's going on up above, so take the feet hip distance apart or possibly slightly wider if you are in the second trimester or later. From the feet, move up to the knees and soften the back of the knee joint. If you are prone to locking your knees, this may feel like having them slightly bent, but ultimately it should be a micro bend, like a secret that only you know about. Yoga Teacher Barbara Benagh often calls this a "natural" Tadasana, which I think is an apt name given it works with the body's natural tendencies.

Now comes the fun part, moving to the connection of the pelvic bowl and thighs. Create some depth to the creases of the groins by gently shifting the femurs back while also dropping the pubis downward away from the navel. Yes you read that right, move the pubis AWAY from your navel. This action will shift the pelvis backwards in space and place the hip sockets more solidly in contact with the heads of the femurs, almost as though turning the bowl onto the legs.

Continue this movement until one of two things happens: either you feel both the thighs and the glutes relax or you feel the deep abdominal muscles organize into support. In fact, these two actions will probably happen simultaneously, as they indicate the pelvic floor has come level with the ground and is now able to come "online." This also means you do NOT need to suck your abs in when your pelvis is in alignment. The transverse abdominals will spontaneously engage and hold the upper body, and the weight of your organs will be borne by your pubic bone and pelvic floor rather than your lower back. This action may also give rise to the thought "I'm sticking my butt out!" For a moment, I'm going to ask you to let go of the judgment around that and stick with me. It's worth it, I promise. Your tail is still grounded, but now, so is your pubic bone.

Allowing your butt to remain "sticking out" (trust me, it's not actually that far back), bring your focus up to your ribs. Think of your ribcage as a bell housing the heart and lungs. With the pelvis tucked under, many of us have compensated by rocking the front side of this ribcage bell forward to try to counterbalance the weight of the upper body backwards. This leads to a forward motion in the ribcage, which is commonly called rib thrust. Rib thrust has two complications when it comes to standing effectively. First, it has the effect of flattening the thoracic spine by moving the upper back forward, which leads to increased tension in the neck and shoulder muscles. But the other challenge is that thrusting the ribs forward puts increased strain on the front line of the body (as does tucking the tail). This means that the weight which should have been borne by the bones (designed for this purpose) is now being born by the muscles and, even worse, by the fascia.

Remember the fascia? If you keep leaning on it, two things happen: it will begin to thin out, and it will also increase its tensile strength by laying down more fibers to share the load. Increased fibers lead to more brittle, rigid fascia. This is especially problematic when we then add the weight of the pregnant uterus and baby into the front connective tissue of the abdominal wall. The surface of the abdominal wall is connected together by a fascia line known as the linea alba (the white line). Lean on this too much, and for too long, and it may separate into something called diastasis recti, a major problem for abdominal and core strength. We'll return to this later on, but let's finish standing up.

To realign the rib thrust, drop your front ribs. You could do this in one of two ways: you could think of weights being attached to your lowest front ribs, gently drawing them downward, or you could visualize the ribcage as a bell and allow the bell to swing backwards, thus raising the back floating ribs while lowering the front ones. No tucking the tail while you do this! The effect will be a widening of your upper back and a small movement of your shoulders forward. Yes, it may feel like you are slouching (again, let go of the judgment around that for a moment). Keeping the ribs heavy, now think about gently lifting and broadening your collar bones and sternum. Keep the ribs down! They don't move much but the action broadens the chest slightly, restoring breath capacity. Finish this alignment by floating your occiput (the back of your skull) back and up, as though someone is lifting you from the base of your skull. Again, the action is subtle, but you'll be able to feel a release in the lower jaw that extends downward throughout the entire spine.

OK, how do you feel? I'm going to take a guess and say…weird. Really weird. Like you are slightly doing everything you've probably been told not to do. The most common comment (or sometimes complaint) I get from yoga students and teacher trainees is that they feel like they are sticking their butt out. Here I have to recall one of my favorite quotes from yoga teacher Judith Lasater: "Don't confuse familiar with correct." The body is made for the weight to be borne primarily through the bones, not in the muscles. But many of us are caught in postural patterns we can't see. Never mind all the other "rules" that yoga sometimes places on our postures.

Over time, the body has slowly recalibrated its internal sensors to believe that where you had been standing was neutral. It's going to take a bit of time before you realize how far out of alignment you may have been standing and for your body to recalibrate. What should you be looking for? Notice the feeling within the feet. Beyond the fact that the weight may have shifted slightly towards the heels, the feet and legs will also feel extremely solid, like tree trunks rooted into the ground, or even like the base of…a mountain (what was this pose called again?).

This solidity is what you are looking for, and it is then combined with a feeling of lightness through the pelvis and upper body. You want to stand on your bones, not your connective tissue or your muscles. This is especially true during pregnancy. Doing so allows the fascia to unwind, creating better room for the baby, and also allows the muscles to do the work of movement rather than being bound up with maintaining posture. All the other structures and spaces in the body are then free to adjust as the pregnancy grows.

You may have noticed that in shifting and balancing the alignment of the pelvis, you are not only affecting the pelvis but all the structures around it. It starts with the pelvis, but the changes we make there ripple outward throughout the body, influencing our overall coordination and balance.

Growing out of the back of the pelvic bowl is the spinal column, the "segmented tent pole,"[9] from which hangs the rest of the upper body and core muscles, bones, and organs. The weight shifts of pregnancy affect not only the pelvic joints but also the overall postural pattern within the body. Understanding these postural shifts and the interplay that happens between pelvis and spine has a dramatic influence on how we practice yoga during pregnancy. So to get the full picture of how the pregnant body is shifting, we have to look at the spine as well.

Exploring the spine

The spine is a series of interlocking vertebral bones which, when put together, make up four curves that allow us to stand upright. The curves mirror one another. The thoracic and sacral curves, sometimes called primary curves, are concave, curving away from the front of the body. These are the curves we had in utero, the ones we were born with. They are easy to see if you look at a newborn baby.

In contrast, the lumbar and cervical curves, sometimes called secondary curves, are convex, curving inward to the body. These develop gradually as a baby learns to exercise their back postural muscles. This is one reason parents are often encouraged to give babies lots of tummy time. Lying prone encourages the baby to engage the secondary curves of the spine by lifting their head and arching the back to look around at their surroundings. As

[9] I first heard this from bodyworker Tom Meyers: anatomytrains.com

the spine comes upright, major muscle groups like the psoas and paraspinals engage to hold the spine in its upright curving positions. The curves allow for mobility as well as stability within the spine. They create a shock absorption system that allows the spine to flex and absorb pressure from above or below, as when one jumps and lands on two feet.

I want you to fully understand that the neutral and intended shape for the spine involves curvature. In fact, the facet joints of the lumbar spine (the joints between the extensions on the back of the vertebrae) lock together best when the lumbar spine is in a curve. This means that when we artificially tuck our tails or flatten our lower backs, we are in fact taking the spinal joints out of their most stable position, the one where the muscles don't have to do excessive work to hold them in place. Think about that with respect to the instruction to "tuck your tail" to alleviate back pain. It may stretch some muscles in the moment, but held in a permanent state, tucking your tail creates more tension rather than less. This is the exact opposite of what we would want for relieving discomfort!

In typical anatomy, the spinal curves are lined up in the way that best balances the body's center of gravity over the legs. For women this means the pelvis (which houses the female center of gravity[10]) is placed over the feet. In contrast, the male center of gravity rests in the chest, making the fulcrum for the male body higher than for the female. This also possibly explains why the male pelvis rises higher and spreads less, as it must accommodate a higher mass above than its female counterpart.

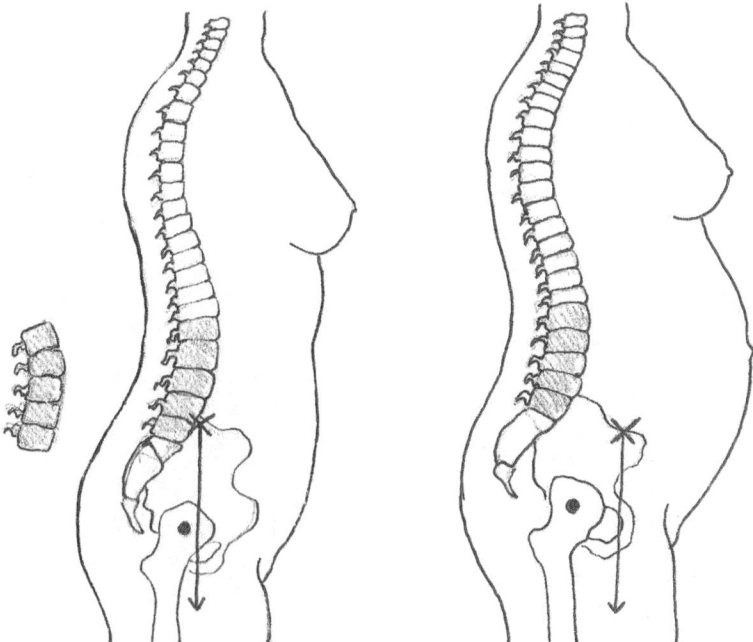

[10] Hall SJ. Equilibrium and Human Movement. In: Hall SJ. eds. *Basic Biomechanics*, 8e New York, NY: Mc-Graw-Hill; . http://accessphysiotherapy.mhmedical.com/content.aspx?bookid=2433&sectionid=191511590.

During pregnancy, the body changes shape, with weight accumulating on the front side in both the belly and the breasts. This results in a change in the placement of the center of gravity within the pregnant body. Look at Figure 3. The arrow pointed down represents the plumb line for the center of gravity. The picture on the left represents a non-pregnant woman, and the one on the right is someone who is maybe in her mid-third trimester. Note how much farther forward the center of gravity is on the right than on the left. By the time mom is ready to give birth, her center of gravity may have shifted as much as four inches further forward. For reference, that would be outside her non-pregnant physical body! This means that without some compensation, the body would topple over by the end of pregnancy. But of course, Mother Nature is smarter than that. She was certainly not going to let evolving human women keep falling over on their bellies every time they carried a baby to term. How could we possibly run away from the mountain lion?

Here comes the fabulous, flexible spine to the rescue! The spinal curves actually deepen during pregnancy, shifting the center of gravity back into the center of the pelvis rather than out over the toes or beyond. And voila! Mom can stand up again! But this shift creates more lower back curvature; in our posture-obsessed culture, sticking one's backside out has long been considered a huge no-no! Herein lies the problem: our everyday postures are not completely neutral to begin with. While the body may be trying to shift, our overly active and judgmental minds often try to maintain our old postural habits rather than allowing things to shift and adjust.

Figure 3

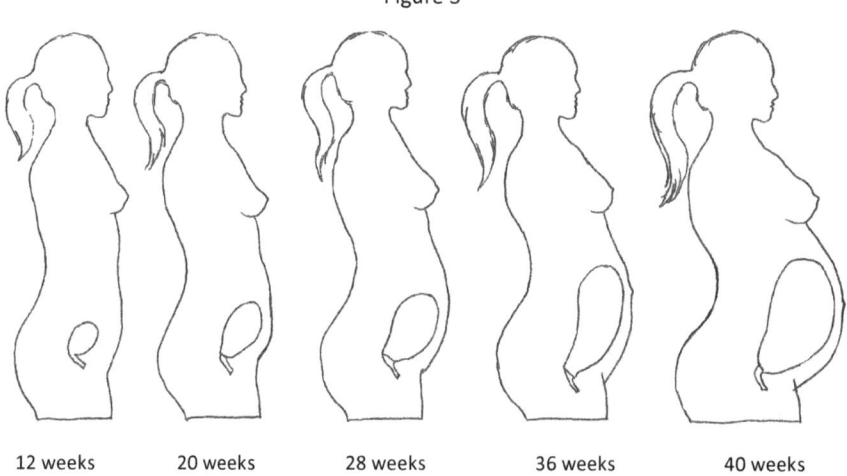

| 12 weeks | 20 weeks | 28 weeks | 36 weeks | 40 weeks |

No, that 40-week-pregnant woman is not *necessarily* overarching her back! We have to look deeper.

Over the course of our lives we have each developed certain postural habits from the balancing act that standing upright requires. We began by simply feeling for where the body stayed upright, with the goal being to keep a plumb line that comes down over our feet. You can see this in babies learning to walk. Shift too far forward or back, and baby goes bump on their bum. But now add the complication of adult movement patterns. If you spend a lot of time either pitched forward or leaning back, then the body may adjust the position of your pelvis and create chronic muscle tension to hold what it perceives as upright.

For example, consider high heeled shoes. Wearing heels moves your center of gravity forward and up, leading to less stability. The result of having the center of gravity shifted forward is a corresponding pelvic shift forward, accompanied by a tucking of the tailbone. This shifts the pelvic bowl literally underneath the abdominal organs in order to "catch" the weight of the upper body and transfer it down to the legs—in this case specifically, into the toes, which are the point of contact with the ground.

The result is a pelvic position commonly called a posterior tilt, or a counter-nutation of the pelvic bowl. The knees try to lock back to create a counter balance to the forward shifted pelvis; with the head of the femur shifted forward by the pelvic tuck, the bottom of the femur (which is also the top of the knee joint) shifts backwards. Remember that old song, "the hip bone's connected to the knee bone…"? At the top of the balancing act, the rib cage gets thrust forward, with the shoulders rolled down and back to compensate for the forward shift of the pelvis below. Furthermore, the head is thrust forward with the chin lifted, compressing the back of the neck.

If this posture sounds familiar, there's a reason. This is what I have found nearly ALL of us are doing to one degree or another! Yes, even the guys! Yes, even the yogis who have been told their lower back curve is too deep or that they have lordosis. Why? One reason could be that almost all shoes have an elevated heel! Even sneakers have more padding under the heels than under the toes, shifting the body's weight forward on the feet and pulling the center of gravity out of alignment with the arches of the feet. Do this long enough, and the body begins to think this is the neutral position it has always been in. Proprioception (the awareness of where your body is in space) recalibrates to consider this posture normal, and the muscles follow suit, locking in postural habits which may or may not be helpful in the long run.

Leslie Howard,[11] renowned pelvic floor yoga teacher in Oakland CA, suggests we are all a nation of "mother tuckers" and that we need to let go of this habit. I couldn't agree more, and this goes double for when we are pregnant. We have built up a series of habits over years from media images, comments people have made, and our own internalized ideals about how we want our bodies to look. Pregnant people come to yoga class with all the postural habits of their pre-pregnancy lives still ingrained. But they have an opportunity to undo these bad habits as they adapt to changes in the body's shape. At the very least, it's possible to better balance the body during pregnancy to have less pain. At best, maybe this shift in awareness can be applied beyond pregnancy to create a better functioning and more lifelong supported body structure.

Anatomy exploration: seeing the pattern
(recording available at www.ombirths.com/ombirthsbook/seeingthepattern)

If you are lucky enough to have several yoga friends who want to explore their own postural patterns, try this exercise together.

---

[11] www.lesliehowardyoga.com

Partner up, getting permission to touch one another in the process. Then using your fingers, locate the ASIS points on the front of your partner's pelvis. Then feel their Iliac crest around towards the back and see if you can locate their PSIS and, right next to it, their SI joints. Place your hand on their sacrum and note if it has any angle relative to the floor. Now using the tips of your fingers, run your hand upwards from their sacrum to their occipital ridge (the base of their skull) and back down. Take note of what their curves feel like.

Now place your hands on the top of their iliac crest and lightly press down. You are looking to see if their pelvis feels tucked under or tilted. For the moment, resist the inclination to make a diagnosis. Just get some information into your fingertips. Now repeat this exercise with several other people, ideally at least four. What do you notice? Is everyone the same? What marked differences did you observe? What conclusions have you already begun to draw? I know I said don't make any, but you can't tell me you didn't anyway.

Want to assess where you are standing? Again with your partner, stand as "normally" as you can, and have your partner put a gentle bit of weight on your shoulders. This should be maybe 5-10 lbs, enough that you can feel it solidly but not so much that you are actually knocked over. If you are aligned over your bones, then without much additional muscle engagement, you should feel your feet press strongly into the floor. When I have done this exercise in training after training, what I have found is that most yogis have hips that are too far forward or tucked underneath, and the result is that almost everyone nearly falls over backwards when I apply even a small amount of weight to their shoulders. And most of these people have been told they had a lower back curve which was too pronounced, and that they should be tucking their tail to get rid of it and reduce back pain! Those who look like they are sticking their tail out like a duck often also have locked knees, which is one way of compensating without releasing the tail tucking.

Now, if you want to explore what solid alignment feels like, go back to the instructions for Tadasana, align the body, and then repeat this exercise. You'll be amazed how much more solid your pose feels.

Postural influencers (not the social media kind)

The bones are the form, but function in posture comes from the muscles. Postural muscles are so deep in the body that we may not be able to feel their tension or release them easily. If we have been unknowingly holding our weight in our muscles rather than our bones, our postural muscles will have shortened and hardened to maintain that posture. Shifting back to neutral, even if it brings the weight more fully into the bones, may be challenging. Chronic muscle and fascial tension will keep trying to pull the bones back to what feels familiar. Add a changing center of gravity during pregnancy, and you see how trying to maintain an old postural pattern can actually become detrimental when the body is no longer the same shape that pattern has been serving. And if the muscles are not strong enough, they may tighten down to brace and stabilize instead of remaining supple and mobile. Certain muscle groups impact the placement of the pelvis, the spinal column, and the body's ability to shift during pregnancy.

The psoas

The psoas is one of the largest and strongest muscles of the body (and if you are a fan of steakhouses, it is literally the filet mignon). The psoas is a major flexor of the hip, but it originates much higher than the hip, on the front side of the 12th thoracic vertebra (T12). Feel on your back, just under the bra line where the floating ribs attach, and you've got the origin point for your psoas muscle. (This is also the attachment point for your abdominal diaphragm, which comes into play during *pranayama* and pelvic floor work.)

From there, the psoas also attaches to the front side of each of the subsequent vertebrae, comes down through the pelvis, and merges with a second hip flexor called the iliacus. This muscle fans out from inside the wing of the ilium on each side. Both the psoas and the iliacus attach to the lesser trochanter, or the deep side of the inner thigh. Given that these two often fire together, they are sometimes referred to as the Iliopsoas muscles.

Why start our inquiry here? Because the iliopsoas dramatically influences spinal posture. If the trunk is fixed, the psoas is the muscle that will raise the leg and swing it forward. But if the leg is fixed in place, then the psoas will pull on its other end and drag the spine forward. This is how it stabilizes the lumbar curve so the spine can stand in relative ease. But if there is excessive muscle tension (say from sitting a lot or being athletic without stretching afterwards) then the lumbar spine is drawn forward, creating a compressed and excessively deep lumbar curve. As a result, the space around the pelvic organs can also become compressed.

The forward pull from the psoas tries to tilt the pelvis forward. But what if our postural pattern insists on continuing to tuck the tail? The body develops a deep groove along the lower back where the psoas is dragging the lumbar spine forward, but the hip and back muscles fight this movement to maintain an upright position. Now imagine additional weight being applied to the front of the body by the growing baby, uterus, and breasts. The pelvis wants to tip even further forward, but the glutes and posterior muscles resist even harder. This tension creates even more strain on the trunk muscles and psoas and, unless something shifts, will lead to increased back compression (tucking the tail further isn't going to relieve the pressure in this situation).

If that weren't enough, the uterus sits directly between the two psoas muscles, as though cradled by them. As the uterus and baby grow, chronic tension in these muscles will affect how much space is available for the uterus and baby. Cue a possible breech problem. Two tight psoas bands wrapping around the back of the expanding uterus can create internal constriction and less space for a baby to rotate head down when the time comes. We'll cover postures for releasing the psoas in the Practice section of this book, but for now, know that stretching a set of muscles which crosses multiple joints is not as simple as pulling the two end points apart. While backbending can stretch the psoas, it won't be an effective technique for a psoas in chronic lockdown; the psoas will simply "borrow" the desired movement from the already compressed joints. Is it any wonder that so many yogis have a common aversion to backbending postures? No one likes to be in pain. Note that in addition to psoas tension here, we are also increasing tension throughout the glute and hamstring groups. This has dramatic implications for the stability, comfort, and potential mobility of the pelvis throughout pregnancy and birth.

The pelvic stabilizers

At the risk of repeating myself, I want to make it clear that the pelvic bowl is not a single unit. While the SI and pubic joints are stabilized by thick sheaths of ligaments and fascia, they are also supported by the external rotators of the glutes and piriformis. These external hip muscles originate from the inside and outside of the sacrum and ilium and extend around the outer hip joint to attach to the greater trochanter of the femur.

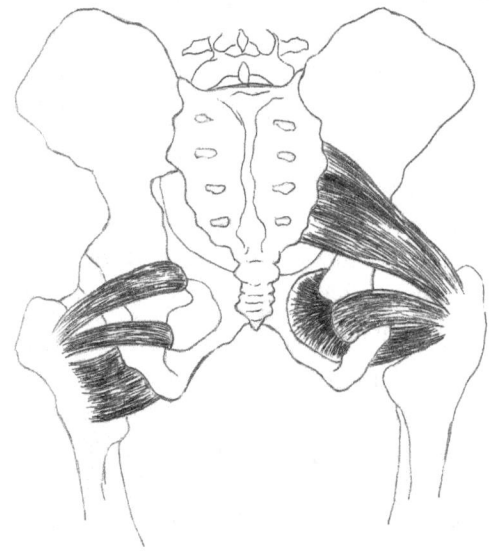

If you run your fingers down from the iliac crest to the outside of the thigh bone, you will be able to feel a solid bony point sitting just under the globe of the buttocks. This is the greater trochanter. When the glutes and piriformis contract, they squeeze the side of the pelvis against the sacrum in the back, possibly also externally rotating the femur bone. This action stabilizes the SI joint, preserving the pelvic bowl during actions such as walking or running when the weight must transfer through the legs down to the ground. Because of their position on the back of the pelvis, the glutes are also involved in extending the hip (meaning they draw the femur bone back and propel the body forward, or, if the leg were fixed, they would rotate the pelvis backwards, tucking the tail.)

It may seem like we would always want to engage the glutes for stability, but recognize that what makes a muscle strong is its ability to release as well as contract. Tense muscles are in fact quite weak. The glutes and other external hip rotators need to be able to both stretch AND contract. So while it might feel good in the moment to do those deep Pigeon or Fire Log postures to stretch the glutes, if we don't then also strengthen these muscles, we will ultimately destabilize the pelvis further. The same is true for the hamstrings and calves, which have a fascial connection into the posterior ligaments on the sacrum. Too loose, and the sacrum is unstable. Too tight, and the sacrum cannot swing backwards as it needs to during the birth process, which may obstruct the baby's pathway. The movements a pregnant person makes during pregnancy, and the ways in which they hold their bodies, impact the pelvis' ability to open as well as recover following pregnancy and birth.

The trunk muscles

The psoas and glutes aren't the only muscle groups involved in supporting the spine and pelvis. Migrate up from the glutes and posterior pelvic stabilizers and we find the posterior chain muscles of the paraspinals, multifidus, and quadratus lumborum. These spinal extensors, while not as massive as the psoas, are responsible for helping hold the spinal column upright and provide additional support for spinal movement. They also bear the increased weight on the front body as the uterus and breasts grow during pregnancy. If we add the tension of the psoas drawing the lumbar spine forward, we may find further compression around the lower back as the muscles become contracted and shortened. This contributes to tension in the lumbar spine, but without internal balancing, the overuse of the back muscles can also have a dramatic impact on the muscles on the front of the trunk: the abdominals.

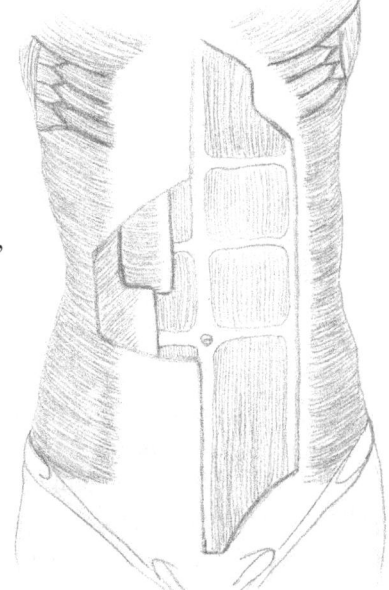

I find that in yoga, the abdominals are often either overlooked or overworked during pregnancy. This muscle group is composed of four muscle layers, each of which can be affected by the expanding uterus. While we are not seeking to maintain a flat stomach, ignoring the front abdominal muscles is one key mistake in practicing yoga during pregnancy.

The deep transverse abdominis (TA) muscle runs sideways, wrapping around the internal organs. Ultimately, it is this muscle that needs both strength and suppleness to be able to support the ones above it. That said, the TA also compresses the internal organs if too strongly engaged, so it's not as simple as solely focusing on TA exercises.

Above the TA are the diagonal layers of the internal and external obliques, and superficial to the obliques rests the "six pack" or rectus abdominis muscles. This most superficial muscle layer is made of two vertical-fiber muscles that run from the base of the ribs to the top of the pubic bone, connected in the middle by the fascial line of the linea alba. As the baby grows during pregnancy, all these muscles must continue to support the front weight of the body while also stretching to accommodate the changing body shape.

So why does posture matter for abdominal integrity? Well the trunk of the body could be thought of as a sort of flexible soda can. There is a wall all the way around, as well as a top and base, and the contents inside are under pressure. Lean too much on one side of the wall, and that wall could fail to support the "soda" inside. We've all seen what happens if you puncture the side of a soda can: the contents then leak out! How we hold our bodies, and how we move them, impacts how well our tissues support the function of the organs within our bodies.

Remember the pregnancy hormone relaxin? It causes the linea alba to gradually widen as pregnancy continues. This expansion is normal up to a point. But if a pregnant person's standard posture has been to tuck the tail and then thrust the ribs forward (as is often cued in Tadasana when we "roll the shoulders up, down, and back"), the weight of their body shifts forward into the pubic symphysis and the linea alba fascial line for abdominal support. The body responds to the stresses we give it over time, and constantly stressed fascia will either become stretched out or hardened and more brittle, depending on the load placed on it. Remember that overly tight psoas muscles often accompany this type of posture. If the linea alba, the line connecting the two halves of the abdominal wall together, is already thin and stressed due to chronic postural habits, movements like aggressive backbends (presumably done to open a tight psoas) or movements that contract the vertical core muscles (rectus abdominis) without proper support[12] could actually cause a separation between the two halves of the rectus abdominis!

This condition is called diastasis recti, and it affects nearly 60% of women in the US[13] (and I suspect even more in the fitness community). Since there are no sensory nerves in the linea alba, many women will not feel this separation happening unless they are extremely sensitive to feedback from the rectus abdominis. Any postural habits that lean into connective tissue rather than directing the weight through the bones carry a risk of damaging areas

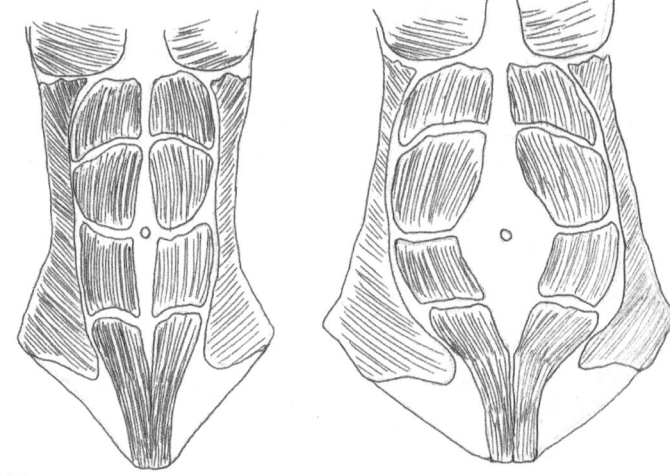

that are intended to provide support, leading to compression, imbalance, pain, and possible injury. Once again, finding good balance has effects which ripple throughout the body.

When balancing the body as we do in Tadasana, consider that the front of the body needs to move into the back as much as the back into the front. The pubic bone needs to dip. The groins deepen. The pelvis tilts slightly forward to place the weight into the legs and the feet.

---

[12] Actions which actively flex the spine could be crunches, sitting straight up or lying straight down, or even active pushing in labor for a prolonged period of time (we're talking multiple hours here)

[13] Sperstad, J. B., Tennfjord, M. K., Hilde, G., Ellström-Engh, M., & Bø, K. (2016, September). Diastasis recti abdominis during pregnancy and 12 months after childbirth: Prevalence, risk factors and report of Lumbopelvic Pain. *British Journal of Sports Medicine.* https://www.ncbi.nlm.nih.gov/pmc/articles/PMC5013086/

In the trunk, the ribcage floats over the bowl of the pelvis. This means the front ribs often need to drop and move backwards rather than thrusting forward and up, and the back ribs need to lift and spread, as though unfurling a set of wings from the mid-back. The irony is that when I have instructed students to float their back ribs and allow the pubic bone to drop slightly away from the navel, they report feeling a subtle organization in their lower abdominals. As one student described it, "It's as though something just came online inside my body. And it seems to extend down to my pelvic floor, too!" If we allow the body to align with the field of gravity, the deep core instinctively responds—without us having to actively engage anything.

A note about fetal positioning: If preserving abdominal integrity and finding a fluid spine throughout pregnancy weren't enough motivation to stop the tucking epidemic we seem to be caught in, there is a further benefit to finding balance in our standing postures. The baby's position towards the end of pregnancy is mostly guided by gravity and the internal tone in the muscles and fascia surrounding the uterus. By 28 weeks, the heaviest parts of the baby are the spine and the back of the head, so all things being equal and aligned, those parts would move to the lowest point in the uterus due to gravity. Ideally, the baby would spiral to face its mother's right side with its spine curved to the left as labor begins, unless something gets in the way.

But of course, not everything is balanced and equal, and our habitual posture often does not encourage optimal positioning of our connective tissues. Constantly tucking the tail makes the back of the pelvis the lowest point, which could contribute to a baby facing forward, not back. This positioning changes how they might move through the pelvis and can dramatically change the sensations of labor for mom (Ever heard of "back labor?"). The simplest way a pregnant woman can be proactive in helping her baby position itself is to find an overall balance in the body, which automatically puts the lowest point of the pelvis at the front of the pelvic bowl. The belly rests softly away from mom's spine, encouraging baby's spine to drop to the front side, thus orienting them to face backwards to begin labor. Easier and more comfortable for everyone.

If we return to Cyndi Lee's assertion that Tadasana is the foundation for every standing pose, how does that change the way we think about pelvic and spinal placement in the various yoga shapes? In Warrior 1, it means no more tucking the tail. In High Lunge, it also means no tucking; instead, find ways to float the back ribs to relieve lower back compression. In Warrior 2, draw that back groin in, rather than splaying it out, to bring the pelvis into neutral. And Trikonasana? Oh, there's so much to explore in that one, and we will in the Practice section of this book. For now, just think about how to keep the creases of the groins deep and align the body so you don't lose the connection to the earth underneath.

Given the increased mobility in the female pelvis, the hormonal changes during pregnancy, and the potential postural habits that people may bring to the yoga mat, we need to remember the significance of the pelvic placement in the body and treat it with the reverence and respect it deserves. This is the crystal bowl holding both the vital organs and the baby. It is not meant to be cracked open like a book, tipped, or twisted like a washcloth. As we shift into different asana shapes, we need to think of the pelvis and the pregnant belly as the cradle for the baby. When it comes to asana, there is a sort of middle ground we are seeking: not too tight, which would restrict adjustments to the weight changes of pregnancy and limit baby's available movement, but not too loose, which would lead to instability, pain, and overcompensation. The trick is to find the balance of strength and flexibility, movement and stillness, support and effort. In this way we can restore the balance needed while still navigating the ever-changing shape of the pregnant body.

Shavasana: lying down

There is one family of postures where the considerations around pelvic and spinal alignment during pregnancy shift dramatically because of a fundamental change in the orientation to gravity. This is the restorative family of yoga postures.

Rest during pregnancy is a key component both in overall comfort and in preparation for labor and birth. Ultimately the ability to release and relax during the labor process is what allows a laboring woman to stay energized and be able to manage the varying sensations of labor and birth. As I often remind prenatal students, birth is the most profound letting go we can do.

But when we consider the king of the restorative postures; Shavasana (and the queen, Supta Baddha Konasana) we run into two key concerns regarding a pregnant body. The first is that if we are working to align the body to promote optimal fetal positioning (head down, looking towards mom's back), lying with the navel pointed towards the ceiling is encouraging the exact opposite. As Gail Tully, founder of Spinning Babies® says, "Gravity is 24/7." If the belly is constantly pointing towards the ceiling, this encourages the heavy part of baby to wind up on the back side of mom's body (i.e., baby facing forward). While gravity isn't the only factor in fetal positioning, it is a contributor, so lying flat isn't the best position once baby's head is heavy enough to influence positioning (around 28 weeks).

The second challenge is that the vena cava, the primary vein for returning blood from the lower body to the heart, runs through the back of the pelvis, slightly to the right side of the spine. Since veins do not have the ability to contract and push blood through, compressing a vein will decrease blood flow while the weight is applied. Think how stepping on a garden hose stops the water from flowing. This can lead to a sudden drop in blood pressure, a condition called supine hypotension. But whether this is even a consideration depends on what stage of pregnancy we are talking about. Prior to 20 weeks or so, the considerations for lying on the back are not as involved, and mom can still lie supine if she doesn't feel dizzy, woozy, or short of breath. This is the reason behind two of the major myths in yoga around practicing when pregnant: that you can't ever lie on your back and that you must always lie on your left side. I'll examine these myths a bit deeper in the Practice section of this book, but for now, let's just say they are being applied far too broadly. Beginning some time during the second trimester, some women feel uncomfortable and may need to modify this posture.

Let's start with the challenge of lying on the back. At some point in pregnancy mom will feel uncomfortable in this position due to the compression on the vena cava or the pressure on the lower end of the sacrum and tailbone. Remember, relaxin makes these joints mobile during pregnancy, so for those more flexible bodies, it may be the pressure, not the compression of blood vessels, that signals a need to move.

The initial way to address the vena cava compression is to get the weight off the back of the pelvis. This can be achieved in two ways. First, you could place a rolled blanket or small pillow under the right hip, shifting the body's weight slightly to the left side. Since the vena cava runs to the right of the spine, for some this can effectively remove gravitational compression from the expanding uterus and baby above.

The thing is, lifting one hip inevitably puts a twist into the body's connective tissue, so if we spend an extended amount of time here we are going to promote tightening in one area and overstretching in another. We don't usually practice twisting *asanas* to only one side, right? The solution is to begin to elevate the body so the pressure from the growing belly and baby is directed towards the base of the pelvis rather than directly into the back. This means employing yoga blocks and/or bolsters to create an incline, ideally about 45 degrees, which mom can then rest back against. I always think of this as creating a yoga lounge chair for Shavasana.

If using blocks and a bolster to create the "lounge chair," begin by placing the first block so it supports roughly under the chest, with the second block behind it on the higher height. Lean the bolster against the block while sitting with the pelvis directly against the bolster so the lumbar spine is fully supported. To come down, shift the weight to one side of

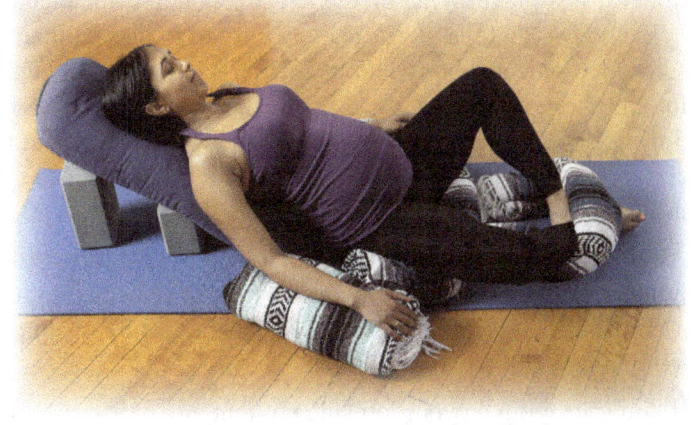

the pelvis, and support the body to lie down slightly sideways before reclining back fully onto the bolster. The slight sideways shift is to preserve the integrity of the front abdominal wall and avoid creating diastasis recti.

If you have extra blankets or pillows available, I recommend placing them under both arms, as well as a rolled blanket under the tops of the thighs to further support and enhance the feeling of being completely supported. Support leads to relaxation. If practicing Supta Baddha Konasana, take the rolled blanket under the thighs and wrap it around the pelvis, bringing the support under the outer thighs. An additional blanket can also be rolled up and wrapped around the feet to support the ankles.

I usually recommend this variation for students looking for classic Shavasana until around the third trimester of pregnancy. After about 28 weeks, while you may still be comfortable lying in a reclined position, we have to begin considering both the impact of this posture on fetal positioning and the stress that putting weight on the base of the pelvis has on the posterior pelvic ligaments. Remember that constantly tucking the tail eventually leads to the back of the pelvis becoming overly squeezed and rigid, and, while comfortable, the reclining position is doing the same action of tucking the tailbone. Remember, those joints are softened by relaxin throughout the pregnancy. Reclining postures should be practiced with caution so as to maintain balance in the SI joints and sacro-tuberous ligaments. And by the end of pregnancy, we need to shift the weight off the tailbone and lower sacrum to allow the pelvis to be supple in preparation for labor and the birth process. For some pregnant people (and I am in this camp), the pressure at the base of the spine becomes uncomfortable long before there are any signals that a blood vessel is being compressed. For these students, we have to shift to a more involved variation, but one which most pregnant people discover on their own for sleeping: Side-lying Shavasana.

Side-lying Shavasana

Shifting Shavasana onto its side has multiple benefits in late pregnancy. The weight can be fully off the vena cava since gravity no longer presses towards the back of the body. Additionally, if we favor lying on the left, we can take advantage of a physiological asymmetry in the body—that the uterus is more curved to the left than it is to the right. A baby which settles its spine and body into its mother's left side will be able to tuck its chin more fully into its chest, which has several benefits for the progression of movements through the pelvis during labor. I'll cover these more in the Birth section, but the main benefit is that a tucked chin presents a smaller circle of the head into the pelvis, so baby is able to move through more easily.

All that being said, the key in restorative postures is rest and support, and if mom is sick of lying on her left side (as many of you may have been told to do), then lying on the right for a time may be more beneficial. Look for the feeling of support and rest rather than always locking into one side over another.

If you start lying on your left side without any props, the curvatures of your body and the weight of the baby will pull the body into a one-way lean that will become uncomfortable over time and also compress certain areas of the pelvis. To alleviate this compression, we have to employ several yoga props to find full support.

Start by placing a pillow or bolster under the top leg so that it rests level with your outer hip. The bottom leg can simply be extended along the ground. It is important that the bolster supporting the top leg supports not only the knee but the ankle and foot as well. The outer fascial line along the leg, if left unsupported, will drag on the upper ilium, leading to tension at the SI and lower back joints. It seems a small thing, but fascial connections can be subtle. With the lower leg supported, roll your weight ever so slightly forward so your belly slightly leans into the bed or floor, re-creating a downward tilt to encourage baby to roll their back into the front side of your body.

Once we have the leg supported, there is also the weight of the belly itself, the curvature of the shoulders, and the angle of the neck and head. To support the neck and head, place another pillow, or possibly a rolled up blanket, underneath the head so the neck rests in a level alignment to the floor. A blanket can be doubly useful to wrap the arms around, hugging it towards the chest as one might do with a teddy bear. This supports both the upper arm and the chest, and for stomach sleepers it can even create the illusion of once again lying on the belly. If the belly is pulling on the lower back, fold up a blanket or towel and place it under the entire waistline of the pose. This raises the lumbar spine back into a level position and re-aligns the pelvis while also supporting the weight of the belly and baby. The intention is to fully release the weight of the body without having additional stretching sensations feeding back to your brain. With the body fully supported, the nervous system has a moment of experiencing less feedback from the body and can enjoy a state of relative quiet. A nice addition to this whole setup can be placing a bolster against your back body. This creates a feeling of containment and safety, and for some, it allows the nervous system to more fully relax because you know nothing is going to "sneak up behind you."

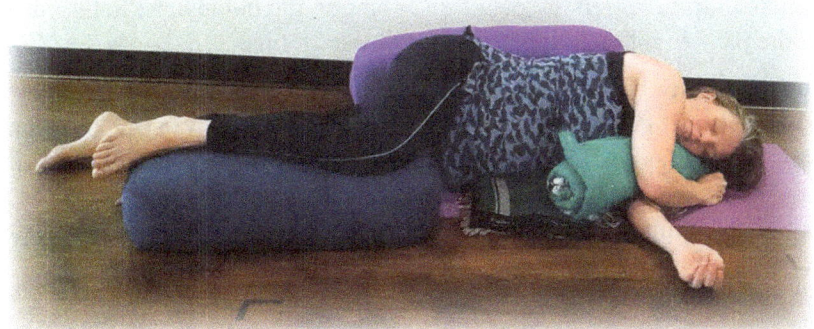

In evaluating whether you are able to practice certain reclining postures, the question is often a matter of degree and duration. How long are we practicing with the belly pointed upwards? How much weight is being applied to the tailbone and sacrum? For something as prolonged as Shavasana (5-10 minutes) it makes sense to modify, but if we are talking about transitional movements, or a pose which might be held for less than a minute, then even late in pregnancy we might be able to practice supine postures, as long as we intersperse some counterposes in between.

With all the changes and possible movement in the pelvis during pregnancy, it would be easy to become overly cautious and create an air of danger for practicing yoga during pregnancy. Indeed, I think many of the restrictions we often hear about for prenatal yoga are brought about by a great deal of fear and misunderstanding about the full structure and function of the pelvic bones and ligaments. Yes, they are more mobile, but that movement has a purpose and should be supported, not avoided. We are seeking a place of middle ground. Too tight, and the body cannot make the postural adaptations necessary for the changes of pregnancy— and ultimately may have trouble allowing the baby out. Too loose, and the body collapses onto itself. And this instability becomes a problem when once again the body must release and open in order to birth. The pelvis is the fulcrum on which the upper and lower body depend, and if we start thinking of how the yoga practice affects this area of the body, our awareness will radiate out to involve everything connected to it.

Key Takeaways

The spine is made of four interlocking curves which create shock absorption for the body. During pregnancy these curves deepen to accommodate additional weight and a shifting center of gravity.

Existing postural patterns can reveal themselves during pregnancy as the body tries to shift but encounters tense muscle patterns. Tucking the tail flattens the spinal curvatures, which reduces their shock absorption and does not relieve back pain in the long run.

The primary muscles which influence the position of the spine (and also the pelvis) are the psoas, the glutes, and the hamstrings. Releasing and balancing these can free the spine to adapt.

When standing (or sitting), align the pelvis and spine so the pubic bone points slightly down to encourage the baby to rotate into better positioning for birth.

The core body (composed of the front abdominals, the back muscles, the diaphragm, and the pelvic floor) must also shift with the weight of pregnancy. Excessive stretching and loading of the front abdominals (as in sitting straight up from the floor or constantly tucking the tail) can weaken the connective tissue line in the center (linea alba) and in some cases lead to a separation in the abdominals. Balancing the body's weight is key to avoiding this.

When resting, the spine, along with the pelvic joints, needs to be fully supported so the muscles can release without sinking into the joints and to avoid compressing the posterior pelvic blood vessels. Elevate the body on props to a 45 degree angle or lie on the side with the legs and head fully supported.

Balanced spinal and pelvic alignment, whether standing, sitting, or lying down, help baby position better for labor and birth.

3 — The Magical Vagina and Her Pelvic Floor

"One of the biggest lies perpetuated by modern obstetrics is that the vagina is inadequate to the task of birthing and thus must be surgically enhanced to accomplish it."

—Debra Pascali-Bonaro, Orgasmic Birth

A note of awareness and sensitivity: For many people, this area of the body is also a place of trauma and possibly shame. From the #metoo movement of 2016, we have become aware of exactly how many women have experienced some sort of sexual assault, trauma, or other abuse. I encourage you to be very gentle with yourself during our explorations, especially if you have had trauma or even a negative experience associated with this area of the body. Notice if there are places or paragraphs that generate feelings for you, and do not feel you must follow any of the exercises or suggested practices if you do not feel ready to do so. Yoga practice is always meant to move at your own pace and be guided by your own inner teacher. That teacher knows your history and your emotions. They will still be with you after you close this book, and they fundamentally love you just as you are—even if you don't fully believe that voice when it comes from within. At the end of the day, I want to remind all of us that we are fundamentally good individuals who are worthy of respect, dignity, and love. So investigate as you feel comfortable, especially as we explore yoga *asanas*. Your vagina and pelvic floor will appreciate the patience and compassion.

A doula friend of mine has a bumper sticker that says "Vaginas are magic!" There are few areas of the body with more nerve endings and sensory awareness than the network weaving throughout the vaginal tube. Radiating and encircling this opening, the surrounding pelvic floor muscle network supports not only the weight of the normal internal organs but also the full weight of a growing baby, uterus, and placenta during pregnancy. And when the time is right, these same muscles guide the rotation of the baby's head and are able to widen and release so much that the baby is able to move through the vaginal pathway and out into the world to be born. With proper preparation, support, and patience, the vagina is able to do this all without damage or dysfunction. It does seem almost magical.

Vagina, *yoni*, vulva, punanni, perineum. There is perhaps no other part of the body that has more names, more mystery, is more maligned or more misunderstood than the vagina. According to a 2016 study by the British cancer charity Eve Appeal,[14] nearly 44% of women in the UK

---

[14] Hinde, N. (2016, August 31). *Nearly half of women can't identify the vagina, so how can they spot cancer?* HuffPost UK. Retrieved September 12, 2022, from https://www.huffingtonpost.co.uk/entry/half-of-women-can-not-identify-vagina-eve-appeal-survey_uk_57c6e0f7e4b085cf1ecccea5

are tragically unable to identify the different parts of their own genital anatomy. Even more stunning, a 2014 study[15] from the Yale School of Medicine found that nearly 50% of American women didn't understand the function of the vagina in reproduction. This area has more shame, fear, and social taboos around it than just about any other. The only one that comes close might be its next door neighbor, the anus. Don't get our culture started on poop talk! There are so many misconceptions around the abilities, function, and structure of the vagina and the surrounding pelvic floor during pregnancy, labor, and birth that it warranted its own chapter.

Books on female spirituality speak of the chalice, the womb, and the cradle of life—which brings a whole different energy into this small space at the base of the pelvis. The Muladhara (root) Chakra is located at the perineum. This is the seat of *shakti*, the Kundalini rising root. No wonder the midwives were burned as witches during the Middle Ages: they were in tune with the primal, feminine, magical energy of the vagina. Or at least we could have some fun thinking of it that way.

While we could go into a vast discussion on sexuality and sexual function contained within the vaginal tissues, that is a topic for another book and outside the scope of a yoga class (unless we want to get into Tantric yoga—which is also another book). Whenever we sequester something away, we give it power by making it secret and restricted. Rather than leaving the vagina to be the territory only of those with medical degrees, let's take a deeper look at this area and the musculature that supports it. In doing so we can reclaim the use and integration of this part of our body, not to mention the energetic qualities of the yogic *yoni*, like mental clarity, that come from having good pelvic floor function.

The vaginal pathway

The word "vagina" itself comes from Latin and means "sheath" (as in the sheath for the "sword"...um). Leaving aside the gender politics around how and why it was named this and whether it should still be called so, I'm going to continue using the word solely because it is the most familiar. Other names, such as *yoni*, have also been applied from the Tantric yoga traditions. Some may feel more comfortable using those terms as they seem less patriarchal. But since vagina is the medical term, I'll continue using it here.

Look in a medical textbook, and you'll probably find the function of the vagina described as a pathway for menstrual blood, a passage for semen, and a canal for the baby to exit through. But there is so much more going on here than simply the functional use of this opening to move and receive things. With its elaborate neural network, the vagina is one physical center for pleasure in the female body and is directly impacted by the tone of the muscles that support this intricate network (A side note: Why the baby's path into the world got a name like "canal," which also involves hard cement sides, is another point I'm not going to fully unpack. There's a lot of baggage here, so we have to step lightly if we're to arrive at a place where our yoga can prove functional and once again empowering.).

---

[15] Peart, K. N. (2014, January 28). The science of baby-making still a mystery for many women. *YaleNews*. https://news.yale.edu/2014/01/27/science-baby-making-still-mystery-many-women

My own experience with the vagina and the birth process came during the first birth I attended as a doula. Apparently my calm demeanor in my support of my client (thank you, meditation practice!) led the attending midwife to believe I had done this before. Thinking I was a seasoned doula, the midwife asked me to come hold my client's leg while she pushed. I had been under the belief that I didn't go near "that end" as the doula, but in the moment, I played along. Sitting awkwardly on the edge of the bed with a foot wedged on my shoulder, I was completely lost about what I was seeing. I heard the midwife say she could see the head, but my only thought was "Really?" What was head? What was vagina? All I could see were folds of tissue expanding and receding. And then slowly and gently, what had seemed like a back wall slid forward and unfurled into a crowning baby head. A small face emerged, the head rotated, and out slid a sleeping, tiny blue human. I'm sure I forgot to breathe. Then, at the sound of her mother's voice this small creature opened enormous blue eyes, turned to look up towards her mother, and let out her first cry. It was all I could do not to leap back from the edge of the bed, screaming "Oh my god! It's alive!"

Despite often being described as a channel or tunnel, the vagina is in fact a soft folding tube surrounded by the layers of muscle and fascia in the pelvic floor. The walls of the vagina are folded like an accordion, with layers of erectile and connective tissue woven throughout. They are capable of both expanding and contracting dramatically depending on what is need-ed. The folds and muscles can contract to create a snug opening during intercourse, or they can expand to create enough room for a baby to emerge, all without any tearing or damage if given enough time and attention. In fact it is the tone of the musculature around the vagina and pelvic floor that guides the baby's head down and through the pelvis during the birth process. So really, when we look at the anatomy of the vagina for pregnancy and birth, we are more correctly examining the pelvic floor that surrounds it.

The pelvic floor

The musculature supporting the vagina and the other two openings in the female pelvis is the pelvic floor or the pelvic diaphragm. This muscle group, which contrary to common depiction domes up, not down, is the support mechanism for the internal organs. The pelvic floor is composed of three muscle layers that weave together in what is called interdigitation. We could think of interdigitation as similar to the interweaving of different fibers in a piece of cloth. The muscle layers of the pelvic floor form the foundation of our core muscles, and when functioning well, they are involved in organ and spinal support as well as maintaining intra-abdominal pressure.

These muscles aid in urinary and fecal continence, and they also assist in moving lymph and blood throughout the body, not to mention pulsing during sexual activity (yes, I'm talking or-gasm here). And the balance of tone and suppleness within these tissues guides the baby's head through the pelvis during the birth process. Quite a lot of complexity for such a small area!

For a better understanding of how the pelvic floor muscles function during pregnancy, and where yoga can help bring balance to them, let's start with the most superficial layer: the muscles closest to the outside of the body. Beginning in the front of the pelvic outlet, along the inside of the pubic bone we find the ischiocavernosus and bulbocavernosus muscles. Moving to the back of the pelvis, we have the fibers of the external anal sphinchter. The bulbocavernosus fibers link with the anal sphincter to create a figure 8 shape that encircles the opening to the urethra and vagina in the front and the anal sphinchter in the back. Where the two circles of the "figure 8" cross, they form an area known as the perineum.

Discovering the perineum (if you're so inclined)

Sit upright, with the weight of your body resting on the front of your sitz bones. Bring your attention to the base of your pelvis, imagining the diamond space between your sitz bones, pubis, and tail. Now imagine drawing a line front to back and another line side to side to intersect in the middle of the diamond. This is roughly where the weight of your body is falling as you sit.

On an inhale, see if you can allow the center of the diamond to expand downward. On an exhale, imagine lifting just the middle upwards. This is the perineum. Notice if you feel more engagement in the front or back of the diamond—or if this feels too subtle. Don't worry if you don't seem to feel any movement. The actions can seem very small at first. But even small movements can have a huge impact.

The perineum marks the space between the genitals and the anus. This area has been called the root, the "taint" (supposedly a contraction of "it" and "ain't," but it always sounded like "tainted" to me). I have also heard it referred to as the "nacho" area (as in, "it's not yo front and it's not yo back") which is at least a bit more humorous. Whatever you choose to call it, the perineum is an area that has been the focus of numerous procedures and practices. It can be massaged for sexual pleasure and to support the birth process. It is where the surgical cut of an episiotomy would be made. It is the physical separation between the opening of the vagina and the opening of the anus. This is also where the first *chakra* (Muladhara), the actions of Mula Bandha, and proper pelvic floor engagement originate.

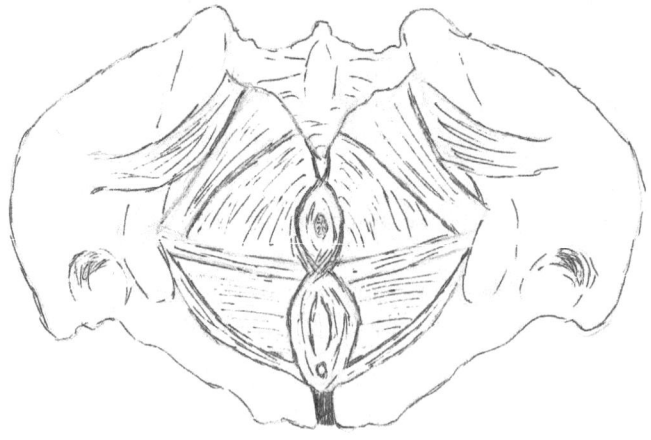

If the fibers of the first layer of the pelvic floor are a front to back figure eight, the second layer fibers are horizontal, running sideways from sitz bone to sitz bone. These initially make up the superficial transverse perineal tendon. Deep (meaning further inside the body) to this tendon, we find the transverse perineal muscles (creative name, eh?) running from the inside of the sitz bones inward and into the central tendon of the perineum. There is also a dense fascial sheath called the pelvic diaphragm creating a platform on which the pelvic muscles can act to lift the pelvic organs.

The interweaving of these layers with the figure eight muscles creates an interdependent and responsive web that can often accommodate for injury to one segment by compensating with another. The intersecting lines of muscle and fascia also make this area extremely rigid. This rigidity is appropriate, as the pelvic floor could be asked to bear intense weight and force from the body (think of the impact of an action like jumping or running). However, it should be noted that excessive toughness of the pelvic floor can become a hindrance during the birth process.

Finding the perineal tendon

Bring your hand to touch your sitz bone. Now bring your fingers to the inside of the sitz bone, onto the pelvic floor (be gentle here!). If you are inclined, try lightly massaging the tissue on the inside of your sitz bone. You may be able to feel a ropey line extending towards the other sitting bone, running into the perineum we discovered in the last exercise. Try exhaling and lifting the perineum as your fingers press the tendon. Did it firm up? Did it drop down? Notice how your own body responds. These will be subtle movements, almost imagined rather than palpated from this far outside. But you may begin to get a sense of how the pelvic floor fits together.

Finishing our exploration into the layers of the pelvis, we come to the deepest and largest group of muscles in the pelvic floor known as the levator ani (Latin for "anus lifter"). Attached to each side of the pelvic outlet and mid-pelvis, this set of muscles is responsible for the lifting of the internal organs, the rotation of the baby's head during the birth process, and—as its name might suggest—the regulation of peeing and pooping in everyday life. The muscle group is subdivided into three segments depending on which opening they connect with: the puborectalis for the rectum, the pubo-urethralis for the urethra, and the pubococcygeus, which encircles the opening to the vagina in women—and obviously doesn't in men (although men have all these muscles, too!). These three layers of the pelvic, combined with the coccygeus muscle, which connects the coccyx to the ischial spine, make up the majority of the pelvic floor.

External pelvic floor massage (if you are so inclined)
(recorded instruction available at www.ombirths.com/ombirthsbook/external-pelvic-floor-massage)

Take an upright posture, either in Sukhasana (crossed legs), Virasana (kneeling) on the floor, or seated in a chair. Bring your pelvis upright so the weight rests on the front edge of your sitz bones. Lean to your left and feel your right sitz bones with your fingers. Now bring your fingers just to the inside of your sitz bone, onto the muscles in the middle (This is over clothing people—we're not getting that personal yet.).

Press and gently massage the tissue on the inside of the sitz bone. Does it feel tense? Squishy? Tender? Is there a feeling like a ropey line anywhere? Be gentle, as this is a very sensitive area, but take note of whatever sensations you might encounter. What do things feel like if you move closer to the pubic bone? Or towards the tailbone? Continue to massage for about a minute.

Now replace the right sitz bone back on the chair or floor. What do you feel now? Does the right feel different from the left? I often find after a self massage that the massaged side feels lower and softer than the other. Take note of your own experience.

Now repeat the massage on the left sitz bone and the left side of the pelvic floor. Are there differences from right to left? Does one side feel more tender than the other? Or tighter? Or looser? Because both the first and third layers of the pelvic floor run front to back, it is not uncommon to have one side be more involved than the other. In fact, this combination of tension and laxity can sometimes make it tricky when working to balance the pelvic floor in yoga practice, and excessive tension can be almost more problematic than not enough tone.

It should also be noted that while most pictures of the pelvic floor show it as a bowl or a cup contained within the pelvis, the pelvic floor actually domes subtly upwards, similar to the respiratory diaphragm.[16] This common misunderstanding came about because dissections are always done on cadavers, and upon death, the pelvic floor releases and falls into the cup shape. When alive, far from being a sagging hammock, a well-toned pelvic floor is like a gentle upward dome, ready to bounce the weight above it back upwards.

This upward dome allows our pelvic floor to constantly shift and adjust to keep our organs from sliding down, and there is quite a bit of weight to lift. Even without pregnancy, we have the weight of the internal organs, the upper body, any food or drink we consume, and bouncing or jostling brought on by movement. When you jump, or run, or cough, or laugh, your pelvic floor muscles respond to the changes in pressure within your abdominal cavity. When pressure is exerted downward (as when we cough), the pelvic floor reflexively lifts up to prevent something from falling out of the base. If this action isn't coordinated, or if the muscles in the pelvic floor are too underdeveloped, then it's possible something might come out when we did not intend it to. A pelvic dome lacking strength may result in an inability to hold urine or poop, or even in the pelvic organs descending into the pelvic bowl and sometimes out of the body (called organ prolapse).

To squeeze or not to squeeze?

Medical professionals have for years understood that developing tone in the muscles of the pelvic floor could be helpful both during pregnancy and birth as well as in postpartum recov-

---

[16] Hjartardóttir , S., Nilsson , J., Petersen , C., & Lingman, G. (1997, July). The female pelvic floor: A dome-- not a Basin. *Acta obstetricia et gynecologica Scandinavica.* https://pubmed.ncbi.nlm.nih.gov/9246965/

ery. After all, these are the muscles which regulate the pelvic organ function. The common medical wisdom for creating tone in the pelvic floor muscles has been to instruct women (especially during pregnancy) to perform pelvic floor toning exercises. These exercises are often referred to as "Kegels" after Dr. Arnold Kegel, who developed the Kegel perineometer and Kegel exercises as non-surgical treatment of urinary incontinence from perineal muscle weakness. While Kegel exercises can increase muscle engagement in the pelvic floor, they are not as precise as we can be with our yoga practices.

Kegels are often taught with imprecise instructions such as "Squeeze the muscles like trying to stop a stream of urine while peeing." While accurate in terms of engaging part of the pelvic floor, this instruction often misses several key points about good pelvic floor function. First, it assumes the person performing the Kegels has an awareness of which muscles to engage—which you may have just discovered is not always available. One may think they are squeezing the correct muscles but may actually be engaging auxiliary muscle groups such as the gluteals or transverse abdominals.

Second, the focus of Kegels is usually on tightening. What if the muscles need to release (as they will need to during the birth process)? An overly tight pelvic floor can actually be as problematic as one that is overly loose. In these cases, performing Kegel exercises may simply exacerbate the underlying problem. And third, Kegel exercises assume the pelvic floor is engaging to the same degree in all parts, when in fact it may be tight on one side but loose on another. Dr. Kegel did find a highly useful tool for combating incontinence if the only other alternative is surgery, but given that the pelvic floor muscles not only control bladder function but also play a key role in pelvic health, we need a more nuanced approach which finds the "yoga" between too tight and too loose.

Pelvic floor breathing
(recorded instruction available at www.ombirths.com/ombirthsbook/pelvic-floor-breathing-discovery)

Sit upright on your pelvis, with the weight on the front of the sitz bones. Take a few deep abdominal breaths and see if you can feel the movement of your pelvic floor without pre-determining whether it should be going up or down. What happens on your inhale? Do the muscles between the sitz bones descend or lift? What about on the exhale? If you can't tell, don't fret. These movements are subtle, and for some we have never truly put our attention into this area of the body. It is also possible that these muscles have become confused, due to a popular fitness trend of sucking in on the inhale, and have forgotten their intended function of providing bouncy support.

As a further exploration, try putting your attention into the pelvic floor. Take a deep breath in. Now, focusing on the feeling within your pelvic muscles, cough. Try it a few times and notice what you feel during this sudden increase of intra-abdominal pressure. Do things lift? Do they drop? (hopefully nothing is leaking out—but if it is, go use the bathroom, and then return to this book). If you now feel more confused than before, take a deep breath and relax. We'll come back here after we look at why too much tension can be as problematic as too little.

What's wrong with being too tight?

Ever try to carry something heavy, like a stack of books? Think about how much your arm muscles were able to respond to changes in movement and weight shift while carrying the books. I'll bet not as much as other times—because they were holding the books. Now imagine adding several more heavy books, say a couple volumes of those old encyclopedias, onto the stack. Your arm muscles would become further restricted, and if you then needed to respond quickly, such as to dodge someone who nearly walked into you, it is quite likely that you might drop one or all of the books.

This is effectively the situation that occurs when the pelvic floor is too tight, also called hypertonic. Instead of acting as a nice springy trampoline, the levator ani muscle group has spent so much time contracting and lifting that it has become rigid, with very little bounce available. Further contracting the pelvic floor muscles compounds the problem instead of helping it. A pelvic floor accustomed to constant contraction (Long distance running? Cycling? Constantly holding Mula Bandha?) can be just as dysfunctional as one that holds no tone at all.

Fortunately, yoga can offer a perfect solution. Before we can strengthen tense muscles, we must first release them. For all the yoginis who have an underdeveloped pelvic floor, I am willing to bet there are twice as many who are overly tight or, even more confusingly, have one muscle set in contraction while the others are undertoned! Add the weight of a growing uterus and baby to the load and we can begin to understand why so many women describe challenges with having to pee or aching in their backs later in pregnancy. It is important that the pelvic floor muscles are able to not only engage but also to stretch and lengthen. Think of the exclamation if one has a full bladder, "Don't make me laugh! I'm going to pee my pants!" or the experience of going for a run with a full bladder. A tense pelvic floor can't contract further when placed under stress, which is one reason bladder leaks are so common in pregnant people and those who have given birth.

A proper "Kegel"
(recording at www.ombirths.com/ombirthsbook/a-proper-kegel)

I will add the disclaimer here that if you are truly dealing with a hypertonic (overly tight) pelvic floor, this exercise is not for you, not yet. At the end of this chapter we will cover ways to open and lengthen the pelvic floor which can assist in promoting good muscle balance and health. But if you must practice Kegels, this exercise will at least promote using a full range of motion.

Sit upright or lie down with the spine in neutral (you should have a lower back curve). On an INHALE, allow the abdomen to expand and see if you can feel the breath dropping into the pelvic bowl, so that the muscles of the pelvic floor spread and release. On an EXHALE, try to contract the muscles around the perineum so that it lifts upwards within the pelvis. If this is too subtle at first, try drawing the walls of the vagina together. Another way of accessing this muscle group is to lift from the floor as though trying to avoid passing gas in yoga class (we've all done it), and then let the movement sweep forward to also lift the muscles involved in stopping urination. The muscle group fully engaged by these two motions is the pelvic floor.

Now, on an INHALE let these muscles release and even spread a bit, as though the pelvic dome were flattening slightly. If we do not release the muscles, we cannot build strength, so allow them to let go before trying to engage them again. On the exhale you may then find that the muscles almost reflexively lift, as the respiratory diaphragm draws the abdominal organs upwards again.

Continue this process of lifting on the exhale and spreading on the inhale for several breaths, then pause and notice the natural responsiveness in the pelvic floor.

For those thinking I have mixed up my inhales and exhales in the exploration, I have not. To do a Kegel exercise that promotes the functional movement of the pelvic floor, you need to release on the INHALE and lift on the EXHALE. I like to think of the movement of the pelvic floor as being similar to how a jellyfish swims in the water. First, the center of the jellyfish spreads out, then the dome actively contracts upwards, moving the jellyfish forward in the water. In the same way, the pelvic floor might spread for a moment under pressure but then rebounds upwards as it responds, lifting and supporting the internal organs. If you find that your inclination is to do the opposite (meaning you are squeezing on the inhale and releasing on the exhale), you may be one of the thousands of people who are caught in reverse breathing. The constant focus on sucking in during the inhale, especially in the fitness industry, has led to many people developing confusion in their pelvic floor muscles.

If this is you, remember that this discovery is an immense opportunity to develop health and function within your body! And if you can actually feel when the muscles contract, you at least are able to contact them. Practice slowly shifting from squeezing on the inhale to doing so on the exhale. At first it may feel like patting your head and rubbing your stomach, but with patience, these muscles can develop better and more responsive function, which will help overall health throughout life.

The pelvic floor during labor

There's another reason beyond good core support to tone the pelvic floor muscles during pregnancy. As I have said several times already, toning these muscles so they can both contract and release influences the baby's pathway during the birth process. Here's how. The opening of the pelvic floor and its muscle fibers create a space inside the pelvis which is longer front to back than side to side. Conversely, the bones at the top of the pelvis are wider side to side at the pelvic inlet. This mismatch means that during the birth process the baby does not simply drop through the pelvis. They must make a 90 (or 270) degree turn when they reach the mid-pelvic level so their head can spiral through the pelvic floor, like a button fitting through a button hole. The ease or resistance to baby making these movements is guided in part by the relative tone of the pelvic floor muscles.

Called internal rotation in medical circles, this turn in the mid-pelvis is part of a larger set of motions the baby makes during labor known as the cardinal movements. These movements involve the baby first engaging in (i.e., settling their head into) the pelvic inlet, then descending into the mid-pelvic region, rotating on the pelvic floor so the head can move through the opening of the muscle fibers. Once through the pelvic floor, the baby extends their neck to draw their head under the pubic arch to crown and be born. I will discuss cardinal movements more fully in Chapter 12. For now, know that the central movement of baby's rotation through the pelvis is guided by the muscles of the pelvic floor, and if we are looking at the different levels of the pelvis, we are generally talking about the mid-pelvis area here. If the pelvic floor is too tight or too loose, it can either restrict movement or give no guidance for when and how baby should rotate, which can translate to a slower birth process.

Even worse, if the muscles are out of balance (common in highly flexible bodies), the head may turn, but only one side of the head moves downward, thus bending the neck to the side and causing a position known as asynclitic presentation, in which the baby's head is tilted to the side and moves asymmetrically into the pelvic bowl. It probably goes without saying that a head presenting in this way creates a larger shape than one entering the pelvis aligned symmetrically, and thus such a presentation can lead to a longer and more complicated labor. This also illustrates one of the many reasons why good, balanced tone of the entire pelvic floor is crucial not only for good pelvic function and support but also to better prepare the body for the birth process. Simply put: balanced pelvic floor tone contributes to a more comfortable pregnancy, a possibly faster and easier birth, and a smoother postpartum recovery. It all really does start with the pelvis.

Yoga pelvic exercises

Many of the initial exercises around connecting to the pelvic floor involve recruiting the breath. That's because in many ways, the movements of the pelvic diaphragm mimic the motions of the abdominal diaphragm above it. Like a piston moving up and down within a tube, or a balloon stretching and contracting as pressure is applied to various sides, the pelvic floor is constantly responding to the changes in internal abdominal pressure from breathing. This makes the breath a powerful tool in connecting not only to our nervous system but also to our root.

Pelvic floor breathing
(recording available at www.ombirths.com/ombirthsbook/pelvic-floor-breathing)

This exercise is designed to improve general pelvic floor awareness as well as help release excessive tension if it exists. The key here is to balance the abdominal and pelvic diaphragms over one another, so the downward motion of the respiratory diaphragm can be felt in the lower pelvic one.

Sit so the pelvis is balanced over the sitz bones, or even slightly to the front of them, and bring your awareness to the diamond between the sitz bones, pubis, and coccyx.

On an inhale allow the breath to move down into the abdomen. At the same time feel the pelvic floor releasing and expanding downward, like a jellyfish widening outward. On the exhale allow the pelvic floor to be drawn upwards like the contracting movement of the jelly-

fish swimming upwards. This movement is quite subtle, and for the moment this motion in the pelvic floor is primarily passive. The movement is simply a mirroring of the motions created by the abdominal diaphragm during relaxed breathing. During relaxed breathing the diaphragm moves downward on the inhale and upward on the exhale. This upward movement creates a vacuum effect which draws the pelvic floor upwards along with it.

In contrast, "reverse breathing" involves the abdomen sucking inwards on the inhale while the ribs expand, then dropping outwards on the exhale. Such breathing can contribute to confusion in the pelvic floor, which gets a lifting motion on the inhale and then a release on the exhale. Many people caught in this type of breath pattern wind up creating a host of pelvic challenges, as the muscles are unclear on when they can release and when they should support. Relaxed function is ideally: inhale, release and expand; exhale, draw upwards and engage.

Practice several minutes of relaxed pelvic floor breathing. Focus on simply feeling the movement of the pelvic floor without trying to increase it or force it. This exercise can help to not only rewire confused musculature but also assist in releasing excessive pelvic floor tension.

Additional variations of this breath can also be done in Shavasana, Supta Baddha Konasana, Balasana/Child's Pose, and Tadasana. Different orientations to gravity can sometimes increase the sensation within these muscles, contributing to greater awareness.

Pelvic exercises from the Kundalini tradition

To find yoga exercises speaking specifically about the pelvic floor muscles, I had to leave my Vinyasa yoga roots and venture into the world of the Kundalini tradition. As someone not fully trained in this tradition, I will beg forgiveness from experienced Kundalini teachers if I deviate from the classic teaching of these *mudras*. The exercises described here are intended to focus on developing pelvic function and balance, not necessarily on moving energy (though I have definitely found they do that too).

I also recognize that these are not hand *mudras* with which yoga teachers might be more familiar. Since my excursion into the Kundalini traditions, I have since discovered some hand *mudras* can also be used to bring better breath and movement into the pelvic floor; I have included those later in this chapter. *Mudra* ultimately means "gesture" in Sanskrit, so some of these movements are named for the movement which comes reflexively in the pelvic diaphragm after relieving the bladder or bowels. The instruction given here is intended to help gain awareness and function within the different segments of the pelvic floor.

A note: if you suspect your pelvic floor tends to be on the tighter side, be sure to do the stretching movements at the end of this chapter before practicing these muscle tightening actions. Remember, you can't strengthen a muscle that is already contracted.

Sahajoli Mudra (the clitoral tickle) ;)
(recording available at www.ombirths.com/ombirthsbook/sahajoli-mudra-the-clitoral-tickle)

This *mudra* brings awareness and engagement to the front triangle of the pelvic diaphragm, especially the muscles of the ischiocavernosus and the bulbocavernosus. In truth, this *mudra* is probably referring to the reflexive motion which comes following urination where the muscles draw upwards after releasing the stream of urine. Given the proximity in the female pelvis to the clitoris, however, there can be some pleasurable stimulation as well.

Sitting in an upright position with the pelvis balanced on the sitz bones, bring your awareness to the space between the sitz bones and the pubic bone at the front of your pelvis. On an inhale breathe down and allow this front triangle to release downward towards the floor. On an exhale gently draw the muscles around the urethra and clitoris upwards just behind the pubic bone. The action is one of lifting the urethral and vaginal walls but mostly leaves the rectum alone, so it primarily engages the first and second layers of the pelvic floor. Squeeze and lift until you feel a slight tickling at the front of the pelvic floor. Release on the inhale, allowing the whole triangle to descend. Do not hold the breath. Rather, allow the muscles to pulse in time with it. Be sure to allow the muscles to fully release before lifting on the next exhale. Practice several times (up to 10 at one sitting).

Ashwini Mudra (the back squeeze)
(recording available at www.ombirths.com/ombirthsbook/ashwini-mudra-the-back-squeeze)

This *mudra* is technically focused on the reflexive reengagement of the levator ani and anal sphichter muscles following defecation, but I have modified it here to also begin bringing awareness and tone to the back pelvic triangle. The difference is that rather than being a totally spontaneous motion, we begin adding some deliberate contraction to engage and tone the muscles.

Sitting with the pelvis upright on the sitz bones, bring your awareness to the pelvic floor. Focus on the space between the sitz bones and the tailbone. On the inhale, allow this back area to relax and open outwards, possibly bulging slightly but not exerting or bearing down. Feel the release and opening of the anal sphincter. On the exhale, draw up the muscle around the anus and tailbone. This is similar to the action we might use when trying to stop ourselves from passing gas in yoga class (we've all felt it—let's be honest here).

Holding this contraction, feel the strong lift in the back of the pelvis. On the inhale, allow these muscles to release and feel the dropping and spreading. Depending on your mobility and awareness, you may even feel the sitz bones spreading slightly. Practice several rounds in time with the breathing. Do not hold the breath; rather, allow it to dictate the tempo.

Pelvic exercises from the Ashtanga tradition

Mula Bandha (the root lock)
(recording available at www.ombirths.com/ombirthsbook/mulabhanda-the-full-lift)

The only pelvic *mudra* commonly used in Ashtanga and the more commonly practiced Vinyasa schools seems to be Mula Bandha. From what I have found, there are varying degrees of understanding of how this *bandha* is actually supposed to be performed—if indeed it should be performed at all, since *bandhas* are technically spontaneous according to yogic tradition. As long time Ashtanga yoga teacher Richard Freeman once said at a workshop I attended,

"When you come into this posture (Crow) don't forget to engage Mula Bandha—whatever that is." (I'm willing to bet Richard knows exactly what Mula Bandha is and is fully able to engage and release it, but his comment speaks to how elusive our awareness and engagement of the pelvic floor has become.) Here again, I find it is helpful to adapt the spontaneous engagement to a more conscious recruitment of the muscles to develop both awareness and tone.

Mula Bandha is probably what Kegel exercises would have developed into had Dr. Kegel been a yogi. Technically, the *bandhas* are spontaneous lifts located in each of the main diaphragms of the trunk: pelvic, abdominal, and throat. When the diaphragms in each of these areas are aligned, there is a spontaneous engagement which can be felt if focusing on the breath. While they are spontaneous, there are active ways to engage them, and it is this more active movement which I employ in my prenatal yoga classes. Active Mula Bandha involves a gentle but consistent lift and then a deliberate release of the entire pelvic floor front and back.

Beginning with the pelvis upright, once again bring your attention to the space bounded by the sitz bones, pubis, and tailbone. As with the relaxed pelvic breathing, on an inhale, allow these muscles to relax and expand downward—possibly feeling the sitz bones widen slightly. But rather than remaining passive, on the exhale actively draw all four points of the diamond towards the middle while lifting in the center at the perineum. The motion involves a contraction of the vaginal, anal, and urethral sphinchters. We could think of this motion as a forceful contraction of the "jellyfish," or as though we were picking up a pearl with the walls of the vagina. On the inhale, allow the muscles to release the pearl back downwards, feeling the pelvic floor spread once again.

Advanced variation

Having found the engagement of the entire pelvic floor, front to back and side to side, we can begin to investigate the relative responsiveness within the pelvic floor muscles. Rather than simply engaging the entire pelvic floor as if picking up a pearl, try this more subtle exercise:

Begin as for Mula Bandha, but instead of drawing up the entire diamond, imagine simply drawing the left side of the vaginal wall in and upwards on the exhale. How does this feel? Can you conceive of this side of the pelvic floor narrowing? Now inhale to release and try moving to the right side. What is the responsiveness here? More? Less? If you return to engaging the entire pelvic floor do you have a feeling of more movement from one sitz bone or the other? What about pubis towards the tail? Or tail towards the pubis? Try doing the sitz bone massage from earlier, then repeat the exercise. Was there a change?

In my experience teaching and talking with pregnant women and new mothers, it is actually quite common for there to be better responsiveness on one side of the pelvic floor than another. This can sometimes correspond to increased tension in other areas such as the glutes, hamstrings, or psoas muscles, or it can indicate an imbalance in the pelvic floor muscles themselves. The body is ultimately extremely smart and has learned how to compensate for our asymmetrical movement patterns. The resulting muscle patterns can sometimes be completely functional for everyday life but, when examined further, reveal massive imbalances in our tissues that become more apparent as we add the hormonal and physical changes and demands of pregnancy and birth. With the body in a state of transition as it is during pregnancy, there are opportunities to create better biomechanics in daily movement to help pregnant bodies manage the internal and external changes they inevitably encounter.

A postural note

In Chapter 2 I covered how ideal alignment for the bones in Tadasana orients the pelvis in a slightly forward rotation but moves the thigh bones back to remove excessive tucking of the tailbone. This same posture also promotes functional engagement of the pelvic floor.

When the pelvic bowl is tucked under (rotated posterior or "nutated"), the angle of the pelvic floor changes relative to the plumb line of gravity. The weight shifts towards the posterior pelvic triangle, making it more challenging for the full pelvic diaphragm to effectively engage and lift the internal organs. The backwards rotation also puts the pelvic floor out of alignment with the abdominal diaphragm, which reduces the strength it can exert during motion. Like a trampoline with one side overly stretched out, the muscles may begin to slacken when they should be toned and responsive.

Proper alignment of the pelvis isn't just for the benefit of the bones. When the pelvic outlet is angled parallel to the earth—or, more to the point, perpendicular to gravity—the natural response of the pelvic floor is to tone and lift in response to the increased pressure. Bottom line? Backing the pelvis up and dropping the pubis down not only distributes the bones effectively, it also assists the pelvic floor in maintaining good health and function. This is true no matter what position the legs are in. Sitting or standing, if we want the pelvic floor to be responsive, we need to have the bowl in its slightly forward rotation to neutral and the weight on the front of the sitz bones (if sitting). Think of this position as bringing the pubic bone down but then at the same time also bringing the tail towards it, the two points drawn to the earth like anchor lines on a ship. And just like the anchored ship, the pelvis is not fixed in this position but rather breathes and bobs as the body moves.

Exercises for freeing the pelvic floor

Because of the close relationship of the breath and the pelvic floor, the first step in releasing the pelvic floor is to get it moving in time with the breathing.

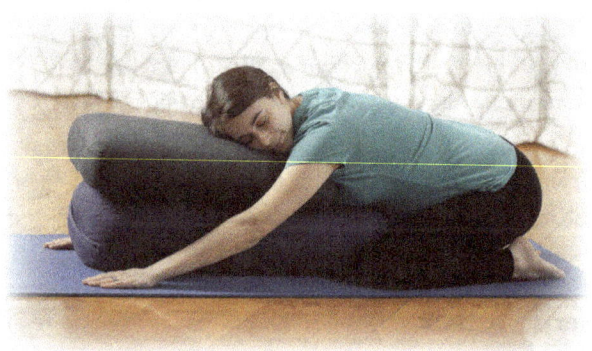

Child's Pose pelvic floor breathing

Begin in a wide knee Balasana (Child's Pose), with a bolster under the chest to bring the spine to neutral rather than being rounded and possibly a blanket beneath the hips to untuck the tailbone.

The exact propping will vary person to person, so the primary thing to focus on is how much movement you can feel within the pelvic floor and whether more padding increases or decreases it.

Taking the knees wide, tilt forward from the hips, focusing on spreading the sitz bones without excessive arch in the back. Bring the chest to rest comfortably against the bolster. Send the breath down into the lower abdomen and see if you can feel the pelvic floor release on the inhale. If not, add more padding to better support a neutral spine (I usually use two or more bolsters). Once you can feel the breath moving in the pelvic floor, rest forward and continue breathing for several minutes (honestly, you could rest here as long as you feel comfortable). The stretching downward on the inhalation helps to release tense muscles between the sitz bones.

This is effectively the same exercise as the seated pelvic floor breath, but the support from the props may assist both in staying longer and getting a deeper release.

Child's Pose pelvic floor release

Once you've become familiar with the movement in the pelvic floor muscles, try this exercise to feel the movement a deeper release allows.

Exhale, drawing the pelvic floor muscles into the body. Feel whatever level of lift you are able to. Then inhale, allowing the pelvic floor to widen. On the exhale, see if you can leave the pelvic floor relaxed. Repeat the inhale two more times without drawing up on the exhale, allowing the pelvic floor to spread further—even mentally imagining can be helpful here. After the third or even fourth inhale, try actively drawing in with an exhale and then releasing once again. Do the muscles seem to lift further?

Stretching the pelvic floor

We can release to a certain degree with the breath, but as we know as yogis, stiff muscles can also benefit from gentle stretching. When it comes to stretching the pelvic floor, we have to focus our attention on specific movements of the pelvis and also consider which layer of the pelvic floor we are trying to access.

Internal pelvic floor massage
(For external massage, see the pelvic floor anatomy exploration on pg 45)

For many people, the relative tone within the pelvic floor muscles is something of a mystery. Even in yoga, we often fail to focus on the sensations between the sitting bones, sometimes referring to them as the general "down there" area. Unfortunately, this leads to both a lack of awareness and a lack of empowerment as to how to fully prepare the body to be strong throughout pregnancy, birth, and afterwards.

The pelvic floor massage described on pg 46 can bring a general awareness as to the relative tone and sensations located within the pelvic floor. For many, this external self-massage may be enough to awaken awareness and feel the impact of the different practices described below and in the practice chapters of this book. For others, it may be beneficial to get even more familiar with this muscle group, and the vaginal and other structures supported within it, by practicing some internal pelvic floor massage.

Let me give a few disclaimers around this exploration. If you prefer not to engage in or even read about this practice, feel free to skip to the next exercise. No judgment at all. Also, I am not going to attempt to describe with medical accuracy exactly the musculature you might feel. If you wish to gain this level of discernment, I recommend seeking out a pelvic floor physical therapist who can do some personal work in a private and safe manner to help you gain understanding. I am only going to describe this practice broadly, since my aim is that we become more familiar with both the muscles and this area of our anatomy.

Lastly, if you are doing this as part of birth prep, let me stress you are NOT trying to stretch the walls of your vagina! There is no need, and in fact for some, doing so can cause the tissue to toughen rather than release. I find myself constantly reminding students in childbirth education classes that the vagina is made of folds of tissue which do not need active stretching. Do you have to stretch an accordion to make it expand? Think of this as simply a more involved exploration and possibly a way to gain some feedback from your own body about your muscle patterns. It should probably also go without saying that we are NOT doing this in a yoga class, but I think you knew that already.

This is where you get personal with your own body (if you want). Find a place where you can be alone, ideally with a lock on the door and at a time when you won't be disturbed. Have some oil or other lubricant so you can make your fingers slippery. Find a comfortable position which will allow you to reach the vagina (when pregnant, I sometimes found it easier to reach from behind the pelvis rather than in front around my belly).

Dipping your fingers into your preferred lubricant, gently slide them into the vaginal opening. You can think of the opening as a clock, with 12 o'clock at your pubic bone and 6 o'clock towards your tailbone. Beginning around 1 o'clock, gently press your fingers outward, feeling the walls of the vagina. You may do this at whatever depth and pressure feels comfortable to you, and it should not be painful. Take a moment and experience this area, the relative tension or softness. Now with that information in your fingertips, shift your fingers to 2 o'clock, then 3, and so on. As you move from one number to the next around the clock, notice if you encounter different levels of muscle tension, softness, tenderness, or any other sensations.

It may be that the sensations are hard to categorize—especially if this is the first time you've felt these muscles. If this is the case, don't try to diagnose; just get to know what is there. This complex network has been holding up your internal organs and body since you learned to stand upright. Be very gentle with and give yourself space to discover where things might be starting out. This information will always be helpful.

If you are interested, you can check the relative coordination of the vaginal and pelvic floor muscles by drawing in Mula Bandha while your fingers are in the vagina. Do the muscles squeeze your fingers? Do they pull them inward? Or do they seem to push outward when you thought you were lifting? If the last case is true, then you may have discovered you are one of the 1 in 3 people who are caught in reverse breathing, exerting downward when they thought they were lifting. Discovering this is crucial to regaining good pelvic floor function and better body balance, not to mention better function during pregnancy and birth!

When finished, gently remove your fingers and rest for a moment. Note any sensations within the vagina or pelvic floor. Also bring your awareness to any emotions or thoughts arising. This network is strongly tied to our nervous system and our emotions, and stimulation, especially combined with release, can result in strong feelings. Again, gaining awareness of these things is a key part of healing and holistic health, but we must always be gentle and compassionate with ourselves and our bodies, especially any part of the body as sensitive as the vagina and pelvic floor.

Having gained some awareness of the relative strength, tension and softness within our own pelvic muscles, we may now be better equipped to bring them into balance.

Yoga postures for pelvic floor stretching

Given that the first and third layer of the pelvic floor run from the front to the back, stretching often involves finding ways to take the tail subtly away from the pubic bone—but doing so without displacing the ribcage, which would decouple the movement of the abdominal diaphragm from the pelvis. For the second pelvic floor layer, we focus on the adductor and inner thigh muscles, whose fascial fibers thread into the transverse perineal tendon.

Prasarita Padottanasana with bent knees and internal femur rotation

A movement which widens the sitz bones and can also incorporate the adductor muscles is a variation of wide legged forward fold, or Prasarita Padottanasana.

Begin by stepping the feet wide apart (perhaps 3-4 ft), turning the toes slightly in and the

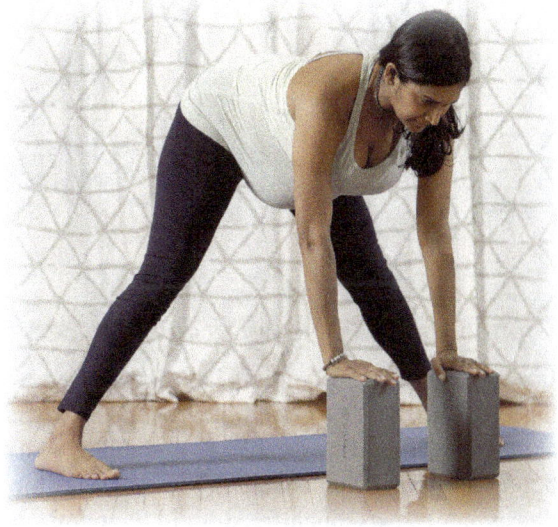

heels out. Bend the knees and hinge from the hips to place the hands on a tall support. Unlike the Prasarita postures which are done in a general population yoga class, the goal here is not range of motion (i.e., being able to touch the floor) but maintaining a neutral spine and moving solely from the hips. This will mean elevating the hands on either tall height blocks or, often, a chair.

With the back long, focus on lifting the sitz bones without dropping the front ribcage (flexible yoginis, I'm looking at you here!). Focus on the feeling between the sitz bones, and allow the tissue there to soften and expand on the inhale. From here, deepen the inhalation, focusing on the sensation of the vaginal and pelvic muscles spreading and opening. On the exhale, let these muscles remain open. The stretch here is done with the breath, not the bones. If no movement is felt, check if the ribcage is hanging towards the floor or overly rounded—both of which would misalign the abdominal and pelvic diaphragms. If you can't feel the breath in the perineum, check the alignment of ribcage to pelvis, and try bending the knees a bit more while lifting the tail slightly.

To come out, hug the legs towards one another and exhale to walk the hands back to the legs, bringing the pelvis upright. Step the legs together and balance the pelvic bowl on the thighs (No tucking!!!). Notice if any sensations have changed.

Downward Dog with bent knees

Downward Dog has the benefit of being able to stretch both the hamstring and calf muscles when the knees are extended and also to access movement within the pelvis when the knees are bent.

To practice Downward Dog with a focus on the pelvic floor, begin on all fours as you usually would. Inhale to lift the sitz bones slightly (Cow tilt); on the exhale, press into the hands, lifting the knees and extending the hips up and backwards into the familiar upside down "V".

Here's the difference with this variation: Keep the knees bent and focus on the lift of the

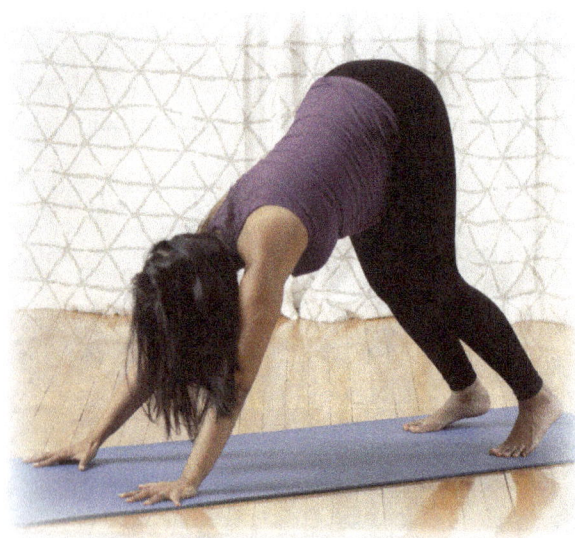

sitz bones towards the ceiling or, even better, towards the back corner of the ceiling and wall. At the same time, maintain a lift through the ribs so the spine makes a straight line rather than hanging into the ribcage and shoulders. This is both so the pubis and tail can be better drawn away from one another and so you maintain the alignment of abdominal and pelvic diaphragms. This alignment allows for better movement in the pelvic floor while holding the pose. Hold this posture for several breaths or as long as is comfortable for the arms. Come out by lowering the knees to the floor and sitting back on the heels in either Child's Pose or Vajrasana.

Variation for sensitive wrists and shoulders or tight hamstrings

It's not uncommon for moms later in pregnancy to feel sensitivity in the wrists. Increased blood volume leads to swelling around the carpal tunnel nerve. In these cases it may be more appropriate, and comfortable, to practice Downward Dog against the wall rather than on the hands. This variation is actually often easier for feeling the spreading of the pelvic floor, as it doesn't require as much freedom in the hamstrings to be able to move the pelvis.

Begin facing a wall, with the hands about hip height. Pressing into the wall, walk the feet back until the spine comes parallel to the floor, creating an "L" shape in the body. To maintain the focus on the pelvic floor, soften the knees while maintaining a lift in the ribcage and armpits, and gently lift the sitz bones away from the heels while keeping the knees bent. As with the classic variation, maintain a neutral spine with the ribcage and pelvic floor mirroring one another. Breathe fully, feeling the breath in the space between the sitz bones. To come out, walk the feet forward to the wall and stand up.

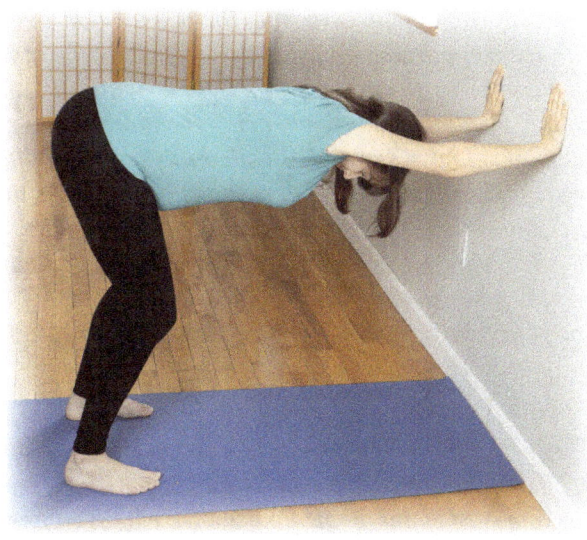

In both variations of Downward Dog, the aim is to feel the breath moving between the sitz bones and have a sense of the pelvic outlet widening. This widening can be further enhanced by inwardly rotating the femur bones, either by turning the toes inward or by drawing the upper inner thighs backward. In both cases keep the knees bent so as not to be distracted by the possibly strong stretch of the hamstrings. Focusing on stretching the hamstrings or straightening the knees will tend to draw the sitz bones down, tucking the tail and decreasing rather than stretching the front to back fibers around the vagina.

Malasana (Squat) with anterior pelvic tilt

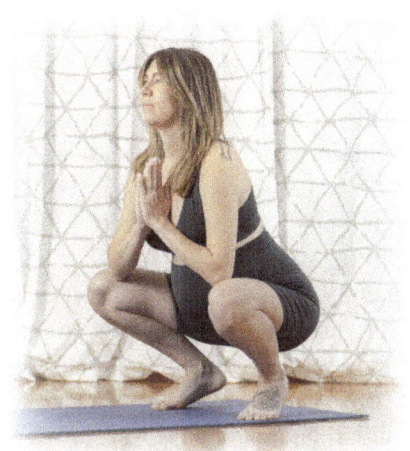

There is a good reason why Malasana is often associated both with the birth process and with defecation. As we saw in the chapter on pelvic structure, the movement of bringing the femur bones up against the top of the pelvic bowl can have the impact of widening the sitz bones and creating more movement in the pelvic outlet. Additionally, when we internally rotate the femur bones we further widen the outlet, and if we externally rotate them we widen the inlet (the top) of the pelvic bowl. Since our bodies are interconnected systems, not just separate bones, muscles, and fascia, if we are moving the bones we are also moving and stretching the surrounding connective tissue. Put together, this means squatting can be extremely helpful in the overall toning—that is, stretching and strengthening—of the pelvic floor, but as always, how we practice has a huge impact on the effectiveness.

To squat with a focus on toning the pelvic floor, begin with the feet parallel and slightly wider than the hips. Inhale to bring the pelvis into a light forward tilt, and exhale, bending the knees to bring the forearms to rest on the thighs. I have sometimes called this posture half squat or camping squat. While here, sit the weight back in the hips, allowing the pelvic bowl to tip forward and feeling the sitz bones moving away from one another. Maintaining this forward tilt, bend the knees further, seeing how low your body is able to go. Resist the urge to turn the toes out more than a few degrees and instead focus on maintaining the forward pelvic tilt.

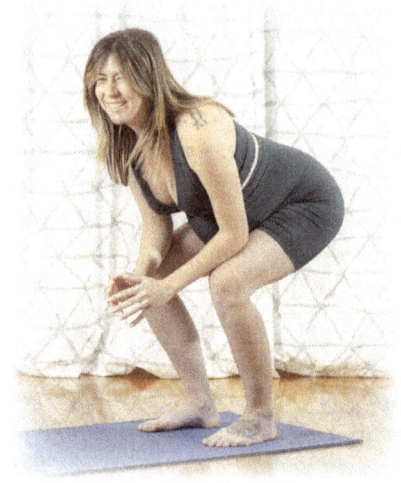

The heels may well need to lift, and you can also place a rolled blanket under the heels for support if desired. The aim is to maintain the anterior pelvic tilt rather than dropping the heels to the floor. Dropping the heels often leads to rounding the lower spine and tucking the tail, which again decreases the stretching of the pelvic outlet and pelvic floor. It is also worth noting that if mom were using a squat during pushing and birth, this would be the squat we would want, rather than one with the knees splayed wide apart. The parallel feet and anterior pelvic tilt create an internal rotation of the femurs which widens the sitz bones, which would be useful if a baby were trying to move through them.

Stay in the squat for several breaths, feeling the expansion of the sitz bones as well as the area around the vagina and anus. To come out, bring the hands to the floor and lift the hips up before walking the palms up the thighs and returning to standing. If you are also looking to strengthen the pelvic floor, coming out would be a good time to practice engaging the perineum, as the action of the glutes and inner thighs can also activate the pelvic floor.

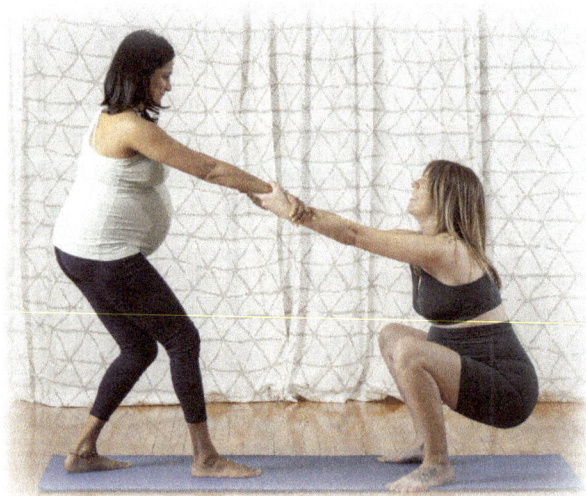

Partner Squat Variation

While the squat can be very helpful for stretching and toning the pelvic floor, it also requires a lot of flexibility, which our chair-sitting culture is often lacking. In yoga and childbirth classes, I frequently suggest students practice their forward tilted squats using either a partner or a solid support to focus more fully on the pelvic movement without having to contend with lower back and knee tension.

For a partner squat, have your partner stand facing you with their feet planted and their weight grounded—ideally in a back foot so you do not pull them on top of you. Clasp one another's wrists (not hands as sweaty palms are slippery). Begin by leaning back to give your partner a sense of the weight they are about to hold and to let them get their own foundation. Then sit back first into the camping squat variation, leaning away so they hold most of your body weight. (Note: if either party is bending their arms, be sure to straighten them before going further. This is a counterbalance, not a biceps exercise.)

Having confirmed that your partner can hold your weight, continue to sit back, focusing on opening the space between the pubis and tail. Mom's weight will almost certainly be on the heels, and if either partner were to let go, you would both fall backwards (please do not test this). Both partners should breathe fully. When ready to come up, say so to your partner, and allow them to pull you back onto your feet, bringing your body upright as the weight shifts. Stand for a moment and feel any changes within the pelvic support.

Side Lunge

Another way to access the two sides of the pelvic floor is to practice a gentle Side Lunge with the front leg at a 45 degree angle. Because this movement can pull on the connection of the pubic symphysis, this action should be done very gently, without a goal for deep range of motion. If mom has been experiencing pubic bone pain, this exercise may not be appropriate until things rebalance (possibly with professional help).

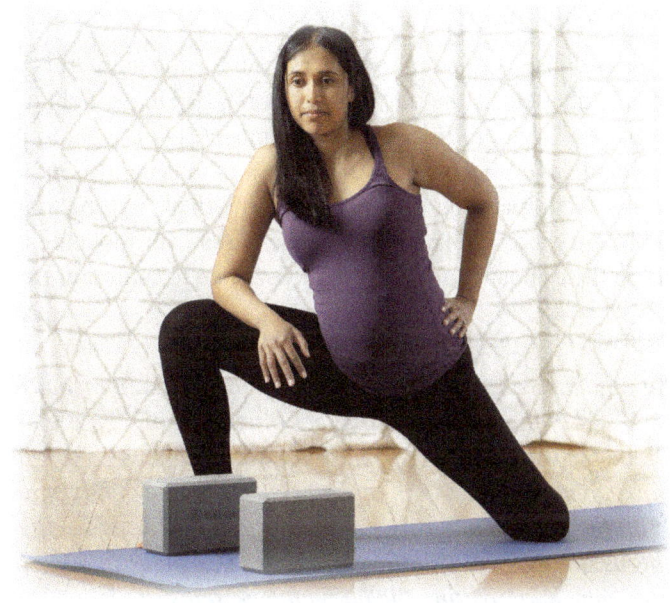

Beginning in Table, step one foot forward and walk the front foot outwards until the thigh points about 45 degrees off the front of the pelvis. Turn the toes and knee to align with the femur bone. Walk the hands up onto the thigh and gently lunge towards the front knee, maintaining the open turn of the belly away from the thigh. Feel the subtle spreading of the walls of the vagina and sitz bones as you move back and forth. This pose can also be an interesting place to explore hip circles to bring release to the whole arc of one side of the pelvic floor. Explore the sensations in the base of the pelvis. To come out, return the knee to table pose and feel any changes before shifting to the other side. Be sure to practice both sides.

This movement can also be helpful during labor as the baby rotates through the middle of the pelvis and the opening cervix. For some birthing people, this movement may create the space for an asynclitic head to drop into a vertically aligned position, allowing labor to progress smoothly.

Toning the pelvic floor during pregnancy

All of the previous exercises are designed to lengthen the pelvic floor muscles. If you find upon examination that the pelvic floor is more lacking strength than overly tense, then practicing postures which encourage pelvic floor engagement would also be appropriate. Practicing a balance of stretch and strengthening will help bring elasticity and awareness to the network of pelvic fascia and muscles that surround and support the pelvic organs and the vaginal opening. When done to their full expression, both active Mula Bandha and the anterior tilted Squat can be helpful for both strengthening and stretching.

To further tone the pelvic network, we can take advantage of the fascial connection between the adductor muscles and the second layer of the pelvic floor as well as the interplay between the glutes and the deeper third layer fibers. Here are two more possible exercises which could bring tone to the pelvic floor muscles.[17]

Seated hip toning

This exercise is done in two parts, one for the adductors (the inner thigh muscles) and one for the abductors (the outward rotators). Begin on a chair to ensure a neutral position for the pelvis and to more fully isolate the muscles you want to recruit. From there, you can increase the challenge by removing the chair and making this exercise resemble Utkatasana (as shown in the accompanying images). For some there will be more response from the pelvic floor with one exercise than another. Use whichever movement brings more response—but be sure to do the opposite movement at least once to maintain balance in the hip joints.

Adductor engagement

Sit on a firm chair or yoga ball, with the knees at or below the level of the pelvis and the feet planted firmly on the floor. Place the weight on the front of the sitting bones so the pelvic bowl comes into neutral, and stretch the spine gently upwards. With the pelvis balanced, place a yoga block between the inner thighs. In your own time, lightly pulse the knees against the yoga block, activating the adductor muscles of the inner thighs. The goal is to pulse for about 60 seconds to begin, then give the legs a break.

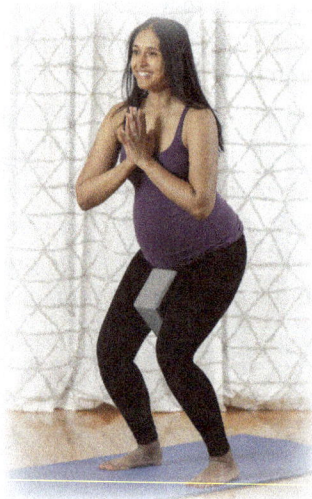

Keep the toes relaxed on the floor. Relax and inhale, allowing the pelvic floor to drop, then exhale and engage upwards, as though lifting something with the walls of the vagina, or like a jellyfish swimming upwards (whichever image works better for you). What sort of response do you get? Repeat this exercise two or three times.

---

[17] For those interested in taking a deeper dive into the full function of the pelvic floor, I recommend looking at *Pelvic Liberation* by Leslie Howard for an exploration of the pelvis outside of the confines of pregnancy and birth. Leslie Howard Yoga; 1st edition (October 12, 2017)

Abductor engagement

To tone the glutes, sit once again on the chair with the weight forward on the sitting bones. Take a yoga strap (or a scarf or belt if you lack an actual strap) and buckle it into a circle around the mid-thighs so it provides some resistance to the outsides of the legs. It's important not to place the belt too high or too close to the knees.

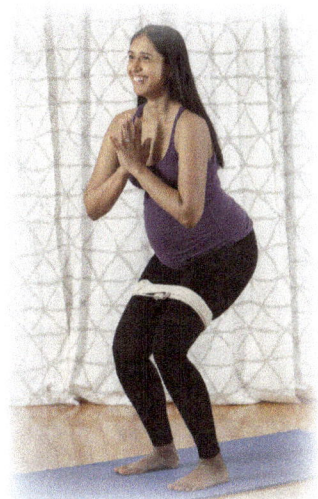

Gently stretching the spine upright and relaxing the toes, begin to pulse the thighs outwards into the strap. Try and focus on moving the upper thigh bones apart, as though trying to fit a yoga block back between the legs rather than simply pushing the knees apart against the strap. It may also feel as though the sitz bones are trying to spread apart. Pulse out with about 50% of the effort you think you could, then relax and repeat. Pulse for 60 seconds, then rest. Again try inhaling and letting the pelvic floor drop, then exhale and actively lift up and in, like the jellyfish swimming up through the water. What do you feel here? Repeat this exercise two or three times.

Utkatasana squats

We can also use the squatting action to tone the pelvic floor and surrounding hip muscles.

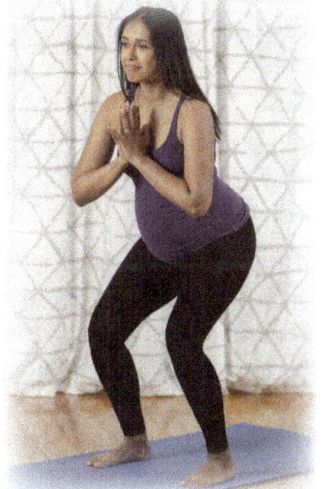

Coming into Utkatasana or Chair Pose in yoga practice, the focus should be on how far back the pelvis can move rather than on how low it can go. Do not overdo this one. I have found that many seasoned yoginis like to "go for the burn" in strengthening postures, and while this may be useful occasionally as a way to develop mental stamina, overall tone will be better achieved by giving the glutes a chance to work and release over multiple repetitions.

Stand with your feet hip width apart, with the toes pointed forward. On an inhale, bend your knees and sit your hips back. Sit back as much as you can without falling over. On an exhale, push down with the feet and activate the glutes and pelvic floor muscle to return to standing. Remember not to tuck the tail once upright. Repeat this motion 5-10 times depending on how your legs and hips feel.

Goddess Squats with pelvic floor focus

Jaiasana, sometimes called Goddess Squat, can be a great place to develop greater pelvic tone and, depending on which direction you focus, can both stretch and strengthen the pelvic floor muscles.

Turn to the side of your mat and step the feet wide apart. Find whatever is comfortable for your body, bearing in mind that anyone with discomfort in the pubic bone may want a narrower stance. In general, four feet apart is a good benchmark. Turn the thighs out so the toes rotate outwards to about 45 degrees. Check that the pelvis is still in a neutral position,

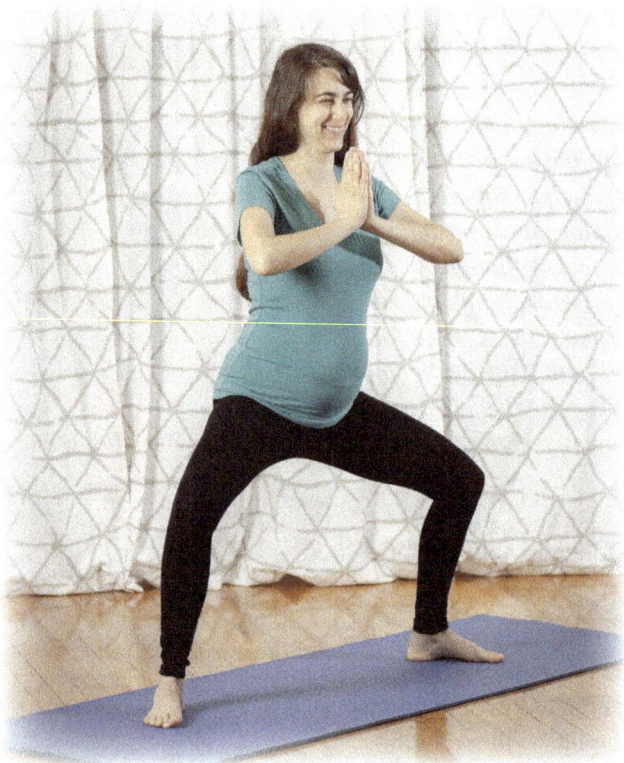

with the pubic bone and tail both anchored towards the ground and the navel pointed forward or slightly down. Bring the hands to the hips.

On an inhale, bend the knees to lower down into the squat. Be sure the knees track towards the toes, and activate the glutes by pressing the knees out while isometrically spinning the heels forward (they won't actually move due to the sticky mat). Feel the sitz bones spread as you descend. On the exhale, push the feet outwards against the mat and draw the pelvic floor up in the middle to rise back to standing. Repeat this action 5-10 times, focusing on feeling the dynamic opening and then lifting between the sitz bones, pubis, and tail.

The pelvic floor is often ignored or dismissed in yoga practice, but this area is vital both to overall pelvic function during pregnancy and to the ability to release during the birth process. The pelvic floor is the gateway from the womb to the world, and the way we prepare these muscles dramatically impacts the progress of both pregnancy and birth. The balance between the sides of the pelvic floor and the layers of muscle can determine the space within the pelvis for baby during birth. The uterus contracts to pull the cervix open, yes, but the head moving down is what actually opens the cervix, and how the muscles guide that descent influences how well baby's head moves during labor. Careful exploration and self discovery during pregnancy can restore the open path through the pelvis and possibly set the body up for a smoother progression in labor, birth, and postpartum recovery.

Pregnancy offers an incredible opportunity to regain understanding and connection to these subtle but powerful structures, but we have to go beyond simply doing Kegels. Pelvic floor preparation for labor begins during pregnancy, with the way our movements load and unload the different muscles around and within the pelvic floor. Discovering how to properly engage and release the entire pelvic floor and being able to relax the walls of the vagina increases connection to these muscles. This strengthens and enhances mom's ability to work with the process of labor and birth.

Moreover, having an elastic pelvic floor is the key to the body recovering after birth. This is something which the body is meant to be able to do. Far from needing to be massaged, stretched, or cut, the vagina and surrounding tissue are completely capable of opening and birthing without even a scratch or tear, if given enough time, patience, and respect. The key is not just tightening the pelvic musculature but learning to release it as well to bring back the overall state of balance and harmony. With this balance, women not only have smoother births, they can even find the process enjoyable depending on the frame of mind. We have not even touched the magical qualities of female sexuality, Shakti and Shiva energy, but pleasure and even orgasm are possible during the birth process. But that is a subject for another book.[18]

Key Takeaways

The pelvic floor is a network of three layers of muscle which interweave between the sitz bones, pubis, and tailbone. They support the weight of the internal organs and control voiding from the bladder and rectum.

The pelvic floor actually domes upwards, not down, as is often seen in graphics.

In good alignment, abdominal breathing stretches and tones the pelvic floor because of its relationship to the abdominal diaphragm.

The muscles of the pelvic floor guide the baby's head to rotate through the pelvis during labor because of their orientation front to back within the middle of the pelvis. The tone of the overall network is what guides the head into and through the pelvic bones.

Pelvic floor muscles can be too tight, too loose, or a combination of both. Simply squeezing them, as in Kegel exercises, is not always the best way to bring overall tone and balance.

Certain yoga postures can be used to help stretch overly tight pelvic floor muscles. In good alignment, internal rotation of the femur bones can stretch the pelvic floor while external rotation can help engage it.

Activating pelvic support muscles such as the glutes can help reduce the action needed in the pelvic floor, allowing it to find a nice balanced tone of not too tight and not too loose.

---

[18] For more information about sexuality and the birth process, look at *Orgasmic Birth* by Elizabeth Davis and Debra Pascali-Bonaro, Rodale Press 2010.

4 — Fascia, the Interconnected Web of Motherhood

"We are here to awaken from the illusion of separateness"

—Thich Nat Hahn

You started as one cell. That cell divided into two, then into four, and continued dividing. Along the way it began differentiating cells into various body parts: this one a skin cell, this one bone, this one contractible fibers in our quadriceps, and this one a neuron in the brain. At the end of the whole process, you emerged as a complex set of systems comprising a human being. It is certainly easier to talk and think of the body in its requisite components. You have a muscular skeletal system, an organ system, a nervous system, each performing certain functions within the whole of your body. But those systems didn't emerge fully formed and then attach themselves together; they grew with and from one another. Just as a hand can be seen as a connected set of digits or as four fingers, a thumb, and a palm, your body systems have individual functions but are also interwoven by a complex and dynamic network of fibers that bridge the gaps between them.

In Chapter 1 we looked at the structure of the pelvic bowl and how that bony cradle supports and impacts the entire postural structure within the pregnant body. In Chapter 3 we looked at the pelvic floor and how this intricate network of muscles and ligaments supports and guides both pregnancy and the process of labor. As we saw in both chapters, hormonal changes during pregnancy shift the integrity of the body's connective tissue. This pliability has to be taken into account not only while practicing yoga asana but also when thinking of the overall body balance for birth. When we speak of connective tissue being softened by hormones like relaxin and estrogen, we are speaking about the network of fibers interweaving between the various systems of the body. This network is called fascia. It is this fascial pliability which both makes the body more susceptible to overstretching and also creates an opportunity to restore harmonious function throughout the body with mindful yogic movements. Fascia doesn't just connect body systems; it is a system of its own that is instantaneously responsive to its own structure and the forces applied to it, both from without and from within.

Fascia needs to be able to resist forces in certain places to provide structural support, as with ligaments and bones, and also yield and slide when needed, such as when the uterus grows and moves the other organs upwards. The yoga *sutras* speak of a posture as being a balance of effort and ease, *sthira* and *sukha*, where we apply enough effort to hold the shape but not so much that the posture becomes rigid and locked. In the same way, the tone throughout our body's fascial network is a dance of *sthira* and *sukha*. Too much stiffness, and the fascia becomes brittle and the joints compressed, but too little, and the body collapses. Especially during pregnancy, seeking this balance both on and off the mat can be a key component to finding overall body balance and to promoting a smoother birth.

Fascia has only recently started getting the attention it deserves. Originally, dissection classes focused on separating out each bodily system for individual examination. As a result, dissection meant cutting and scraping the fascia away from the muscles or nerves so they could be viewed in isolation. Anatomists then sought to determine what each single component's function might be. But just as a single individual has an impact on their entire community, each system of the body impacts and interconnects with the others. Researchers are now discovering that fascia responds not only to muscular and postural tension but also to inflammation, diet, and even emotional stress.[19][20] As the ancient yogis pointed out via the *koshas*, the body is made up of multiple layers which interweave with one another. Emotions born from thoughts can manifest in physical adhesions and tension within our fascia, thereby impacting other organ systems. Bodyworkers like Tom Meyers have begun exploring how releasing fascial adhesions in one area of the body can begin to restore function in seemingly unconnected parts.[21] Carrying and giving birth to a baby involves far more than the physical structures directly connected by muscles and ligaments, and fascia is at play in more ways than just supporting the pelvic joints during pregnancy. The saying goes that "it takes a village to raise a child," and I would add that it takes a whole body to birth a baby. And that whole body includes the fascia.

So what exactly are we talking about here? If we move back in our assessment of pelvic bones and muscles, we might notice that the muscles are each encased within sleeves of silky, sliding connective tissue. (Ever cut the silver-skin off a piece of meat or found some gristle in a steak? That's fascia). Fascia spreads out across the body's systems, linking muscles to nerves and bridging from organs to bones. Where fascia encases the muscles, these sleeves taper into the tendons, which thread into the attachment points on the bones. The bones in turn thread into ligaments which run into organs and other bones, providing stability and tensegrity (stability through balanced tension). Each layer of fascial connection lays and glides alongside the next one, adjusting to the movements and weight loads applied to our tissue. How smooth or sticky the fascia is within a certain area can determine the ease or stiffness of that area of the body.

Jiggling your fascia
(recording available at www.ombirths.com/ombirthsbook/jiggling-the-fascia-the-leg-shake)

Stand on both feet in a relaxed Tadasana position. Put your attention on the sensations within your legs: the quads, hamstrings, shins, and calves. Initially there may not be much

[19] B., B., & Marelli, F. (2017, March 10). [*emotions in motion: Myofascial interoception*]. Complementary medicine research. https://pubmed.ncbi.nlm.nih.gov/28278494/

[20] Tozzi, P. (2014). Does fascia hold memories? *Journal of Bodywork and Movement Therapies*, 18(2), 259–265. https://doi.org/10.1016/j.jbmt.2008.09.001

[21] *Anatomytrains.com*

sensation to notice. Maybe some feelings of slight tension left over from whatever posture you were sitting in while reading this book. Technically speaking, some of that residual tension is the imprint of your previous alignment on your body's fascia, but by adulthood, many of us have become so accustomed to this general state of body feedback that we no longer notice it.

Now try shifting your weight onto one leg (hold onto something if you feel unstable) and moderately shake your free leg. Don't worry about doing this perfectly; simply shake your leg so that the muscles and tissue of the quads and calves begin to jiggle and flop like Jell-o (and please let go of any self judgment about body image right now—we want to jiggle). Continue shaking gently for about a minute, then replace your foot on the floor and shift your weight back to a balanced Tadasana (No tucking!). Notice the sensation in the shaken leg vs. the other one. Do things feel softer? Looser? For many there is a sense of spaciousness or ease in the jiggled leg and an almost lack of sensation in the unshaken leg. This spaciousness is the feeling of released fascia! Rather than continuing to hold the tension lines imprinted from sitting, we have somewhat restored the body's suppleness—at least in this specific area. This is not a permanent state: even now, the fascia is adjusting to support the weight in this new orientation of vertical standing. But just as a simple jiggle can help restore a creased piece of fabric, gentle stretching and wiggling, and sometimes massage, can help to ease out bound areas in the body's fascial system. Now go shake the other leg before it gets jealous of the relaxed one!

Fascia is like the body's memory. Everything we have done and experienced is imprinted somewhere in our connective tissue network. Like constantly shifting water balloons, our organs and body systems overlay and glide subtly against one another. But leave them resting against one another for too long and the balloons will eventually begin to stick together; the same is true of our fascia. Trauma, overuse, inflammation, prolonged tension, and compression can affect the fascia's ability to be supple and glide.

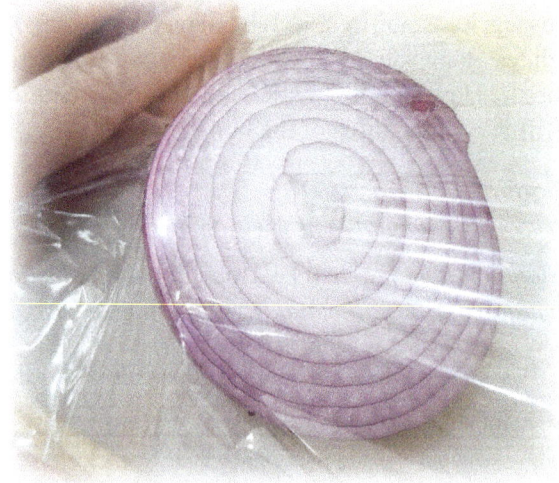

Think of a sheet of plastic wrap when it first comes off the roll; it's smooth, stretchy, able to adapt and adjust to whatever you might be wrapping it around. But unwrap it from, say, your sandwich and it retains the creases and wrinkles from whatever it was last around. In the same way, when we are first born our fascia network is stretchy and clear of adhesions, torques, and tensions. It is ready to respond to whatever we want it to do.

But as we move into adulthood, the movement patterns we have imprinted on our fascia remain, just like the imprint of the sandwich. The fascia network is constantly adapting to our current movement diet. Fall down and bang your tailbone, and the fascia in the back of your pelvis binds around itself to protect against further injury. Train for a marathon, and the ligaments of the pelvic floor will reinforce to support the added downward pressure from all that running. Cut the network, and the fibers twist and bind against one another to maintain as much of their original form as they can, resulting in scar tissue. Scar tissue creates a place in the web where the threads move less freely. The impacts on the rest of the system can range from subtle in some places to dramatic in others.

Yoga and gentle stretching practices have the ability to restore the pliability of the fascia as well as the muscles. If you spend some time each day gently stretching and unwinding tense areas in the body, the fascia remembers that you want to move those areas. However, if those movements are done too aggressively or without awareness, they exacerbate rather than alleviate existing asymmetries in the body. Our bodies are constantly adapting and adjusting to the movements we ask them to perform and the loads we ask them to carry. Think about the change to the body's shape and its shifting center of gravity during pregnancy. How might moving the center of gravity forward change the load on these connective tissues? What if those tissues have existing twists or stiff spots?

The relative tone of the fascia impacts the amount of space within the joints, but it also affects the balance within the pelvic structure. These factors in turn affect the space surrounding the growing uterus in pregnancy, the loads placed on the pelvic ligaments, and the body's ability to adapt during and after pregnancy. The uterus and other pelvic organs don't just magically float in the middle of the pelvic bowl. They are supported not only by the musculature of the pelvic floor but also by a web of pelvic ligaments, like a dreamcatcher inside the lower pelvis.

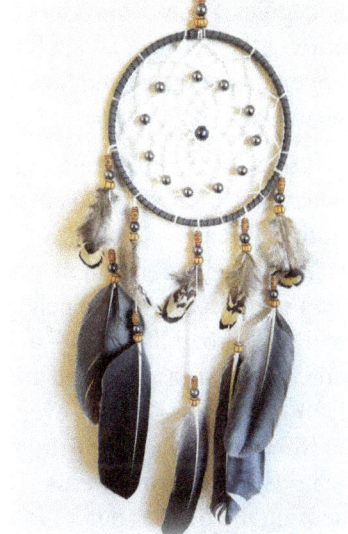

I first encountered these Native American ritual objects when decorating my college dorm room. The circular hoop was interwoven with a latticework of crisscrossing threads, at the center of which was suspended some ritual object—usually an arrowhead. When I looked more closely at the fascial fabric supporting the base of the uterus (the cervix) within the pelvis, the image of a dreamcatcher sprung to mind. In the center we have the opening of the cervix, but just as the arrowhead rests centrally within the balance of the dream catcher's woven network, the cervix sits in the interconnected web of internal pelvic ligaments. Ligaments running from the uterus to the internal border of the lower pelvis provide a network for the support of the lower uterine segment.

Let's back up a moment for those unfamiliar with pelvic organ placement. Ideally the cervix—the base of the uterus—rests in the middle of the pelvic bowl. Extending from all sides of the cervix, the fascia network spreads out, maintaining the cervix's central placement through balanced tension and suppleness. From the back of the cervix, the two wide utero-sacral ligaments run from the lower uterine segment to the border of the sacrum. From the front, the pubo-cervical ligaments attach the anterior border of the cervix to the internal border of the pubic bone. These two ligaments also spread around the bladder, located just in front of the cervix, in the same way the utero-sacral ligaments wrap on either side of the rectum just behind the cervix.

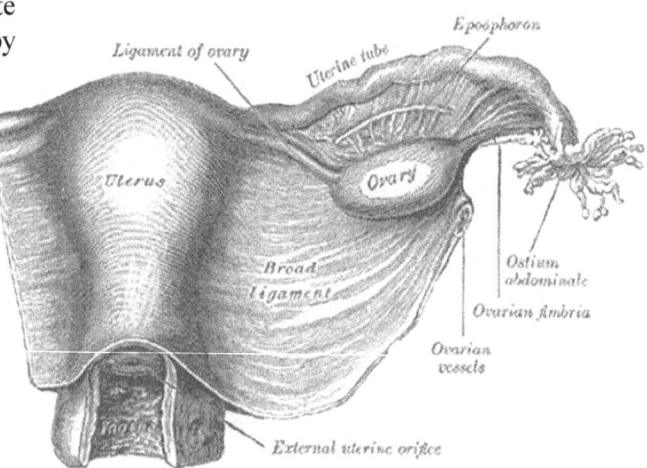

Pubic symphisis
Pubo-cervical ligaments
Bladder
Cardinal ligament
Cervix
Rectum
Sacro-tuberous ligament
Utero-sacro ligaments
Vertebra
Sacrum

Running laterally from the cervix, the cardinal ligaments connect the side borders of the cervix to the interior of the pelvic wall. Additionally, beyond the specific connections to the cervix, the sacro-tuberous and sacro-spinous ligaments connect the sides and back of the pelvic bowl together. As we saw in Chapter 1, the sacro-tuberous and sacro-spinous ligaments reinforce the structure and integrity of the pelvic bowl and can also be responsible for the degree of pelvic movement available during crowning and birth. The relative tension and laxity of the cervical and pelvic ligaments impacts how easily the cervix and pelvis are able to open during labor and how much space is available for the baby's head to slide and rotate downward.

As if these structures weren't intricate enough, the uterus is also encircled by multiple threads and bands of fascia that help maintain its position in the center of the pelvic bowl. The broad ligament—a wide sheath of fascia in the middle of the pelvis—drapes over the front of the pelvis and around the midsection of the uterus, encasing the ovaries before following the line of the utero-sacral ligaments and attaching into the sacral border.

This fascial band both supports

Ligament of ovary
Uterine tube
Epoöphoron
Uterus
Ovary
Broad ligament
Ostium abdominale
Ovarian fimbria
Ovarian vessels
External uterine orifice

Image by Henry Vandyke Carter - Henry Gray (1918)
Anatomy of the Human Body, Plate 1161

and protects the uterus and, as it grows during pregnancy, buffers the jolts and tugs brought on by the body's movements. Above the shawl of the broad ligament, the round ligaments run from the midsection of the uterus over the exterior of each pubic bone, attaching to the anterior pubis symphysis (and for some women, even into the lips of the vulva). The pelvic organs are not simply suspended by a series of tension lines; rather, they are interwoven with one another in an interconnected abdominal network.

Why does all this matter? First, if we are practicing yoga with an eye towards creating better space and more ease during pregnancy, then we need to be conscious of how each asana pulls not only on the muscles but on the totality of the pelvic structure. Second, the network of fascia woven into the base of the pelvis provides support for the cervix to be able to open evenly—and for a baby to spin into optimal position before and during the labor process. When in balance, the birth pathway is open and supple. Out of balance, the pelvic structure eventually develops a twist that carries the uterus and cervix along with it. The cervix may be drawn off to one side or put into a twist and thus unable to open evenly during labor. Or the bones might be drawn out of alignment, leading to a possible restriction that could cause the baby to be unable to move down through the pelvis after the cervix has opened. Simply put, a balanced body may be able to birth more easily, and yoga practice can affect that balance!

Going back to the analogy of the dreamcatcher, if the internal fascial web has developed a chronic twist (say, from constantly crossing one leg over the other when sitting?), this can put a torque into the outer ring of the pelvic bowl … aching SI joints anyone? Or, the result could be an imbalance in the pelvic floor or lower back muscles … pelvic incontinence or low back pain?

Far from being inevitable, the aches and pains commonly felt during pregnancy can be windows into where the body is out of balance. They are effectively the body speaking to us directly, asking for some attention and space to be brought into an area—though not necessarily the one that is aching. Relieving these imbalances doesn't just create greater ease and comfort during pregnancy; it may also help restore the open channel inherent within the female pelvis and even create more space for the baby to descend and rotate during labor.

Working with the fascia network

The solution isn't as simple as finding the right stretches and yoga *asanas* that will help everything unwind. Each body carries its own memories, and not all of those memories are physical. Remember that fascia doesn't only respond to bumps and pulls but to emotions as well. As a yoga teacher, I have often heard colleagues talk about how certain memories are stored within our bodies, and research is finally beginning to confirm that feelings are quite literally reflected in our tissues.[22] It may be a bit far to say that the specific childhood incident with your mother is stored in your piriformis muscle, but emotional energy and resistance has literally been shown to be present within the fascia network. When interacting with fascia, we must therefore allow for the full range of emotions which might be impacting the subtle

[22] B., B., & Marelli, F. (2017, March 10). [*emotions in motion: Myofascial interoception*]. Complementary medicine research. https://pubmed.ncbi.nlm.nih.gov/28278494/

as well as physical body. The yoga space needs to be safe (as does the birth setting). We need to feel seen and respected. And we have to allow the body to guide and get curious about sensations and discoveries.

I will always remember one of my mentors relating a birth story told to her by a midwife. The midwife noticed during a vaginal exam that the mother's sacro-tuberous ligament was very thick and ropey. After gaining permission, she held the ligament with her fingers (yes, we are talking internal touching here) and "talked" to the ligament. After a little time, and with an emotional release from mom, she felt the ligament release and become more pliable, and out popped a 10 pound baby! The physical can impact the emotional, just as psyche affects soma. The two are inextricably linked.

So, how do we go about beginning to connect with the fascia network? We could start by simply focusing on the muscles, since the fascia is connected to them, but this approach misses the subtleties involved in balancing this interconnected spiderweb. Especially during pregnancy, fascia is capable of responding to more subtle and gentle touch than we might initially apply in the usual *asana* practice. Far from finding a good stretch—which inherently pulls the network in one direction or another, gentle release work can actually be equally or more beneficial for restoring balance and thus creating better overall harmony. The postural changes that a pregnant person makes as the center of gravity shifts are subtle but create profound ripples throughout the body. The reverberations gently release those ligaments that are holding excessive tension and help to tone those areas which are overly lax. Postural shifts begin by developing an awareness of where the body is tense versus where it seems to sag or collapse, then looking for the place which I often call the "goldilocks zone." Not too tight, not too loose—just right.

The fascial system is highly sensitive and highly responsive—in fact, its response rate is four times faster than that of the nervous system! Keeping this in mind, we might start by using a light and respectful touch on the body, feeling how we respond internally to physical contact. I often find that pregnant students like to place their hands directly on their bellies, feeling the gentle rise and fall of their breathing and connecting to the baby growing within. We then begin moving the hands around, simply sensing the connective tissue that holds the body together.

The following exercises are ways to explore and connect with the fascial system and possibly bring greater balance to it overall. As you move through different areas, notice if there are tender spots or places where things seem soft. These are relative areas of tension or suppleness, and they can then inform where tissue needs to gently stretch or where it might need to tighten. Allow the breath to keep moving, and be mindful not only of physical but also emotional reactions which might arise. It's all connected after all. (Note this is subtle work and not something everyone is able to immediately feel; stay present with whatever sensations arise.)

Breathwork for abdominal release
(recording at www.ombirths.com/ombirthsbook/breathwork-for-abdominal-release)

This very gentle meditative exercise can help with relieving tension in the round ligaments and the broad ligament across the front segment of the uterus. Round ligament pain can sometimes feel like a sudden, strong cramping along the mid- or lower abdomen or a twinge-y sensation when quickly twisting or walking fast. Tension in the broad ligament can sometimes show up as discomfort along the front of the belly when baby moves—especially when kicking. It can also manifest as aching in the SI joints at the back of the pelvis since both the broad and the utero-sacral ligaments attach to the anterior border of the SI joint. Imbalance in either of these fascial supports can lead to an altered position for the uterus and thus change the space available both for the baby and for the uterine muscles that will be working during labor.

From a comfortable reclining position (be sure to prop at least at a 45 degree angle if past 25 weeks or short of breath), place the hands gently on the abdomen, feeling it rise and fall with the breath. The hands do not apply any pressure; they simply hold the belly as though holding a delicate Easter egg.

Begin by imagining the space between your hands, softly breathing as you would in Shavasana. At your own tempo, begin gently sliding your fingers from one side of the belly towards the navel. Feel for tender spots or areas of increased sensation. If you feel one, pause the movement of the fingers and simply rest the hands on the tender area, gently moving the breath down into your touch. Imagine your fingers are lightly holding the fascial "plastic wrap," giving it time and space to unwind. You may find that using your hands to gently draw the belly in a direction creates a sense of greater ease. If this is the case, lightly support that ease for a few moments.

After about a minute (the time will vary person to person) you may find that the sensation has either lessened or that the area has softened. This will not be a stretch feeling, more a feeling of letting up or slacking instead. Once the area has released, continue moving along the belly, connecting and talking to the fascia (and the baby). It's also common that as the tissue releases, the baby may shift and move as there is more space for them. This exercise can be helpful in releasing the abdominal diaphragm as well, leading to greater breath capacity and better movement in the pelvic floor.

As with all body self-care, pay attention not only to physical but also to emotional sensations. Bringing attention to different areas of our bodies can stir up strong feelings if we have held emotions or trauma there. Allow yourself time and space to experience what comes up in the amount you feel comfortable working with.

Jiggling Bum[23]

This one can be done on your own or with a partner. Given the hand placement, I would suggest this partner be someone you are very comfortable with.

Note: If you have had bleeding, a history of preterm labor, or are still in the first trimester, skip this practice until you have conferred with your care provider.

Twisted, tense fascia responds well to gentle ripples, especially if we can find the internal

---

[23] This technique is adapted from the work of Jenny Blyth, (*birthwork.com*) whose attention to overall body tension and function is now one of the principles involved in the Spinning Babies® childbirth preparation program.

wave rhythm of the "water balloon" in the muscle fibers. In general, this very gentle jiggle can help balance some of the lateral cervical ligaments deep within the pelvis and pelvic floor. Given that it's all connected, this movement can also soften the fascial network running into the lower back and around to the lower abdomen. Release in one area can have an impact on others, and the gentle jiggle sensation can help activate the parasympathetic nervous system, encouraging deeper relaxation and ease throughout the body.

Partner variation

Begin with mom lying on her side, supported as for Side-lying Shavasana or resting on hands and knees with the arms over a chair or birthing ball. Have your partner place their hands gently on the ASIS points at the front of your pelvis and also on the sitz bones near the base (no, this is probably not one for a standard yoga class unless you are really getting to know one another personally). Take a moment and breathe together, as your fascial networks are now in contact and will respond to one another. Remember we are talking about light touch here, not deep massage.

With the hands resting on the pelvic landmarks, begin very gently jiggling the tissue of the buttocks back and forth. This action will initially be mild, like making a Jell-o mold wiggle. What the partner is feeling for is a wave where the fluid seems to be sloshing from one hand to another. For some this wave will be vertical, from hand to hand, and for others it will be more horizontal to the line of the pelvis. Remember that less is more. The goal isn't to create a huge movement and definitely not to shake the pelvic bones but more to find the sort of motion you might use in soothing a fussy baby.

Give the glutes and pelvic area a chance to unwind. The jiggle may also "want" to move down into the thighs or up into the lower back. If this is the case, simply follow whatever feels good to mom. Continue jiggling for as long as it feels good to both of you. Ideally 5 to 20 minutes (in my experience, the partner will often tire first, and partner work must accommodate both people).

To finish, slow the jiggle down until the hands once again simply rest on the body. Take a deep breath. Then remove the touch and pause a moment for mom to feel the impact. Though the entire network will unwind from just doing one side, it's usually nice to flip over and jiggle the other hip as well.

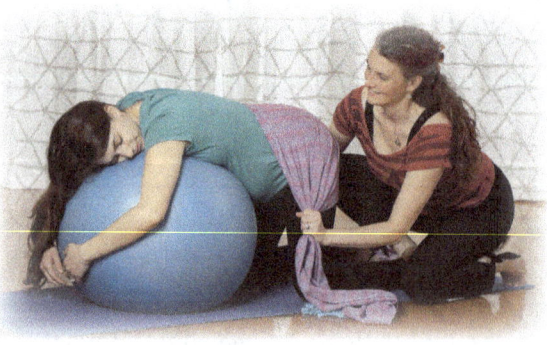

Hands and knees variation

If resting on hands and knees, have a partner drape a shawl or sheet across the bum. The ideal implement for this variation would be a Rebozo, a woven cloth from Mayan and Mexican traditions by midwives specifically made for birth work.[24]

---

[24] Visit *www.spinningbabies.com/pregnancy-birth/techniques/other-techniques/rebozo-manteada-4/* for more information about Rebozo

With the Rebozo draped across the hips, gather the sides of the fabric together and softly press down, anchoring the fabric to the hips. With very soft, gentle movements, begin jiggling the skin of the buttocks, allowing the waves to gradually ripple their way through the body. Continue jiggling for several minutes, then gradually slow to stop.

Practicing alone

For practicing alone, the impact is a bit less on the nervous system since you have to remain active rather than being able to fully release into the shaking, but the effect can still be of benefit to the connective tissue.

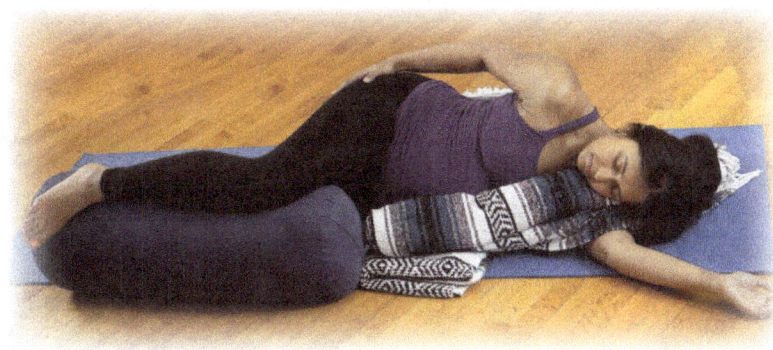

Begin either side lying or seated comfortably. Take the top hand and cup the globe of your gluteal muscles between the ASIS and your sitz bone. Beginning gently, start to jiggle this side of your bum, trying not to contract any muscles that would restrict the movement. Feel for a gentle but deep shaking in the connective tissue, and notice if a specific direction feels easier or has more movement. Continue in the way that has more ease. When I practice this on myself, I sometimes also feel a coolness within my SI joint, or sometimes a sense of warmth within the gluteus muscle as things begin to release. Continue jiggling until either your arm begins to fatigue or you feel satisfied with the practice. Then gradually slow the movement until still and switch to the other side.

Tennis ball release[25]

For myofascial release during pregnancy, practice these techniques with a tennis ball on your bed or another soft surface. It is important not to practice these on such a hard surface that the fascia—which is already pliable from relaxin—begins to bind or reinforce because of excessive strain. The explorations listed here are not exhaustive in any way but are offered as a place to begin. From here, feel free to explore any places that could benefit from a little love and attention.

Piriformis/glute release

Glutes and piriformis are muscle groups which can often hold a lot of tension during pregnancy, from the increased mobility and their role in stabilizing the pelvis and also from the weight gain that leads to more work in the outer hip muscles. Balancing this fascial network

---

[25] These exercises are offered from Dina Abbondante, LMT, Myofascial release body-worker and massage therapist

can have an impact on the pelvic floor as well as the lumbar spine and all the structures connected thereto.

Sitting on the bed, lean back on your hands and cross one foot over the opposite knee to create a figure 4 position. Place a tennis ball beneath the working hip (the one with the crossed leg) so that it rests into the globe of the buttocks. Allow the weight of the body to sink

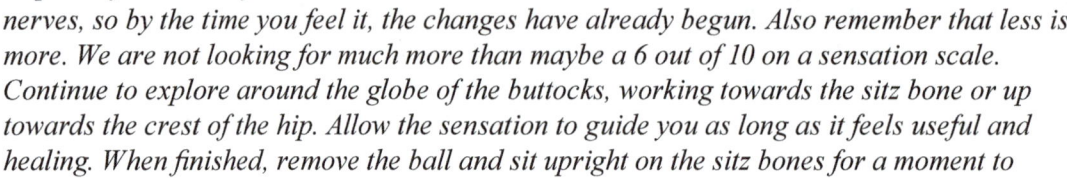

into the ball. Feel for a gentle softening within the tissues as you apply pressure. Then, with gentle awareness, begin to shift the body around, rolling the hip on the ball beneath. Follow your intuition, feeling for places of tenderness or tension. When you find one, see if you can linger there and allow the ball to sink further into the tight spot, as though the knots were gradually melting away.

Remember the fascial network responds faster than your nerves, so by the time you feel it, the changes have already begun. Also remember that less is more. We are not looking for much more than maybe a 6 out of 10 on a sensation scale. Continue to explore around the globe of the buttocks, working towards the sitz bone or up towards the crest of the hip. Allow the sensation to guide you as long as it feels useful and healing. When finished, remove the ball and sit upright on the sitz bones for a moment to observe the impact. Then switch to the other side.

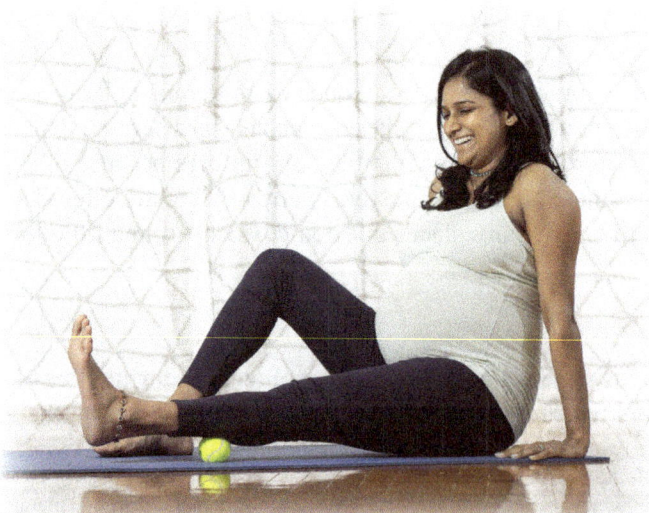

Calf release

The fascial line in the calf connects up the backside of the leg and eventually runs into the pelvic floor and sacrum. Loosening the calves can be one of the simplest changes we can do to help with both pelvic balance and lower back discomfort.

Sitting on the bed, extend one leg out in front and place the tennis ball at the base of the calf, by the heel. Allow the weight of the leg to drop onto the ball, inviting it to sink into the tissue of the calf. Breathe gently and allow the calf to relax, then shift the hips forward so the ball rolls slightly higher towards the middle of the calf. Repeat, possibly rolling the ball from side to side.

Continue moving up the calf, pausing anywhere there seem to be pressure points which can yield to the ball. When you are finished with the exploration, pause and feel the difference from one side to the other. This exercise can also be done with the tennis ball under the arch of the foot against the floor to complete the fascial line. Be sure to do the other leg as well. This exercise can be done daily, especially if you spend more than 3 hrs a day on your feet (mothers of small children or yoga teachers, I'm looking at you here!)

Pelvic clock: cervical ligament variation[26]

Unlike a core-focused pelvic clock from the Alexander technique[27] where the pelvic bowl moves (see Chapter 15 for a pelvic clock description for postpartum), this exercise is almost an internal meditation, though it can feel very similar to a gentle engagement of the pelvic floor. Those muscles are, after all, encased in the dreamcatcher of the pelvic ligaments. The aim of this exercise is to bring awareness and balance to the entire network of ligaments which support and extend from the cervix. Unlike a Kegel, however, this exercise functions primarily in the horizontal plane of the pelvis rather than actively lifting the muscles upwards towards the heart. This exercise is probably most effective after 28 weeks, when there is enough downward pressure to bring the pelvic ligaments under tension from above.

If we return to the picture of the ligaments radiating from the cervix at the center of the pelvis, we imagine on top of that network an analog clock, with 12 o'clock located at the pubic symphysis, 6 o'clock at the sacrum, 3 o'clock at the right hip where the femur bone connects and 9 o'clock at the junction of the left hip and femur. The rest of the numbers would be arrayed around the clock face. This version of the pelvic clock exercise involves mentally imagining contracting from the border of the "clock," the pelvic rim, in towards the cervix at the center. The pelvic floor muscles will certainly engage, but the key is to use the mind-body connection to subtly impact the balance of tone within the entire pelvic network.

Standing in Tadasana, with the pelvis in good alignment (so no tucking!), bring your hands gently to the pubic bone at "12 o'clock." The hands do not need to apply any pressure. As with the breath release for the abdomen, the simple contact is enough to bring awareness to the fascia.

With the mind focused on the line from the pubic bone to the cervix, exhale and contract the front muscles of the pelvic floor, visualizing them moving horizontally into the center. There will be other muscle contractions involved; this is OK for the moment. Keep the mental attention focused on the line you are intending to activate (in this case the one at 12 o'clock).

---

[26] I first learned this exercise at a Spinning Babies® virtual conference from Australian midwife Fiona Hallinan. Subsequently I began exploring it with yoga students and found it was extremely helpful in developing awareness within the deep segment of the lower pelvic bowl.

[27] *alexandertechnique.com*

Hold this contraction for a moment, then fully release. Repeat this action, moving the hands and focusing to rest at 1 o'clock. Repeat the horizontal contraction and release around the full pelvic clock circle until you return back to the 12 o'clock position at the pubic bone.

Initially, this exercise can feel very uncoordinated and confusing. I have had students say they didn't think anything was actually happening or that they were just imagining things. But with consistent practice (maybe a few weeks), awareness of the space within the pelvic bowl and connective tissue begins to increase. During labor, the mind is then more open to examining sensations within the pelvis, which is where the business of labor occurs. Of course there are multiple factors involved, but bringing awareness into the fascia and pelvic ligaments is one of many ways to empower a pregnant woman during the birth process.

In addition to these exercises for developing awareness and sensitivity in the overall body fascia network, gentle rocking movements can help to hydrate and mobilize fascia, relieving sticky spots. Think of movements such as Cat/Cow, done either on hands and knees or standing upright. The gentle, rhythmic motion of the pelvic bowl in conjunction with the lower back and hip muscles helps restore the sliding quality of the myofascial structure throughout the lower body. As with the release and awareness exercises above, these movements are done in the 50% range. We're not looking for extreme range of motion but rather a gentle massaging of the tissues.

Another variation on this movement which incorporates the legs is Chakravakasana, or the rocking Child's Pose sequence of moving from Table back to Child's Pose, then forward again. Moving back and forth not only creates a subtle and rhythmic arching and rounding in the lower back between the lumbar spine and sacrum but also squeezes and releases the calves and knees, helping to move fluid back into the circulatory system.

The interconnected web

When seeking body balance in yoga during pregnancy, keep in mind that any imbalances are pre-existing. A stretch may need to be held longer on one side than on the other, or there may need to be more attention paid to feelings arising as well as sensations from certain *asanas*. No one exercise will work for every single pregnancy, just as no single asana is beneficial for every yoga practitioner. At some point, each yoga practice needs to become personalized if it is to restore the balance needed to manage the intensity of labor and birth. Developing a sense of curiosity about sensation can be the window into restoring better birth function and finding greater comfort throughout pregnancy. We need to think of the pregnant body holistically, maintaining the elasticity of both the muscles and the fascia so the body can shift as it needs to during pregnancy and recover after the baby has been born.

In the same way that our bodies are interwoven by and from our fascia, the experience of motherhood is an interconnected one that develops with no clear moment of beginning (or ending for that matter). While some might argue that motherhood begins at the moment of conception (if we can even determine exactly when that occurred), there are others who might say it is at the moment of birth.

And then there is the idea of matrescence,[28] first coined by anthropologist Dana Raphael in the 1970s and more recently popularized by psychologists Alexandra Sacks and Aurelie Athan.[29] Matrescence acknowledges that there is a physiological shift in a mother's body which does not occur at one time but is rather a process. Similar to the progression of adolescence, where the body and mind go through dramatic changes and carry a series of social and physical expectations and understanding given to those going through them, matrescence recognizes that mothers do not suddenly emerge fully formed but rather grow into the people they become. Along the way, they are shaped by the people and societies who surround them, their own personal and cultural backgrounds, and the specifics of their birthing experiences.

Motherhood is ultimately a process of becoming that is connected to body, mind, and society. While we will revisit the social implications of this interconnectedness in later chapters, it is worth noting that in the fascia network, we have the perfect analogy for the progression into motherhood and the physical apparatus for creating greater ease during this time. What is the point of practicing yoga if not to create more harmony off the mat by balancing the microcosm of body and mind while on the mat? We can start this balancing by examining how each part is interconnected through our bones, our muscles, our minds, and our fascia. Then, armed with this knowledge, we can open where we can to find that ever-changing balance of effort and ease.

Key Takeaways

Our bodies are connected via an interlocking network of connective tissue known as fascia which influences the space between our bones, muscles, and organs and also impacts how much room the baby has to rotate and position during gestation.

The base of the uterus is supported in the center of the pelvis by the fascial network. Tension can lead to twists in the uterine placement.

The tension in our fascia comes from the movement patterns in our daily lives as well as emotional stress.

Releasing fascia can be done through jiggling, gentle massage techniques, or careful yoga movements.

Releasing fascia can help to restore space for baby and also bring overall balance and ease to the body.

---

[28] The transformation involved in becoming a mother physically, socially, and spiritually

[29] *www.matrescence.com*

5 — The Subtle Body During Pregnancy

"As to the subject of matter, we have all been wrong. What we have called matter is energy whose vibration has been so lowered as to be perceptible to the senses."

—Albert Einstein

From the point of view of the medical and anatomical world, the human body is composed of blood, muscle, bone, and various connective tissues. It functions as a series of interconnected systems which support one another to keep the larger human being alive and functioning. During pregnancy, this physical body is said to undergo major medical changes in order to support the growing embryo. At the appropriate time, the body moves through a series of actions to birth the baby and placenta, then gradually restores its internal functions.

This is the Western medical view, and it works fine if we are only focused on the physical body itself. But yoga views the physical body as one of multiple layers which comprise the full entity called our "self." Each of these layers is said to surround the deeper, eternal essence, which some refer to as our true nature or being; the part which reincarnates (if you subscribe to such beliefs), and the part which we are ultimately seeking to know through our yoga practice.

I have to be honest, the subtle body was always the aspect of yoga of which I was most suspicious. I prided myself on being a yoga teacher who was fully grounded in this plane of existence, and the very mention of "energy" within the body always left my skin crawling just a bit. While I enjoyed the idea that we were more than our physical selves, and maybe that meant there were literal energy centers within the body, I held these notions in the same category I held astrology: fun to think about, but were they really true?

Like many yoga teachers, my teaching centered on feeling the physical placement of the body and calming the nervous system through breathing and mindful awareness. Nothing esoteric here, I thought. We can't actually work directly with our *koshas*; they're just nice ideas…Then I became pregnant, and while I was still dubious about the *koshas'* existence, I had to admit that there was an overall change within my body. Sometimes clear, more often quite muddy and vague, there was a definite shift in awareness. And even if it was solely in my mind, it was no less real than the physical changes to my body's shape and metabolism. I discovered I had been working with the more subtle layers of the body throughout my whole life. I'd simply misunderstood what they were.

The conventional yogic view of the subtle body is as a series of sheaths or *koshas* that surround our true inner self. These layers are usually represented as a series of concentric circles, with the physical body at the outermost ring, and the Atman, the true and indestructible self, at the center. Between the physical body and the true self are the rings of the energy body, the mind, wisdom, and bliss. The concentric circle graphic gives the impression of the body being an onion, where each layer could be peeled back to discover another deeper one.

While this wasn't the exact intention of the graphic, this was how I tended to conceive of it—and, as I discovered, so did many other yoga teachers. The image becomes further confusing when we hear that each *kosha* can also be in or out of balance, and their interplay impacts how each *kosha* expresses itself. So much of the yoga and fitness world focuses on the physical body that while there is discussion of deeper states of awareness, the *koshas* are often abandoned in favor of more attention on the placement of the feet or the release of a specific muscle or fascial system. The *koshas* seem relegated to the periphery of the yoga practice, with primary attention focused back onto the physical body. But the physical body is just one of several layers…

The Koshas
The Five Sheaths of the Human Being

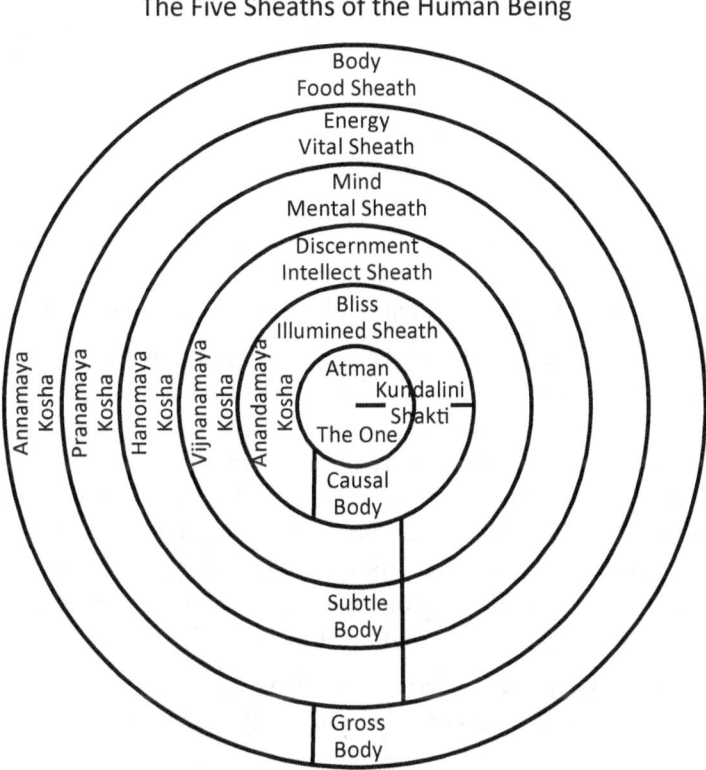

The classic representation of the subtle body

I credit my yoga teacher Barbara Benagh for the image which shifted how I thought about the *koshas* and the energy comprising a human being. "This isn't an onion," she said. "It's like a cloud." Suddenly I saw the misunderstanding. Rather than separate layers, these different "sheaths" were interwoven with one another as different facets of how we perceived our larger selves. From everyday awareness they looked white, the various colors of mist blending together into a seemingly cohesive whole. But given the right angle of light, those colors refracted out to illuminate the full color palate available. But the light had to be at just the right angle and just the right time; otherwise, we would perceive only the whiteness of the full cloud.

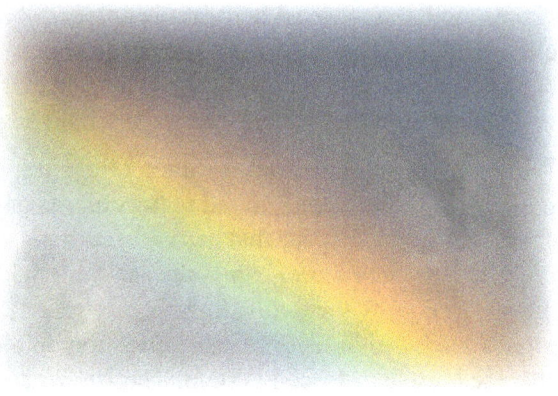

In the same way during everyday awareness, most of what we perceive is our physical body, and this is what Western culture tends to focus on. But go into the field of psychology and we have a completely different awareness of our thoughts and feelings which make up an entirely different side of our "self." While this psychological self may have feelings and thoughts about the physical body and is affected by discomfort or ease, our psyche is fundamentally different from the literal physical muscles and bones that allow us to stand and move. But your psyche is every bit as much a part of you as your body. Awareness can illuminate the different qualities which make up the unique rainbow of experience and existence, and just as the *koshas* can be in or out of balance, so too can the cloud wax and wane in density and wispiness. Seeing the rainbow is challenging in an everyday state of awareness. In this state we may only be able to see/feel the most outer and visible layer of ourselves, the physical body. Drop into a flow state or yogic meditation, however, and the colors begin to refract out.

During pregnancy, my physical body suddenly contained not only my own inner rainbow but also the energy that was creating my baby's body. These two fields began to interplay with one another, imprinting back and forth as they created a new internal balance. I'm not speaking hypothetically here. Medical research has shown how maternal thoughts lead to the release of emotional hormones that cross the placenta and affect the development and composition of the developing baby's brain.[30] Even more amazingly, fetal stem cells and DNA enter into the mother's system and even remain following the birth process.[31] For many perinatal psychologists there is the concept of the mother and baby being not two separate individuals but an interconnected dyad; the *mamatoto* in Swahili.

This interplay is what the yogis were referring to, but as we walk through the different *koshas*, it is important to remember that separating them out is like separating out a single muscle

---

[30] Kinsella, M. T., & Monk, C. (2009, September). *Impact of maternal stress, depression and anxiety on fetal neurobehavioral development.* Clinical obstetrics and gynecology. https://www.ncbi.nlm.nih.gov/pmc/articles/PMC3710585/

[31] Boddy, A. M., Fortunato, A., Sayres, M. W., & Aktipis, A. (2015, August 28). *Fetal microchimerism and maternal health: A ... - wiley online library.* Bio Essays. https://onlinelibrary.wiley.com/doi/full/10.1002/bies.201500059

from the larger human body muscular system. While the biceps muscle may bend your elbow, it is never acting in isolation. Likewise, the different sheaths of your human existence are not separate aspects from one another but an interwoven mist, with each color only able to be perceived when the light of awareness is directed in the necessary angle or flow state.

The *koshas*

Annamaya Kosha: the food body

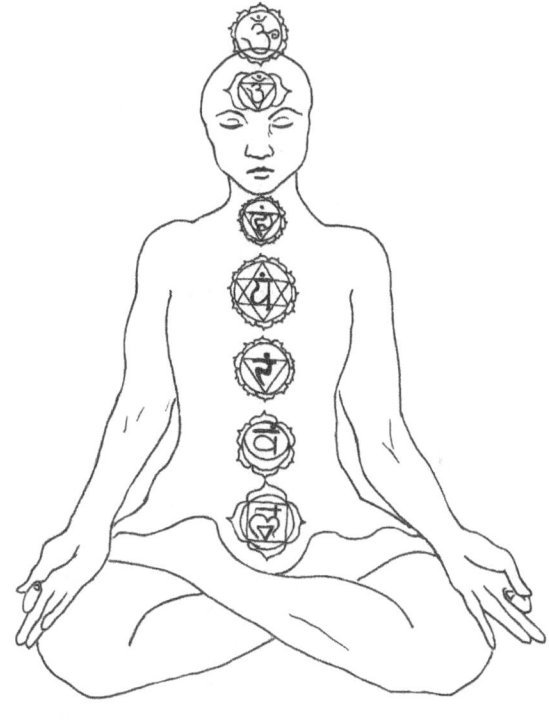

This "mist" is the easiest to perceive. This is the blood, muscle, bone, and connective tissue that makes up your physical body. Since it's the easiest to see and touch, this sheath gets the majority of the attention from both the medical and fitness worlds. This sheath is vitally important. Without it we would have neither yoga nor a meditation practice. During pregnancy of course, this "outer" layer is subject to major changes as the body changes shape, adds weight to support the pregnancy, and adjusts to support the shifting center of gravity.

Imbalances in Annamaya Kosha usually show up as physical manifestations. The shift in muscle tension due to a changing center of gravity can mean that the physical body becomes out of balance. This then affects how the bones sit relative to one another. Additionally, imbalance could show up as too much or too little weight on the body. This is not a comment on needing to be an ideal size or shape but simply refers to states where the physical body is out of balance with the larger "energy" of the whole being. We also see imbalances of Annamaya Kosha manifest as an extreme focus on appearance and perfecting the physical form. Rebalancing involves learning to be comfortable in the form we are in and working with it so that we can function at other levels of the subtle body as well.

In pregnancy there is an acute focus on the Annamaya Kosha. During my own pregnancy, I noted where my muscles grew tense or overstretched. I tried my best to do physical movements which would help create physical strength where I needed it and release tension where I had become overly contracted. I was fortunate that my care providers were relaxed about how much weight I was gaining, so while I did track it, I did not have to be overly concerned about it. Like many of my students, this was also a time when I "indulged" in more physical self care than I would normally, paying for regular massages and body work, as well as yoga practice, with the intention that it would all prepare me for a smoother labor and birth. But while we often focus on the physical body during pregnancy, it is the interplay of the physical with the more subtle layers of experience that can have the most dramatic impact.

Practices for balancing Annamaya Kosha

Ultimately, balancing Annamaya Kosha is what the physical yoga *asanas* are all about. If we want to relieve physical imbalances within the connective tissues, then practicing *asana* is what's needed. We'll delve fully into *asana* practice during pregnancy in the Practice segment of this book. For now, suffice it to say that if the physical shifts in pregnancy lead to aches and pains or other types of discomfort, it's probably time to hit the mat.

Along with physical *asana*, a generally well-rounded diet can also help balance Annamaya Kosha. Nutrition for pregnancy is outside my expertise, but general tips I give to my child-birth education classes are to eat the rainbow (not Skittles!), lean towards whole grains, drink plenty of water, and get enough protein. Another way of internally guiding whether something is beneficial for Annamaya Kosha during pregnancy is to ask, "Would I feed this to my two year old?" If you don't plan to feed it to your two year old, don't feed it to the baby now.[32] In addition, holistic alternative practices can complement the physical changes the body is undergoing. Chiropractic, ayurvedic, osteopathic, and even conventional Western (allopathic) medicine can be helpful in balancing Annamaya Kosha.

Pranamaya Kosha: the energy body

Moving to the next most subtle mist, we get to the layer which I mistakenly took as the whole of the *kosha* family. Our energy body, or the Pranamaya Kosha, is perhaps the layer most talked about in physical yoga practices. I have heard teachers often mention the *nadis*, the channels of energy within this layer, without truly explaining how to conceive of these "little rivers." Especially prominent are mentions of the Sushumna *nadi*, or the main channel running along the spine, and the *ida* and *pingala nadis*, which are referenced when practicing the Nadi Shodhanam *pranayama* (alternate nostril breathing). The whole *nadi* network is often said to contain 72,000 little rivers, which I have also heard noted as the number of nerve channels in the body.

This correlation between Pranayama Kosha and the nervous system is where I believe the misunderstanding about the subtle body originates. I have heard teacher trainees reference the energy body as an ancient way of describing our nervous system, which always left me a bit confused, since the nervous system is clearly part of the physical body. Maybe some ancient yogis meant it this way (and let's also remember how old some of these traditions really are![33]), but we miss a key component of the mist analogy if we hold too closely the metaphor of *nadis* as nervous system.

---

[32] Diet is of course an area of awareness during pregnancy, especially if mom develops a condition known as gestational diabetes. Always check with a care provider or refer students to their own providers if giving diet suggestions.

[33] *The Science of Yoga*, Matthew Broad, Simon & Schuster; 1st edition (December 1, 2012)

The nerves and the network they create are not the energy body; they are part of the physical body and thus part of the first *kosha*. But the electrical energy flowing along them, the literal current without which we would not be a living body, *that* is what comprises Pranamaya Kosha! Without this electricity, this *prana*, we are not alive. Our physical body requires the energy of Pranamaya Kosha to function and thrive, even though we cannot physically touch this electricity with our hands.

There is one place where the Pranamaya Kosha does touch the Annamaya Kosha and where we can physically affect it, which is in the breath. The breath is a physical action of coordinated muscles, but it is also a direct reflection of our overall nervous system. If we make our breath rapid and shallow during yoga practice (or any time in our life), it triggers our body's stress response. The electricity flows more quickly, brain waves shift, and the fight or flight side of our nervous system becomes more activated.

Conversely, if we deliberately slow our breath, as in Ujjayi or Viloma *pranayama*, we send a signal to our nervous system to down-regulate and increase the functioning of the parasympathetic nervous system. Given this connection to the breath, imbalances in Pranamaya Kosha can therefore often be seen in the responses to uneven breathing: anxiety or nervous stress, shortness of breath, depression (the other side of anxiety), ADHD, a general inability to focus the nervous system that leads to overdoing and exhaustion, or the physical results brought on by living in a chronically stressed state.

The vayus

In working with the breath, we encounter another aspect of the energy body, the *vayus*. Related to the *nadi* channels of energy rivers, the *vayus* translate as "the winds" and are usually described as different currents of energy moving within the body. These currents link to different aspects of the breath. Most of the time in yoga classes, the *vayus* are mentioned only in passing as qualities inherent within certain postures, such as backbends being more *pranic* in nature.

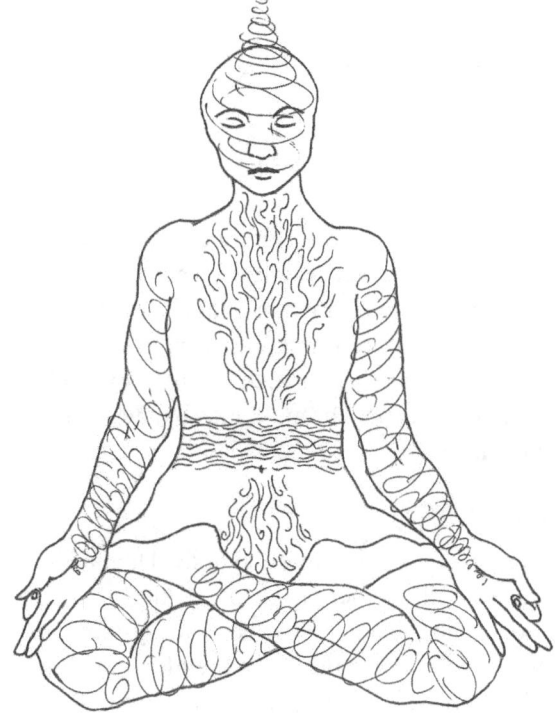

However, a closer look reveals that the *vayus* are correlated with the movement of life force within the body, possibly as an ancient format for explaining how the body continued to function and regulate its inner energy, or *prana*, without an understanding of digestion, the nervous system, or the electromagnetic energy of the brain and body. Through this specific lens, we may be able to learn or intuit something about the energy body itself.

The *vayus* are usually listed as Prana Vayu, Apana Vayu, Samana Vayu, Udana Vayu, and Vyana Vayu. By listing them this way, I believe we have misrepresented how these different currents relate to the daily and even moment to moment functioning of our larger body and mind. Each of the *vayus* are said to govern a certain segment of the body, but for me, like the overall mist of the cloud, each permeates the entirety of our internal being.

Prana Vayu

This is described as an upward moving energy current running from the ribcage to the throat. It is said to govern our respiratory system and represents the absorption and taking in of sensory perceptions and impressions. It is associated with the fourth *chakra* and is said to be "solar" in nature. The Prana Vayu current is said to set things in motion and move us forward in the world. It is our inhalation, and brings in the fuel from which we generate energy and ideas.

Samana Vayu

Samana means balance. This current is said to be a sideways current moving between the navel and the lower ribs. It is often correlated with the core and abdominal-activating *asanas*. Beyond muscular action, Samana Vayu is said to govern digestion and focuses on assimilation and processing of both literal food and any ideas or challenges we might be "chewing on" or working out. Because of its location around the navel and its connection to assimilation, this *vayu* is associated with the third *chakra* and the element of fire. It is the pause between our inhale and exhale, when the body takes the fuel of the breath and begins to work with it.

Vyana Vayu

This *vayu* is usually described last, but I find it fits better into our body flow here. Vyana Vayu is said to be an all pervasive current running throughout the body that enlivens the tissues. It circulates the energy digested from Samana Vayu out through our being and holds the body together (energetically speaking). It is responsible for regulating and coordinating the other currents, which might be why it is often described last. Vyana Vayu is associated with the element of water, and though it pervades the whole body, it is most closely associated with the second *chakra*. Though Vyana Vayu is not associated with a specific aspect of the breath, it can be brought into balance through breathwork such as Samma Vritti or Nadi Shodhanam.

Udana Vayu

As energy moves out into the body, Udana Vayu begins to make use of it. This current, said to be a spiraling energy inhabiting the arms, legs, and head, governs the sensory organs, our actions, and the autonomic nervous system. Udana Vayu focuses on expression and how we interact with the world. For a breath connection, it relates to what some call the "up breath," which I have always understood to be the short, quick inhale we might take before standing up to go do something. The fast inhale up into the chest we take as we reach for our water bottle following a vigorous Sun Salutation? That's what we're talking about. Udana Vayu, importantly, is also the breath a laboring mother might take just before she begins bearing down to birth her baby.

Apana Vayu

And then finally, having used the energy created by the fuel brought in, we are left with waste products and must eliminate them. Enter Apana Vayu. This is the downward moving current of energy said to reside from the navel to the perineum and below. It governs excretory and reproductive functions and is specifically associated with the second stage of labor.

Ayurveda traditions stress the need to keep Apana Vayu in balance during pregnancy, as you need the downward current to birth the baby but obviously do not wish to birth prematurely.[34] Where Prana Vayu is solar, Apana Vayu is "lunar" in nature. It is associated with the first and to some extent the second *chakra*, and it promotes a grounding energy, both mental and physical. As it relates to the breath, Apana Vayu is the outward exhalation where we release the waste products of our respiratory cycle.

So, if we follow the *vayus* as they seem to be connected within our body: We bring in air and fuel through Prana Vayu. It then drops down to our center to be digested with Samana Vayu. Vyana Vayu then moves this new fuel throughout our body to enliven it. Udana Vayu makes use of this energy with the arms and legs as we perform whatever action or posture we are practicing. Then finally, Apana Vayu releases the waste product back out into the environment, and the cycle repeats.

But it is possible to go too far in one direction or another, and here we return to our overall body posture and the intersection of Annamaya Kosha with the more subtle layers. Each *vayu* corresponds to part of the breath, and Prana Vayu and Apana Vayu are also associated with movements related to the breath. The inhalation tends to create an opening movement in the chest, with a slight backbending quality to it; thus many of the backbends are referred to as being *prana* postures (note that "*prana*" here is just the inhale and not to be mistaken for *prana* as life force). Meanwhile, the exhalation is associated with a closing of the chest and slight flexion of the spine. Thus, forward-bending postures are often referred to as being *apanic* in nature. They are more focused on the exhale than the inhale.

If we practice in a way that accentuates the lifting, extending, backbending quality of postures (think about practicing with a wide open chest with ribs slightly flared forward), we increase the intake quality of the *asana*, but we also compress the releasing quality. This can lead to the overall posture being slightly out of balance. While practicing in this way may feel "energizing" in the moment, it is overall depleting.

When the energy is forward and up (and, one might argue, ungrounded and slightly aggressive) in this type of rib thrust posture, it leads to compression in the base of the back ribs.

---

[34] Visco, C. (2014, April 9). *Promoting the health of mother and baby during pregnancy using ayurveda.* California College of Ayurveda. https://www.ayurvedacollege.com/blog/pregnancy/

This is the same area that houses the kidneys and adrenal glands. Does squeezing the back ribs lead to the adrenals squirting adrenaline into our nervous system? I'm not sure that it does in a strict physiological sense, but energetically there does seem to be some correlation. At the very least, creating space in the tissues and fascia around this area could be helpful in calming an overstimulated nervous system. Yoga teacher Richard Freeman of Boulder, CO, has described this posture as "hyper-*pranic*," leading to overstimulation in the *asana* practice. It's an interesting thought given how our culture prizes expansion and activity, but that, too, is a topic for another book.

On the flip side, we could also be practicing in a way which overly emphasizes the *apanic* or flexion movement. In this case, rather than developing hyperactivation of the nervous system, we wind up in a posture I refer to as the "Eeyore" position: shoulders slumped forward, chest collapsed, pelvis tucked. While we aren't looking for the excitement and adrenaline of the constant rib thrust, neither do we want to overly emphasize the downward motion of the *apanic* exhalation. Taken to its extreme, this direction would lead to depression and less air consumption. Rather than shrinking into the back body, we need to find the balance between front and back over the course of our full yoga practice.

If you reflect back on the Tadasana instructions given in the chapter on pelvic alignment, you may notice that there does exist a happy medium. We are not looking to lock into a single shape midway between backbend and forward bend; rather, we want to find the dance between them. As we balance the pelvis on the legs, we have to play with the physical positioning or forward tilt (*pranic*) and backward tilt (*apanic*). And this interplay continues throughout the spine and all the joints. If we find the action of grounding the pubic bone as we place the pelvis onto the legs while simultaneously anchoring the tailbone, we bring the pelvis into neutral position and level the pelvic floor with the earth beneath us.

Paying attention to the action from the pelvic floor, we then discover that leveling the musculature actually leads to activation of both the pelvic floor and the deep transverse abdominals, bringing the engagement of Samana Vayu into the mix. This dance between intake and expulsion functions on both an energetic as well as physical level, and working with that dance, helps regulate the body's larger "energy" state.

In pregnancy, Pranamaya Kosha adapts first to the energetic requirements of the first trimester. Pregnant people often report feeling an energy drain in the first few months, as though their overall state was being taxed without their doing anything further. Step back, and the stress becomes obvious. We're only growing another full human being here! And it's during the first trimester that the highest rate of fetal cell division takes place. The overall demands on the body system are increased, so this is often a time for greater rest and rejuvenation.

Balancing Pranamaya Kosha

Part of balancing the energy body involves balancing the physical body as well. But if we want to impact our breath body, we might start directly with the breath. The connection between the breath and the nervous system means that practices for balancing Pranamaya

Kosha can begin with practicing *pranayama*. Which *pranayama* is needed will depend on whether the nervous system is overly activated or overly lethargic. A simple way to evaluate what's needed is to sit quietly, tuning in to the pace and rhythm of the regular breath. If the inhalation is longer than the exhale, it can indicate the nervous system is in a more agitated state and might benefit from calming *pranayama*. Alternatively, if the exhale is longer than the inhale, then more energizing, "vigorous," or focusing *pranayamas* might be appropriate. The Practice section of this book contains several *pranayama* exercises that are safe and effective during pregnancy, and even some that can be helpful during labor and birth.

We can also access Pranamaya Kosha through the physical body by practicing restorative yoga postures. Supported backbends and forward bends have different impacts, but they both access the parasympathetic nervous system (the relaxation response). Forward bending restorative postures can have a rejuvenating effect on the body and mind, especially during moments of physical exhaustion or shortness of breath. On the other hand, if someone is experiencing depression, supported backbends and other heart opening postures (both physically and mentally) might be more helpful in restoring balance. I do not claim that depression can be treated only with supported backbends, but I do believe they can be helpful as part of a comprehensive treatment program. Acupuncture, *reiki*, and homeopathy can also be complementary practices for balancing Pranamaya Kosha.

Manomaya Kosha: the mind body

Go one layer deeper into our human cloud, and we get to the intersection of our electrical energy with that complicated organ of our brain. Our "mind body" consists of our thoughts, desires, and wishes, which have been shown to have impacts on our physical tissues as well as our emotional state. Our mind body is said to govern the *kleshas*, or the attachments which eventually lead to suffering throughout life: *avidya* (ignorance), *asmita* (over-identifying with your ego), *raga* (desire, or attachment to pleasure), *dvesha* (avoidance, or attachment to not having whatever we currently have), and *abhinivesha* (fear of death/attachment to life). Within each of these is a component of focusing on or being attached to something that is destined to change, leading to suffering when the object of focus inevitably shifts.

The *kleshas* often seem to become heightened during pregnancy and immediately postpartum. Changes in body shape and weight can lead to confused feelings in a culture that prizes slenderness and shuns curves. This is just one way that *avidya* and *asmita* can come into the picture. We may not realize how entwined our egos were to our physical shape until that shape changes without our control. Of course, we know as yogis the body is always changing and that even the lowest weight is not destined to be permanent. But the weight changes during pregnancy are sometimes accepted and not accepted at the same time. We might avoid (ignore) looking at the scale, or we might embrace how things are changing.

I have often heard students comment on their changing body shape during class check-ins. For some this is a source of suffering ("I look huge!"); for others, it can be a celebration ("I'm finally showing!") Either way it is Manomaya Kosha that is shifting and directing the attention. And it doesn't stop with the body: for many pregnant people, pregnancy challenges their entire sense of self. I once had a student say to me, "I feel like I have all these roles I've been playing, and I'm not sure how many of them fit with being a mother."

Attachment to ego—or how you have framed your identity—can become vividly apparent during pregnancy as you navigate the social changes of bringing another human into the world. For some, this is a time of major upheaval; for others, it feels like stepping into who they always wanted to be. Either way, the mind's level of attachment to an old identity influences the mental "mist" we experience.

Of course, the next two *kleshas* are woven throughout the exploration of the first two. Attachment to having what we want (*raga*) or aversion to what we have (*devesha*) are the root of the suffering in the first two *kleshas* and feed into all of the other experiences around pregnancy. It's completely understandable that pregnant women don't want to be in pain: no one wants to feel discomfort. But there is a difference between having discomfort in the body (or mind) and actively pushing it away or clinging to the good moments.

Recently, I had a pregnant yoga student who was brought to tears over pain in her tailbone and back from an unstable pelvis. The sensation she could handle, but she so desperately wanted it to go away that her whole pregnancy was becoming miserable because she was unable to do the things she wanted to do. *Raga* and *devasha* were running rampant. She so wanted to enjoy her pregnancy, but she also wanted to be able to retain her active lifestyle, including biking and running, and didn't want to have to modify or temporarily stop because of instability. We spent several months working with the ways in which she had attached to certain movements and finding ways to help shift her focus to how things were right now, being compassionate with the feelings that arose from being in pain and having to rein in her active lifestyle. (It wasn't until her baby settled lower into her pelvis and filled in the circle of the pelvic bowl that her pain subsided).

Working with attachment and aversion has implications for labor and birth as well. Being able to sit with possibly uncomfortable sensations, without trying to push them away or mentally running from them, gives mom more options to work with during labor. We'll come back to this concept in the Birth section of this book.

Finally, if we look at *abhinivesha*, or the fear of death/attachment to life, we can see where it could become heightened during pregnancy. We know that birth comes with some severe baggage, not the least of which is the adage "Women used to die in childbirth." While this risk is less common in modern times,[35] the thought may be there nonetheless.

For some women, examining the process of birth may also involve contending with a fear of death. Even if the literal fear of death is not present, the changes of pregnancy can make it seem as if the old "self" is going away; for some, this experience is as confusing as facing the possibility of physical death. Additionally, if we consider *abhinivesha* to be the attachment to

---

[35] It should be noted that the United States has one of the highest maternal death rates in the industrialized world, and at the time of this publication it is still rising. Centers for Disease Control and Prevention. (2021, March 23). *Maternal mortality rates in the United States, 2019.*

life, what better exemplifies this than wanting to take care of your child? As my own meditation teacher commented after his granddaughter was born, "I can leave many things behind, but now there is a really strong desire to watch her grow up." Children inherently tie us to this world, which makes it more difficult to contemplate letting go. All of this has an impact on Manomaya Kosha.

Balancing Manomaya Kosha

To balance the mist of the mind, one must first and foremost start working with the mind. The simplest practice for bringing this part of the cloud into balance is meditation—simple, but not easy. I have often found that unless pregnant students already have a meditation practice, this is a difficult time to dive in.

We can be sensitive to this difficulty and begin exploring meditative awareness through *asana*. Ultimately yoga, especially flowing yoga, is meditation in motion. For some, the grounded, tactile quality of focusing the mind on physical sensations can be an easier introduction than simply sitting down and dropping in. Once we have established a base of awareness, we can then shift towards sitting meditation at the end of a practice. Eventually, we can blend the meditative awareness developed on the mat into everyday life as post-meditation practice.

It should also be noted that any practice which focuses on the mind and our emotional experiences would also be helpful in balancing Manomaya Kosha. Thus, different types of psychotherapy, including cognitive behavioral therapy, mindfulness based cognitive therapy, and mindfulness based stress reduction could be of benefit. All of these can assist a meditation and yoga practice and would be appropriate in any case where mental imbalance is more acute.[36]

Vijanamaya Kosha: the wisdom body

Beyond our thoughts and intellectual understanding and knowledge, we also have a felt sense and internal wisdom that seems to come from deep within ourselves. Many of us have experienced this feeling: the lightning strike insight that clears the fog of the mind for a moment. Beyond the realm of the mind body, this primal insight is what yoga refers to as the wisdom body. It is like an intuitive answer or solution that seems to transcend thought processes or the rational mind. This capacity for insight is with us at all times and is sometimes called our basic goodness in spiritual circles.

From the perspective of pregnancy, it is this basic intuition that birthing women and new mothers tap into during labor and the first weeks of the baby's life. This subtle layer of the cloud may only be seen in small flashes between the other, denser colors of the mist, but it guides the larger cloud's position and shape nonetheless.

Vijanamaya Kosha is thought to be the guiding instinct throughout the labor process. In natural childbirth circles, it is often said that the body ultimately knows what to do; the pregnant

---

[36] Perinatal mood and anxiety disorders affect 1 in 5 women and should not be treated solely through yoga.

woman (and her care providers) simply need to listen. In her video "Birth Day," Naoli Vinaver Lopez explains that "Women giving birth, if you just give them the space, they will know exactly what to do. Women have inside the deep knowledge of exactly when to push, how to push. The body that has made this baby knows exactly how to get it out of the body and give birth."[37]

But trusting this insight is not often encouraged by the Western medical community, and so many well-intentioned yogini moms may still feel they can't fully trust that their bodies know what to do. This feeling may result from direct comments or from more subtle experiences around miscarriage, fertility challenges, or family stories that have not been fully processed.

If Vijanamaya Kosha shifts out of balance, we start questioning our own inherent worthiness and instincts, which manifests as a lack of trust. Alternatively, this internal lack of trust could manifest outwardly as arrogance, a lack of empathy for others, or an inability to be alone (because we do not trust and love the person we find when we are alone with ourselves). Healing and balancing this layer is one part of coming into and restoring a pregnant person's power and confidence during the journey to motherhood. Without a sense of yourself, it is far more difficult to trust the choices you need to make.

Balancing Vijanamaya Kosha

Because this *kosha* is often only seen in flashes and moments, balancing this layer of the cloud often involves working with the more visible layers to get deeper into the mist. Sitting and walking meditation, especially when done in nature, can help. Being outdoors may help remind us of our interconnectedness with the natural world and may also help calm Manomaya Kosha. Silent retreats or other practices where we create the space to fall into deeper meditative contemplation and almost literally sit *with ourselves* can help promote a sense of trust and compassion for both the inner and outer selves and ultimately help us find ways to make friends with them.

Anandamaya Kosha: the bliss body

Lastly and on the most subtle level of mist, we come to Anandamaya Kosha. This "bliss body" is often hard to quantify because its experience is so elusive and covered by the other mists. But it might be said to be the feeling of pure enjoyment of the moment. We encounter this mist when we find ourselves in a flow state, when we become fully absorbed in what we are doing, and the boundary between us and the world around us almost seems to dissipate. Being in this aspect of our body is sometimes said to be "one step from enlightenment." When students ask why it's not enlightenment itself, since we feel "at one" with the world around us, my response is usually twofold. First, we experience Anandamaya Kosha only in flashes rather than as a consistent state. Second, while we feel at one with the world when in contact with the bliss body, "we" are still present. There is still an infinitely thin boundary between us and the world around us. Were we to reach enlightenment (so I'm told), this boundary would dissolve and we would fundamentally know ourselves as interconnected with everything around us.

---

[37] Film Australia production company. (2001). *Birth Day.* Sydney.

Just like the other layers of mist, this layer can also become unbalanced. Imbalance displays itself here as being ungrounded or unfocused, as in not having a strong connection to things as they truly are. This imbalance can also manifest as suicidal thoughts due to the misperception that the discomfort being felt could be solved by removing the very being that perceives it. I have often thought of this imbalance as being similar to preferring the dream state to the real world, somehow thinking that if one were to leave the real world, the dream world would become reality. Balancing this layer mostly involves balancing the others around it. When the body is supple, the energy is flowing, the mind is awake and aware, and our trust in our insight is functioning, then the flow state is able to move easily through the cloud.

The Atman: your unchangeable self

At the very center of the cloud, we find the Atman. This concept has been given numerous names—the soul, the self, our inner being—but the consistent aspect of all these names is that this is something which does not change. Regardless of whether you believe in reincarnation or prefer to think of this being the only life you have (or somewhere in between), we can all agree that during our lives we have grown and changed as people. Becoming a mother is a fundamental change and one which can almost completely remake the outermost layers that swirl and bubble up as ourselves. But at the core, there is a piece that remains constant.

During my yoga classes, I often ask students to pause and feel what it feels like to be them at this moment. After the baby is born, we return to this practice. While thoughts may seem completely confused, and priorities and self-identities may have shifted, there is always a felt sense of something "the same" that is still present. In yoga, we seek to ground our identity in this unchanging quality rather than clinging to the titles, shapes, or names we might give ourselves. The irony is that when we truly sit and examine what or who is at the center of this ever-shifting cloud, we find that there isn't anything solid we can hold onto. Rather, there is only the collection of energy that is currently manifesting as "self."

Psyche and soma

During pregnancy, Western medicine focuses almost exclusively on the physical body, but from yoga's perspective, there is no separation of psyche and soma. Each of the five sheaths influences the others. Mental stresses can create physical tension and vice versa. In seeking balance and internal ease, we can sometimes address *kosha* imbalances via the other components of the cloud. Physical ailments can be relieved through mental practices, and mental practices can help balance fascia and muscle tension.

Research has now discovered that during pregnancy, the maternal body provides an environment and nourishment for the growing embryo and also influences the embryo through the hormonal and chemical soup in which the baby is developing.[38] Even more incredibly, the connection runs both ways. Fetal stem cells can enter mom's body to aid in healing during

---

[38] Kinsella, M. T., & Monk, C. (2009, September). *Impact of maternal stress, depression and anxiety on fetal neurobehavioral development.* Clinical obstetrics and gynecology. https://www.ncbi.nlm.nih.gov/pmc/articles/PMC3710585/

injury, and fetal DNA actually remains in the mother's system following birth. Some researchers have postulated that it may even protect against diseases such as Alzheimer's.[39]

Emotions and feelings (Manomaya Kosha) trigger hormonal responses in mom's body, which have been shown to cross the placenta and impact the development of the baby's brain. More stress (we're talking chronic here, not just running for a bus), and the baby's brain gets wired for hypervigilance and quick reaction time.[40] More relaxation, and the baby learns that the world isn't a dangerous place that requires constant alertness. A mother who is chronically stressed about the health of her baby holds that stress somewhere within her body's physical tissue. This can be worked on through physical stretching, or through meditation and trust, or even better, through both! We can learn to cope with the physical changes of being pregnant and find ways to remain mentally calm and balanced rather than stressed and disturbed.

Key Takeaways

Yoga describes the body as being made up of five sheaths or layers: the physical body, the energy body, the mental body, the wisdom body, and the bliss body. The sheaths are called *koshas*.

The *koshas* refer to the more subtle qualities of our being and "self."

Each *kosha* can be in or out of balance. Different illnesses or challenges appear when one or more *koshas* are out of balance. There are also practices to bring each *kosha* more into balance.

The *koshas* can affect one another. From yoga's perspective, psyche and soma (mental and physical) are not separate.

Pregnancy shifts the balance and stresses on each *kosha*. We can address physical stresses through the mental body, or vice versa, through our yoga practice.

---

[39] Chan, W. F. N., Gurnot, C., Montine, T. J., Sonnen, J. A., Guthrie, K. A., & Nelson, J. L. (2012, September 26). *Male microchimerism in the human female brain.* PLOS ONE. https://journals.plos.org/plosone/article?id=10.1371%2Fjournal.pone.0045592
(It should be noted these studies were done on female mice, not humans.)
[40] Verny, T. R., & Kelly, J. (1988). *The secret life of the unborn child.* Dell Pub. Co.

Practice

This is where the rubber meets the road.

6 — Yoga Myths About Pregnancy

What have you heard that pregnant women shouldn't do in their yoga practice?

Ask this question at a conventional yoga studio and you will get a range of partially accurate information, wildly outdated assumptions, and some answers that are not only fully incorrect but are based on superstition and fear of the pregnant body. For every yoga teacher who has a working knowledge of the structure of the pregnant body, there seem to be three or four who have learned, and in some cases internalized, mistaken assumptions about what a pregnant body is capable of. The result is a confusing mixture of conflicting answers, given with varying levels of confidence.

You may have heard some of these answers already:

"Never invert when pregnant!"

"No lying on your right side!" "No, you just have to roll to your left side when coming up!"

"Always lie on your left side."

"No lying on your back."

"No closed twists." "No twists at all."

"No Plank pose." "No Planks in the first trimester...or was it the third?"

"No squatting." "Wait, no, we should be doing lots of squatting!" "Always squat!"

"No balancing postures."

"No backbends."

"No forward bends."

"No breath work." "No breath retentions." "No heating pranayama." "No pranayama at all!"

And the list goes on. To be honest, if pregnant women actually followed every restriction stated about practicing yoga while pregnant, there would be no prenatal yoga classes! All pregnant women would be able to do is sit quietly, lie on their left side, and roll their ankles to avoid blood clots for the full nine months.

Obviously, something has gotten out of hand in the yoga world around what is actually safe in pregnancy versus what should be done with caution versus what is actually contraindicated. On one hand, we can understand where these restrictions came from. Yoga studios are always concerned about students injuring themselves. At the end of the day, yoga is a physical practice and carries a risk of physical injury (so does stepping off the curb into the street). But now add to that anxiety the fear of hurting someone who is also carrying another human being—or even worse, hurting the baby—and we can see how some of these misconceptions developed.

In the same way that some hospitals have taken protocols for high risk women and applied them across the board to low risk women "just to be safe," yoga teachers have given modifications to one student or one group of students, and those modifications have gradually been applied to the entire general prenatal population. There are contraindications that should be avoided during pregnancy, or at least by those with certain pregnancy conditions. However, in most cases we have become far too restrictive in the conventional ideas of yoga and pregnancy. Just as we have made birth more complicated than necessary by putting too many restrictions and judgments on it, so too have we made prenatal yoga too complicated by using rules and conventions that are well-intentioned but ultimately impede true understanding.

Let me also dispel one of the biggest initial fears that yoga teachers seem to have: that something in the yoga practice is going to hurt the baby! There are movements and practices that could adversely affect a baby if done without any awareness. That said, for the most part, babies are very well protected within their mothers' bodies. This isn't to say that the risk is non-existent, but the idea that a *gentle* yoga practice will disrupt a pregnancy that is proceeding well is just not accurate. It really isn't the baby we need to be worried about in the yoga practice, provided that we take some basic precautions. The person we need to be concerned for is mom. Her practice affects the balance and structure of her body, not just while pregnant but, maybe more importantly, after she gives birth.

With that said, let's examine some of the major myths around practicing yoga while pregnant:

Myth: No inversions
Verdict: False!

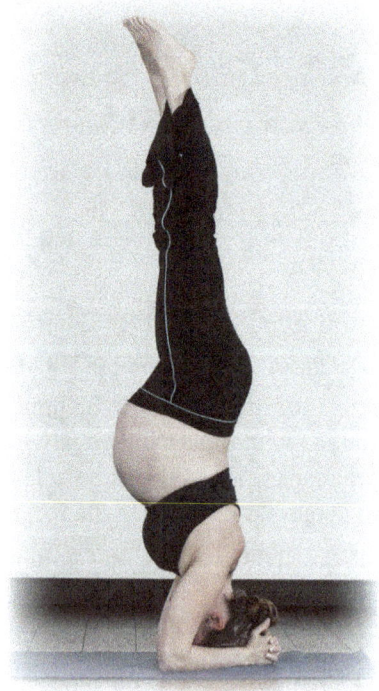

I honestly think this is the most common misstatement I hear when I ask teacher trainees what "no-nos" they have heard about pregnancy: no Headstands, Handstands, Forearm Stands, or Shoulder Stands while pregnant. But for some it doesn't stop there. I have also heard yoga teachers proclaim that pregnant women shouldn't do Downward Dog or even Uttanasana because these poses place the head below the heart, constituting an inversion. By this logic, how on earth is a pregnant woman supposed to pick something up off the ground? Now there are a few caveats, but in general this is one statement which is NOT TRUE!!!

The thing about inversions (excluding the whole Uttanasana/Down Dog thing, and I'll come back to that) is that they are advanced postures. Generally speaking, one does not teach the four primary inversions to beginning yoga students, and definitely not in their fullest form. Instead we build up their body awareness, strength, and foundations so that at a later date they might be able to explore this *asana* family if they choose. The reason to avoid inverting in prenatal yoga isn't because it's truly contraindicated during pregnancy; it's because most students don't know how to do it in the first place. Combine that with the changing center of gravity, the increased relaxin and other hormones softening the connective tissue, and the risk of falling, and this is not the time to learn how to go upside down.

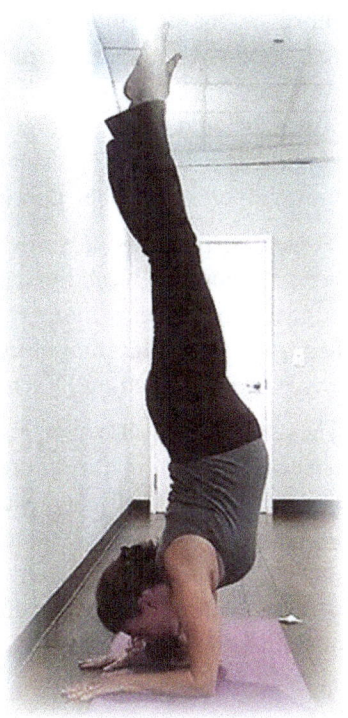

I have a sneaking suspicion that the ban on inverting during pregnancy actually dates back to the "rule" of not inverting while on your menstrual cycle. For years, women were told that doing so would "reverse the flow of energy in your body and possibly lead to endometriosis." Besides my skepticism that a position "reverses the flow of energy" in my body, the claim of causing endometriosis has never been shown to be true.

This strikes me as something stated at some point, probably by a MALE yoga teacher who lacked an understanding of the functioning of women's bodies, which stripped women of their power. The truth is that for some women, inverting during their period feels wonderful, a relief to the heaviness of that time of the month.

There are other reasons to consider gentle inversions. Midwife Gail Tully, founder of Spinning Babies®, has developed a program for helping pregnant women balance their body's connective tissue. It involves what she terms a "forward leaning inversion," where mom kneels on a couch or firm bench, places her elbows on the floor, brings her hips nearly over her shoulders, and tucks her chin into her chest. This position is then held for three breaths, after which mom returns to an upright position. The inversion gently tugs on the utero-sacral ligaments on the posterior lower uterine segment, allowing the ligaments to unwind into greater space when mom turns upright again. But she is nearly fully inverted while practicing this shape. (It should be noted that this position is not done in isolation; for a fuller understanding of the Spinning Babies® program, please visit spinningbabies.com)

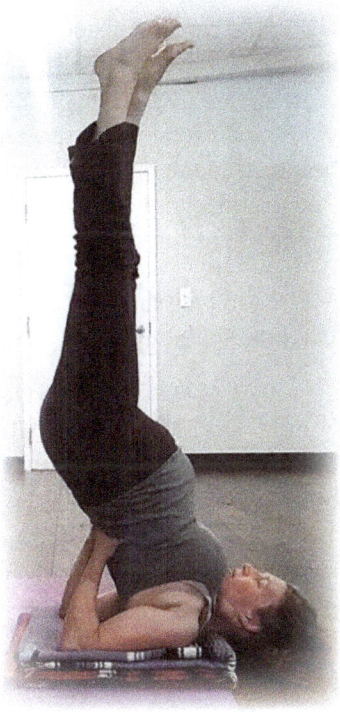

There is something to take into consideration about putting the head below the heart but not to the exclusion of common sense. By the time mom is ready to give birth, the body is carrying nearly 1.5 times its original blood volume. This extra fluid is needed to circulate nutrients through the baby's body as well, and it leads to a change in blood pressure. But this by itself doesn't mean that pregnant women should never put their heads below their hearts. Again, how could we tie our shoes? It simply means we might want to exercise caution and move slowly when leaning forward, or more importantly, when coming upright as we might in a Sun Salutation.

Generally speaking, postures that briefly put the head below the heart are ok, but if someone has pregnancy-induced hypertension, pre-eclampsia, or other conditions where there is a concern about them having their head below their heart for longer than one or two breaths (e.g. glaucoma, placental bleeding), then that individual shouldn't perform extended holds in any position, including Downward Dog and Uttanasana.

These restrictions are also true for the general population, and something like glaucoma isn't more common during pregnancy. They are not a valid reason for all pregnant women to avoid the benefits of Downward Dog. However, we might consider cutting out the extended inversions out of compassion for mom's own comfort. Given a 150% change in fluid volume during pregnancy, most women will prefer to keep their head below heart movements (including advanced inversions) to shorter holds by the second half of their pregnancy, and I encourage them to follow that instinct.

So, can a woman invert when pregnant? Well, did they know how to invert before becoming pregnant? Are they clear of things like high blood pressure, eye problems, or other usual inversion contraindications? Can they place themselves against a wall so there is no risk of losing the center and suddenly flipping over backwards? And has the baby been head down for at least a week after 32 weeks? (Head down is the preferred position for birthing, and most babies will assume a head down position between 30 and 40 weeks of pregnancy.) Then yes, brief inversions are possible. Again, there is a lot going on inside the body: this is not the best time to attempt a 10 minute headstand.

Practice inversions for maybe three breaths or up to one minute at a time.

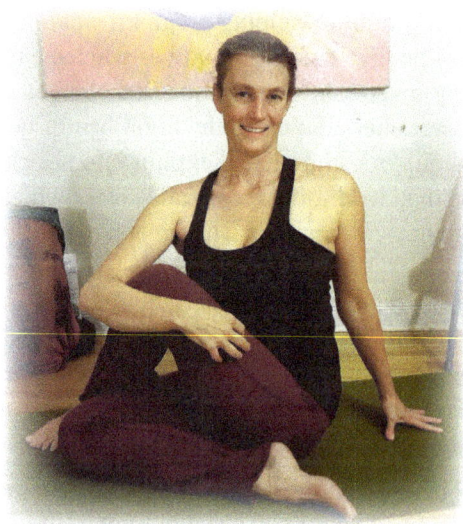

Myth: No twisting
Verdict: False!

Yes, there are certain twisting postures you'd want to avoid as a pregnant person. But as with inversions, we've gotten too restrictive when common sense more readily indicates appropriate limits.

Twisting postures are often said to have two main benefits. The first is mobilization and stretching of the spinal joints and muscles, which is fairly useful to relieve something like back pain. The other benefit is a supposed "squeeze-and-soak" effect on tissues, muscles, and organs that occurs by momentarily restricting blood flow to the twisted area and then allowing blood to return back in after the pose is done. This is especially true of closed twist postures, which press towards the midline of the body and might compress the thigh against the abdomen. Like the water behind a dam being released at greater pressure, the thought is that twisting will help flood the area with new blood, refreshing the muscles, fascia, and organs therein. Setting aside whether you believe in the squeeze-and-soak effect (because I'm not sure it has actually been proven yet), it's safe to say that if it is true, then we should be very cautious about not creating a squeeze-and-soak effect on an area where someone else is relying on that blood supply to develop and thrive. In simple terms: don't wring out the uterus, the placenta, or the baby!

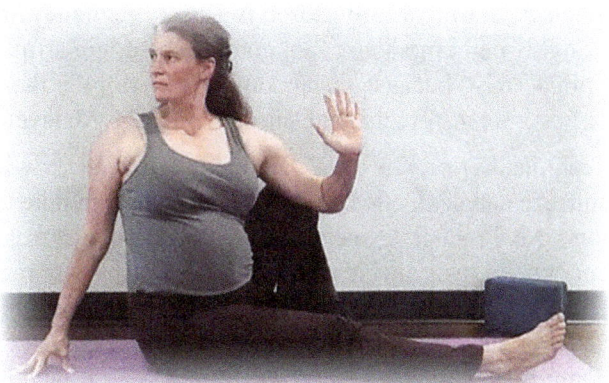

But what about open twists? This is where I think we have gotten a bit too restrictive. Open twists don't create the squeeze-and-soak effect because there isn't anything pressing against anything else. There are those who would say that any twist that reaches across the midline of the body constitutes a closed twist, but again, I think this is too simplistic an answer. If one body part squeezes against another with force, then the position is considered a closed twist. But simply reaching an arm across the midline to hold a knee doesn't rise to that level.

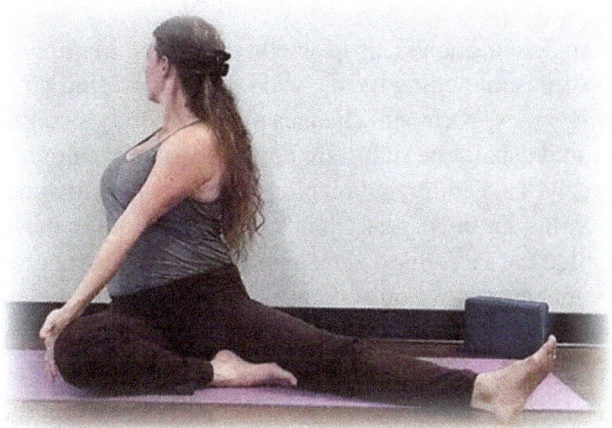

We also have to consider what stage of pregnancy we are talking about

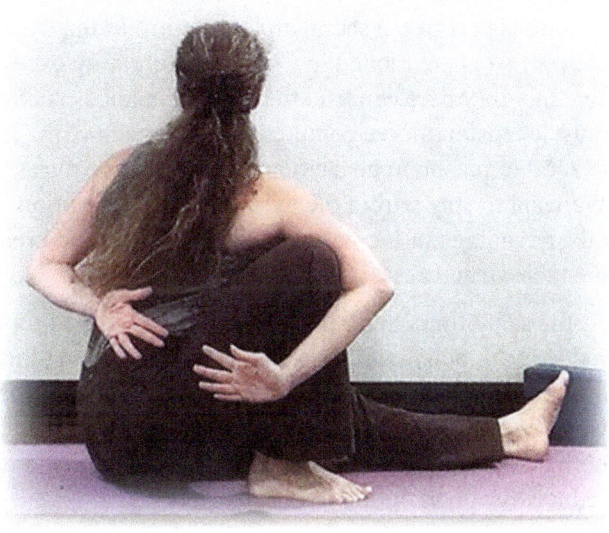

when evaluating a fully closed twist for pregnancy.Someone who is 36 weeks pregnant (roughly eight months) is not going to be doing a full Ardha Matsyendrasana (Half Seated Spinal Twist) because the abdomen is literally in the way. But what about someone who is only six weeks pregnant? Can she do Ardha Matsyendrasana?

Technically, yes, since she's probably not even showing yet, but here is where considering the squeeze and soak effect comes in. Yes, she can take the shape, but she shouldn't "activate" the pose. Practically speaking, this means that she can happily move into the twist until she encounters resistance from her body. But at the point where she needs to force or press in an effort to go deeper, she should stop. The uterus requires steady blood flow during this time, and while gentle twisting within the normal range of motion should be fine, the extreme compression and movement sometimes encouraged in yoga practice is not something to strive for at this time. Take the shape, but don't activate it and compress the belly. And once the abdomen is in the way, twist open.

Range of motion is also something to keep in mind as we move through several families of postures, including twists, wide legged standing postures, and hip openers. Even in early pregnancy, hormonal changes make the body's connective tissue more flexible. Joints that would usually be stable are now able to move more freely. This additional mobility can be especially concerning for those pesky joints in the back of the pelvis called the sacroiliac (SI) joints. These joints are normally meant to move only slightly, but with the increased mobility of pregnancy, they are at risk for hypermobility.

This is especially true in a position such as Ardha Matsyendrasana, where the hip bones are fixed on the ground but the spine is being actively pulled around. The SI joint bears the load of the spinal twist. Given that the SI joint is part of the sacral arch structure in the back of the pelvis (as mentioned in Chapter 1), creating excessive mobility here can lead to other imbalances such as muscle tension, nerve compression, and back pain. This is another reason to be cautious in twisting postures. We want to stay within the existing range of motion, not take advantage of increased flexibility that could create unstable structures.

At the same time, these postures can be modified to reduce both belly compression and sacral torque to make them safer. Staying with the previous example, why not lean the spine lightly away from the leg and keep the twist above the waist so that the pose focuses on twisting the shoulders rather than binding into the hip? The belly maintains space for the baby to rest happily, and the force on the sacrum is dramatically reduced. A good option for all involved!

Myth: No lying on your back; no lying on your right side; always roll to the left
Verdict: False...sort of

In every myth there is a kernel of truth, which is why the myth is perpetuated. This is the case with this whole "no lying on your back" recommendation.

The root of this myth comes from a concern about compression of the inferior vena cava. The inferior vena cava is a large vein running slightly to the right side of the spine in the back of the pelvis. It is the major vein that returns blood from the lower body back to the heart and lungs, and it is vital to maintaining the body's circulation and regulating blood pressure.

Consider the effect of a heavy baby and uterus compressing this vein from above, as is the case if mom is lying fully flat on her back. Since veins do not have the ability to contract as arteries do, compressing one is effectively like stepping on a garden hose while the water is running. The flow at the end of the hose is dramatically reduced, and the water pressure inside the hose increases. Apply enough compression to the vein, and the blood return to mom (and thus to baby) would be constricted. The result is a sudden drop in blood pressure as the body tries to compensate for the increasing fluid buildup below the pinch point. This condition is called supine hypotension or reclining low blood pressure. If mom were to experience this, it might feel like the sensation just before one begins to feel faint: a slight nausea, tunnel vision, dizziness, or shortness of breath. Sometimes the symptoms don't fully appear until mom moves out of the position causing the compression.

So first off, we need to remember that during a yoga class, students are awake and aware. If they know what to look for, they will actually know when they should stop this practice. For most of us, if we began to feel dizzy or lightheaded, we would naturally sit down so we didn't faint. Now imagine you became dizzy or woozy and felt you should lie down, but you were already doing so. This is what mom might feel if she lies on her back for too long. And if she does, then it is the body telling her to move.

In this case, when there are signs of dropping blood pressure, mom should be rolling to the left side. Remember where that vein was sitting? Given its position slightly to the right of the spine, if the vein is in fact being compressed, then rolling to the left would remove the pressure more completely than rolling to the right. This is the science behind the yoga recommendation to roll to the left, and it's also why women are often told to sleep on their left side throughout pregnancy. While there are also arguments that the female energy is more on the left side of the body (the Ida Nadi, or left nostril energy channel, is said to be the feminine side of the nervous system), they don't feel strong enough to start insisting that women roll only to the left. By that logic, women should always be rolling left because of our feminine nature, and this obviously isn't how things are suggested in general yoga practice.

We should also consider these recommendations *vis-a-vis* the stages of pregnancy. During the first trimester, the baby and uterus aren't really big enough to compress the blood vessels in the pelvis. Later on, it can very much depend on where the baby is sitting in the uterus and the specifics of how mom's body is aligned. In general, care providers recommend not lying on the back after 20 weeks, but I have also heard some women being told not to lie on their back as early as 12 weeks, so there is some variation. Also remember that for many of her prenatal check-ups, mom will be lying flat so the care provider can evaluate the size of her belly, listen to the baby, and perform other assessments.

So, if a pregnant person can lie on their back at the doctor, then why not in yoga? Here's the real question: How *long* is the pregnant person on their back? If the duration is a brief moment before going on to another posture, then it's no big deal. But if the position will be held for more than five minutes or so, then at the very least teachers should let students know what to watch for so they can assess whether they need to roll to the side. If mom experiences dizziness, nausea, shortness of breath, wooziness, feeling overly anxious, or just has a sense that something doesn't feel right, she should roll to her left side. But if she still feels comfortable, then it's generally fine for her to be on her back for a short span of time.

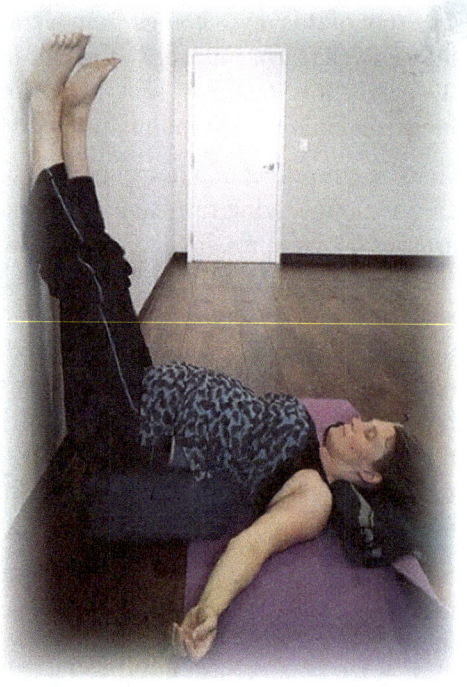

You may have heard about studies that demonstrated an increased risk of stillbirth from lying supine or on the right side. While there were some studies which showed a slight increase when lying on the right or supine,[41][42] further studies showed this risk didn't apply before 30 weeks of pregnancy, and the studies didn't evaluate past then.[43] And we are talking about sleeping through the night here, not practicing a yoga posture for two minutes. The latest conclusions are that after 30 weeks, sleeping supine is not recommended. Prior to that, there does not seem to be an impact on the pregnancy.

This information does not indicate that we need to remove a whole family of postures from our practice. We have to remember these statistics are from women who are sleeping for

[41] Heazell, A., Li, M., Budd, J., Thompson , J., Stacey, T., Cronin, R. S., Martin, B., Roberts, D., Mitchell, E. A., & McCowan, L. (2017, November 20). *Association between maternal sleep practices and late stillbirth - findings from a stillbirth case-control study.* BJOG : an international journal of obstetrics and gynaecology. https://pubmed. ncbi.nlm.nih.gov/29152887/

[42] Stacey, T., Thompson, J. M. D., Mitchell, E. A., Ekeroma, A. J., Zuccollo, J. M., & McCowan, L. M. E. (2011, June 14). *Association between maternal sleep practices and risk of late stillbirth: A case-control study.* The BMJ. https://www.bmj.com/content/342/bmj.d3403

[43] Silver, R. M., Hunter, S., Reddy, U. M., Facco, F., Gibbins, K. J., Grobman, W. A., Mercer, B. M., Haas, D. M., Simhan, H. N., Parry, S., Wapner, R. J., Louis, J., Chung, J. M., Pien, G., Schubert, F. P., Saade, G. R., Zee, P., Redline, S., & Parker, C. B. (2019, October). *Prospective evaluation of maternal sleep position through 30 weeks of gestation and adverse pregnancy outcomes.* Obstetrics and gynecology. https://pubmed.ncbi.nlm.nih. gov/31503146/

hours at a time, not just lying for five minutes a couple of times during a yoga class. There are some postures that can be very beneficial in pregnancy which actually *need* to be done on the back. The point at which vena cava compression would matter is if the baby was being monitored and went into distress. Regarding the lying on the left vs lying on the right, there are small variations in blood flow when lying on the right vs lying on the left, but they are not enough to be a factor in a yoga practice.

In yogic tradition, there are different energetic qualities to the right and left side of the body. The right is more heating, the left more cooling; the right is more masculine, the left more feminine (whatever is actually meant by that). While it's nice to think that we can promote different states of being by turning to one side or the other, I think a far greater impact could be made by simply tuning in to which side of the body is active and following that inner guidance. Which side of the nose is more active? What about rolling to that side to both calm the more active side of the nervous system and to stimulate the quieter side—not to mention maybe opening a blocked sinus passage? It's easy to wax poetic about the energetic qualities of womanhood and pregnancy, but at the end of the day, the best thing we can do is to give the power back to mom (back to any woman for that matter) and allow her to make her own well-informed choices.

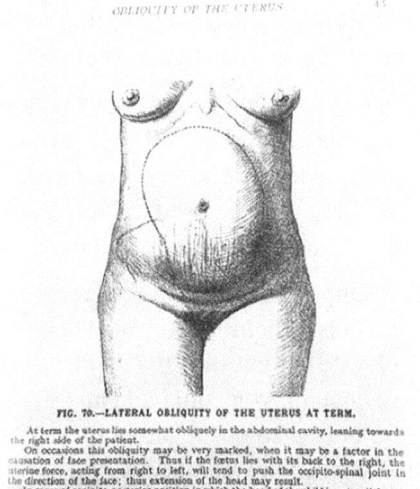

FIG. 70.—LATERAL OBLIQUITY OF THE UTERUS AT TERM.

At term the uterus lies somewhat obliquely in the abdominal cavity, leaning towards the right side of the patient.
On occasions this obliquity may be very marked, when it may be a factor in the causation of face presentation. Thus if the fœtus lies with its back to the right, the uterine force, acting from right to left, will tend to push the occipito-spinal joint in the direction of the face; thus extension of the head may result.
In cases of occipito-posterior position in which the head of the child is not well flexed, by increasing the lateral obliquity of the uterus flexion of the head will be encouraged. Thus, if the position of the head is a 3rd vertex, the patient should be placed on her left side, and if a 4th vertex on her right side.

Illustration: Pictorial Midwifery 1948, Berkeley

That said, there is another reason that a pregnant woman might choose to lie on the left side over the right. The uterus is more curved to the left, and if a baby settles their spine onto the left side of their mother's body, then the spine is generally more able to curve, creating greater ease in flexing the head. A baby with a flexed head (chin towards its chest) will more easily engage into mom's pelvis because the flexed head presents a smaller circle (up to an entire centimeter) than a head positioned chin up. A baby can certainly flex its head when on the right side of mom's spine, but it is slightly more challenging because their spine is in a straighter position. Try sitting up straight and dropping your chin to your chest. Now try slouching and repeat. Much easier from the slouch, isn't it? Given that baby will follow gravity, during the third trimester it's a good idea to lie on the left as much as possible to encourage the baby to curl their spine into the rounded side of the uterus, thus promoting a flexed head position. A baby doesn't position by gravity alone, but maternal position is one of the influencing factors, and an area in which mom can be proactive.

All that being said, sometimes moms are sick of lying on their left or genuinely feel more comfortable lying on their right that day. In this case, let the mom decide! If she has found a place of comfort and rest, don't shift her just because she's not in the "correct" position. May-

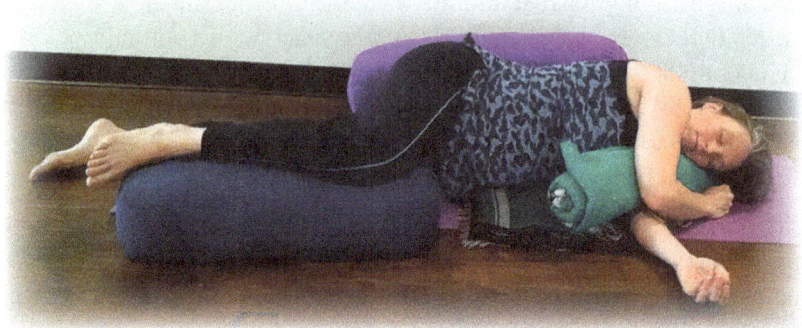

be she knows something we don't. Maybe she knows something she doesn't even realize. The bottom line is, if a student is comfortable on their back or on their side, LET THEM BE!!!

What about yoginis who aren't comfortable on their backs? Are you simply stuck lying on the (preferably left) side? What if you wanted to practice a back-lying sequence for the hamstrings? There are several options for people who don't feel comfortable lying flat on their back. Props can be used to increase the angle of the body so that the pressure of the uterus and baby shifts from direct compression into the back of the pelvis towards the pelvic floor.

The simplest adjustment is placing a bolster behind mom's back to elevate her chest. If that isn't high enough, you could add another bolster to create an incline or place two blocks like a step unit with a bolster leaning up against them. The bolster should primarily rest against the first block, which should wind up

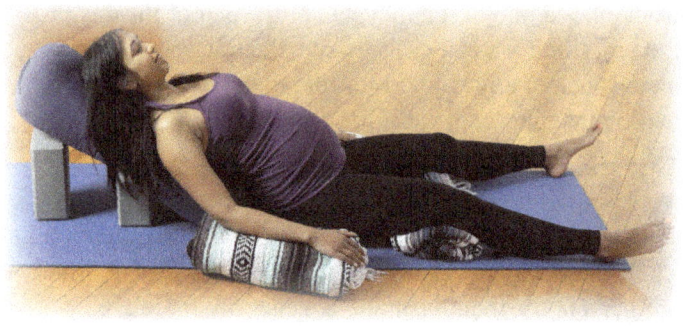

directly under mom's chest. The second block is more for supporting the head and preventing an overly soft bolster from collapsing, putting mom into a backbend.

This configuration brings mom's spine to roughly a 45 degree angle, high enough to relieve most vena cava compression. However, this position does also place pressure on the tailbone and lower sacrum, impacting the SI and pelvic joints. Because of this additional joint pressure, this position could be used for a hamstring sequence or to approximate something like Viparita Karani, but it might be preferable for mom to take long postures such as Shavasana on her side after the 34th week.

Myth: No lying on the belly
Verdict: True...but only after a certain point

While we are on the subject of lying down, let's discuss lying on the belly. Obviously, someone who is 38 weeks pregnant (technically full term) is not going to be comfortable lying on their abdomen because there will be someone underneath them, and we don't want to lie on top of our babies. This part should be self-evident. But at what point in the pregnancy are we talking about mom not being able to do prone postures? There are people who say one shouldn't be on the belly as early as six weeks because it puts pressure on the abdominal organs. Keep in mind that many women may not even know they are pregnant by this time. How is one going to avoid something they don't even know is an issue?

The answer is that, with a few caveats, you don't really have to worry about this until you can feel something while lying on your abdomen. For most students the shift occurs somewhere between 10-14 weeks of pregnancy, when the uterus becomes big enough that you can sense something inside your abdomen when lying on your stomach. The basic rule of thumb is: if you can feel something, don't lie on top of it; if you can't feel anything, then you're clear to keep practicing.

The caveat I will add is around postures where something is pressing into the abdomen or where there would be strong pressure on the internal organs: postures such as lying with a belly bolster, where a student would lie over a folded blanket and allow it to sink into the soft section of their abdomen, or strong prone backbends such as a deep Bow posture (Dhanurasana). Given the direct pressure on organs in a belly bolster posture, and the fact that this practice has a squeeze-and-soak effect for the internal organs, this pose should be avoided at all times during pregnancy—and even during the months before if someone is actively trying to conceive and isn't sure if they might be in the early stages of pregnancy. How would you modify prone back-bends that put strong pressure on the abdomen? As with twists, do them more gently, and maybe start considering why there is such a strong attachment to doing that specific practice right now?

Myth: No abdominals/core work
Verdict: False...sort of

To crunch or not to crunch? That is the question. Actually it's not; the answer is always NOT to crunch. But this question of whether mom can engage her core, and how much, comes up over and over again in conversations around yoga and pregnancy. There are two primary concerns around doing abdominal work while pregnant: strain along the central connective tissue of the rectus abdominis muscle and pressure being exerted on the internal abdominal organs and the uterus.

As discussed in Chapter 2, the rectus abdominis is the "six pack" of the abdominals, and it is actually two vertical bands of muscles running from the lower ribs to the front of the pelvis, connected in the middle by a fascia sheath called the linea alba (literally "white line"). As the belly grows and hormones soften the connective tissue in the body, this central line begins to widen so that the top layer of abdominal muscles can stretch around the baby. But if there is too much force applied to this area, or if the muscles bulge outward due to a lack of deeper core support, the linea alba can actually separate (this separation is called diastasis recti), leading to a compromised abdominal wall following the pregnancy.

Since there are no sensory nerves in the linea alba, you will not feel the separation happening unless you are paying close attention to the sensations around the abdomen. And once separated, there is little we can do to bring the rectus abdominis muscles back together (little, but not nothing) until after the baby is out. Even then, depending on the degree of separation, surgery can be required to repair and rethread the two halves of the outer abdominals together. For this reason, abdominal work which demands intense control of the abdominal complex, such as Navasana or yoga Bicycle, should be avoided during pregnancy.

Next, we must consider how much pressure is being exerted on the internal abdominal organs and the uterus. While the rectus abdominis runs vertically, the deepest layer of the abdominals, the transverse abdominis (TA), runs horizontally in the body and draws the abdominal wall inward to support the internal organs and the spine. This is the muscle that would ultimately need to engage to support the halves of the rectus abdominis staying together as the belly grows with pregnancy. So it seems like a good idea to work the TA to maintain an intact rectus abdominis, right? Well, sort of. The thing is that if the TA is overly taxed or compresses too strongly, it can adversely affect the space available for the growing uterus, restricting the baby's movements. Simply put, this isn't a time in life to try and maintain a flat stomach.

So what's the solution? Tone, not tension. We need the TA to be toned so it can help with back support but not have it so tight that it restricts intrauterine growth. We need to find a balance of strength and softness. So strong abdominal work like Plank, Bicycle, Crow and other arm balances should only be done with extreme caution and really only by advanced practitioners who can gauge how much they are working their core. Also, during the first trimester, it seems prudent (though as yet there is no science to support this) to avoid Plank. The amount of expansion and change happening in the uterus during the first 12 weeks seems like something which would not be helped by a strong upward pressure against the uterus, such as that produced by Plank pose. Following the first trimester, however, gentle engagement of the TA is recommended. As the belly grows, it is quite possible that this engagement would need to be modified by bringing the knees to the floor in Plank, since what is Table if not Plank with its knees on the floor?

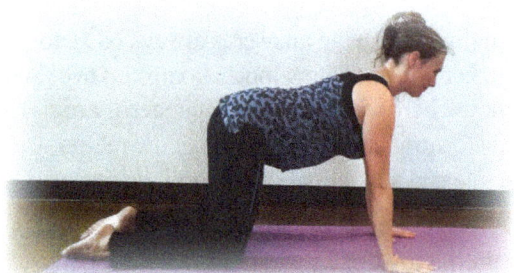
Yes

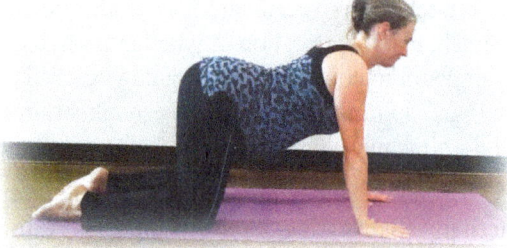
NO! Note the lack of belly support!

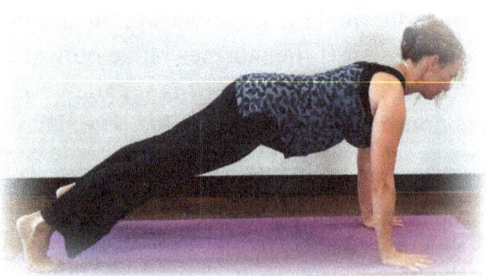

But generally speaking, provided the engagement is moderate and not designed to seek a flat stomach, engaging the abdominals during pregnancy is not only safe but might actually help prevent diastasis recti.

Myth: No *pranayama*, breath retention, or "heating" breathwork
Verdict: True...sort of

The breath is our physical expression of the nervous system. As such, when you change it, you have the potential to access deep places in your neurological wiring. It is for this reason that *pranayama* is usually recommended to only be studied with a qualified and senior teacher. That said, I have found some wildly inaccurate statements about what sort of breathwork pregnant women should or should not be doing. I also find the statement that NO *pranayama* should ever be done slightly comical, given that nearly *every* natural childbirth program involves some sort of breath work or breath awareness. Lamaze, Bradley Method®, HypnoBirthing®, and Mindfulness-Based Childbirth all teach variations on several forms of yoga breathing. So what are we actually talking about when we say that pregnant women should not be doing *pranayama*, especially if this is a time when women want to calm and steady the nervous system as much as possible?

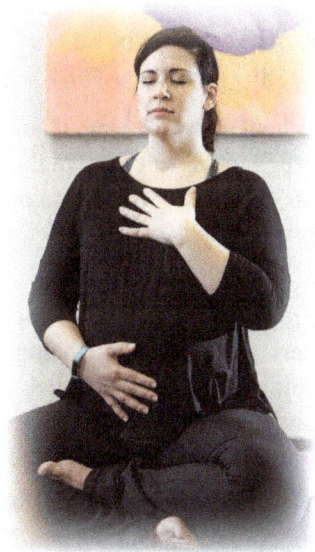

There are two types of *pranayama* to avoid: those which might change the oxygenation level in the blood and those which would require a lot of contraction and movement in an already expanding TA muscle. This means we are talking about *pranayama* like Kapalabhati (skull shining breath), which involves pumping the abdomen vigorously towards the spine while sharply exhaling. Not only is this action too strong and sudden for an expanding TA but if practiced for an extended period it can lead to mild hyperventilation, which is not good when someone else is relying on mom's oxygen (Hi, baby!).

The same goes for Bhastrika, the fast paced breath performed while pumping the arms overhead—and for the same reasons. Other variations include fire breathing and holotropic breathwork. None of these should be practiced extensively while pregnant because of the baby's reliance on mom's blood for oxygen. Likewise, *pranayamas* which involve breath retention, or *kumbhakas*, are not advised for the opposite reason. With the baby relying on mom's blood oxygen levels for their own oxygenation, let's not go cutting off that airflow. The brief pauses between breaths are one thing, but extended *kumbhaka* holds, especially those also involving active *bandhas* (particularly Uddiyana Bandha, which requires the abdomen to be forcefully pulled in) should not be practiced during pregnancy.

But most of the gentle, focusing *pranayamas* are actually useful and even beneficial during pregnancy. Ujjayi *pranayama* in particular is effectively the same breath taught in natural childbirth classes to help moms ride through the intensity of contractions. Other *pranayamas* such as Nadi Shodhanam (Alternate Nostril Breathing) practiced without breath retention would be fine, as would Sitali (Cooling Breath). A basic rule of thumb is that if the breath requires a marked increase or decrease in breathing rate or depth, then it is probably out, but something in the middle focused more on balancing the nervous system should be fine and might even be recommended. See Chapter 8 for instructions on types of breath work that are helpful and safe during pregnancy.

Myth: No backbends
Verdict: False…sort of

Wheel, Upward Dog, Cobra, Camel—these postures often get lumped into the "not during pregnancy" category in the yoga world, but once again I think such generalizations go too far. While some of these postures do call for caution, the general rule of no backbends during pregnancy is overly restrictive and disempowering for those students capable of wider ranges of motion.

Pregnancy puts a lot of additional weight on the front side of the body, leading to the shoulders and upper spine being dragged forward. Not only that, but the increased curvatures in the spine also lead to spinal and hip flexors becoming shortened and possibly tight. Backbends are a wonderful way to relieve some of this pressure and to restore movement and space to the lumbar spine, which can become compressed by tight hip flexors and psoas muscles.

While backbends themselves could be of great benefit, the concern is the stress they place on the linea alba and the abdominal wall. The expanding abdomen is already widening the linea alba, so the thought is that additionally stretching it by arching the spine backwards could contribute to diastasis recti. As a result, I suggest approaching backbends with some caution, keeping in mind whether the weight is falling towards or away from the linea alba. In other words, does the linea alba face up or down, and how deeply is the spine bending? Likewise, is mom able to engage the transverse abdominals well enough to support the spinal extension required without placing the central abdominal fascia in jeopardy?

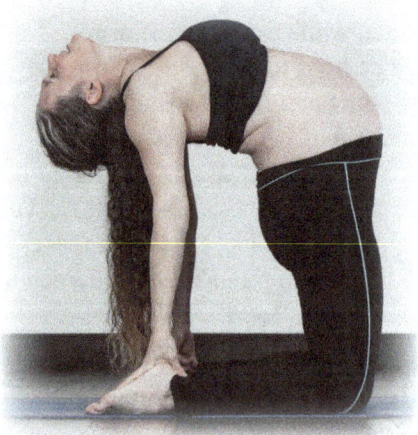 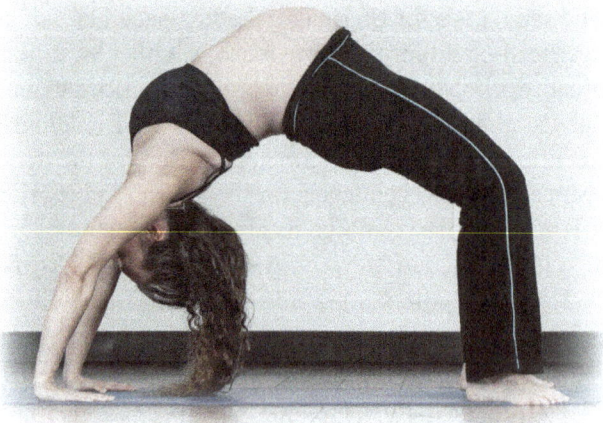

Similar to the rule about inversions, a determination about practicing backbends isn't just about the position of the body but also about how long a student has been practicing. We don't usually teach Urdhva Dhanurasana (Wheel) in a beginner class, and the same might be true for Upward Dog or Ustrasana, depending on your tradition. So the problem with these deep backbends isn't the pregnancy so much as the ability of the yogini and the frequency with which these postures are being practiced. I lump deep backbends into the caution pose family. They are postures which, if done with good warm-up, care, experience, and awareness, could be quite helpful; if they are simply performed for the sake of an amazing Instagram photo, they might not be such a good idea

Note: if the placenta is on the front side of the body (known as an anterior placenta), extremely deep backbends should probably be avoided. The placenta interweaves its fibers into the inner wall of the uterus, and pulling dramatically on the front body also pulls on the uterine wall and placenta. This has the potential to cause part of the placenta to come away from the wall it was attached to (a rather dangerous condition known as partial placental abruption). For this reason, avoid postures that dramatically stretch the front side of the body if you have an anterior placenta.

However, we are talking about postures that are beyond the range of motion of Wheel or Camel—something like the full expression of Kapotasana, where the spine bends backwards to practically bring the head to touch the feet. This backbend is too much if the placenta is in the front because movements this deep will inevitably pull on the uterus and thus the structures contained inside. So once again, we find ourselves in that middle ground. Gentle backbends are fine, mid-range may be fine if your body is accustomed to that type of movement, and super deep ranges of motion should probably be avoided.

Myth: No Forward bends
Verdict: False...with a couple of exceptions

Are you starting to see the issue with many of these "rules" in yoga for pregnancy? What about forward bends? Well, if we are talking about the classic seated forward bend of Paschimottanasana being executed at 35 weeks pregnant, the challenge quickly becomes apparent. The pregnant belly is going to be pushed against the thighs, and mom will not be able to lean forward more than a few inches, if that. In that case, the pose more closely resembles Dandasana than Paschimottanasana (which, in my opinion, is a perfectly fine pose to take during pregnancy or any other time).

But to achieve a true forward fold, this posture requires some modification. In this case, it would mean taking the legs slightly wider apart, leading to something closer to a narrow Upavista Konasana (Straddle Split). This would still be a fully valid stretch for the hamstrings, if a bit more focused on the inner thigh than the outer hamstring line.

The same modification could be done with standing forward bends such as Uttanasana. As the belly grows, a yogini needs to widen her feet, both to create a more stable base and to accommodate a growing belly. If the belly gets to a place where the legs simply cannot be moved out of the way, decrease the angle of forward motion, either by placing blocks under the hands or by resting the elbows on the thighs rather than hanging over from the hips (or simply accept that the posture isn't as deep during pregnancy).

The kernel of truth hidden in this myth relates to deep forward folds such as Kurmasana (Tortoise) or Titibhasana 1 (Bound Firefly). These postures require enough flexibility in the hips, hamstrings, and lower back to allow the ribs and torso to come fully between the knees, so the arms can then be bound beneath or behind the knees. Few yogis actually have this range of motion to begin with, and during pregnancy, the body's joints and connective tissue are softened in preparation for labor. This

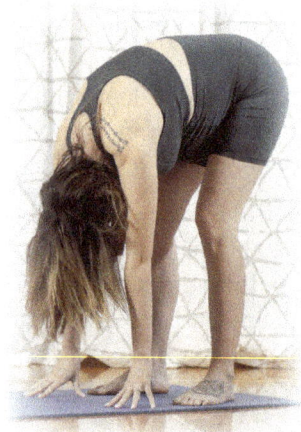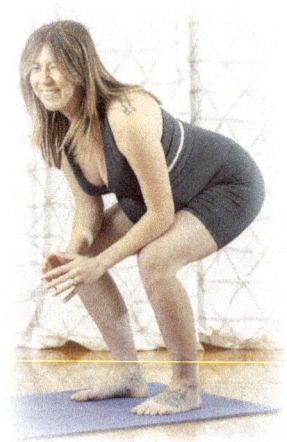

softening starts from the moment of conception, so any pose demanding an extreme range of motion will pull on the joints—unless the range of motion to perform that movement existed before the pregnancy began.

The body is extremely smart when practicing *asana*, and also very sneaky. If we have restrictions in one area, the body first looks for a way to borrow the requested movement from somewhere else, usually immediately above or below the stuck spot. This means that even someone practicing while not pregnant will try to borrow movement from their lower back if their hips are bound with tight muscles. Hip extensions usually borrow from the lower back if the hip flexors are too tight. Upper body backbends borrow from either the lower back or the neck if the thoracic spine won't budge. Hip openers are often rough on the knees since that is the next joint down the chain. Alternatively, students slump into the pelvis, trying to borrow the movement from the lower back.

Consider this last movement, where the pelvis is in a posterior tilt (tucked) while a pregnant woman performs a forward bend. Given the additional flexibility in the pelvic joints, her body might "borrow" more movement from the SI joints to achieve greater depth in the forward bend. Taking a very deep forward fold without the hamstring and hip flexibility to allow for it strains the SI joints. If done repeatedly or aggressively, this stress has the potential to pull the top of the sacrum forward into the pelvis instead of moving the bowl as one unit. Strain the SI joints and you begin to compromise the integrity of the pelvic bowl and the body's infrastructure—not to mention that you close the top opening of the pelvis where the baby's head will need to engage to be ready for birth.

For both these reasons, and because the average yogini doesn't have the range of motion to perform such deep forward bends, stay away from advanced folds unless you know you already

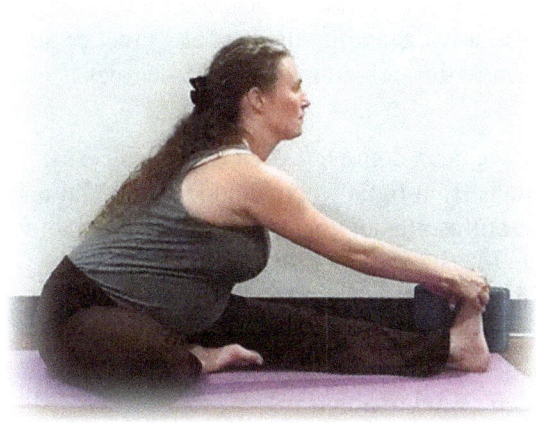

have both the range and the body awareness to perform them safely (and there aren't many of those out there.) If we are talking about something like Uttanasana or a seated forward bend, it's fine to reach forward and stretch your hamstrings. In fact, when practiced with a focus on finding the movement at the hip (instead of the spine) forward bends can actually be helpful in freeing the sacro-tuberous ligaments at the back of the pelvis. This restores the natural mobility to the sacrum, making more space available during the birth process as the baby navigates down.

Yes, stretch your calves and hamstrings. No, don't try to drag the belly through the thighs.

Myth: No hot yoga?
Verdict: True!!!

Ding ding ding ding!!! Sorry, all you hot yoga enthusiasts, but this myth is actually accurate! And yes, it even applies in the first trimester. Here's why: The proteins governing the baby's gestation were intended to work best at body temperature: 98.6 degrees. Pregnant women are told to avoid saunas and hot tubs during the first trimester due to demonstrated risks of neural tube defects and possible miscarriage from the increased heat.[44] If medical advice says that pregnant women shouldn't be in saunas or hot tubs, then being in an artificially heated room, practicing physically demanding postures, should also be reconsidered. The baby can't sweat, so they are taking their body temp from mom's internal temperature. While one hot class *probably* won't adversely affect your pregnancy, we simply don't know what effect consistently elevating the internal temperature a tenth of a degree might have. And it's difficult to find out because it's unethical to do research on pregnant women, especially when we know there is a demonstrated negative outcome that could result.

Some babies might be fine with hot yoga. But the brain is a highly complicated organ, and its development is relational to the environment it is in. The growing field of epigenetics has revealed that environmental factors can play a role in activating or quieting certain genes during development. There is enough uncertainty about how each individual baby is developing that the risk doesn't seem worth it. What if we discover in 30 years that neurodivergent development has something to do with a slightly elevated internal core temp at a specific time in pregnancy? (Note: I AM NOT saying it does, but the fact that we don't know what we don't know seems noteworthy here).

We simply don't have definitive answers, and this is one place where we could exercise

---

[44] Milunsky, A., Ulcickas, M., Rothman, K. J., Willett, W., Jick, S. S., & Jick, H. (1992, August 19). *Maternal heat exposure and neural tube defects.* JAMA. https://www.ncbi.nlm.nih.gov/pubmed/1640616

caution and practice *vairagya* (non-attachment). For the sake of a soon-to-be-born child, I encourage pregnant women to let go of any ego about withstanding the heat of a practice and shift to a room that is at least below body temperature throughout the class. 85 degrees is one thing; 105 is quite another.

Yes, this recommendation still holds true if you have been doing hot yoga for a while. Yes, even if it's a hot day outside. Yes, even if someone is from India where outdoor temperatures climb to 110 in the shade. Women in those temperatures are not voluntarily performing active and strenuous *asana*. They are generally sitting in the shade, hopefully sipping some ice water to stay cool. I have heard all kinds of justifications for not giving up this practice, and they all miss the point. Stepping out of the room to take your temperature and see if you are overheating is not exercising restraint. If you are debating whether you should be in the room, you probably already know the answer and just don't want to admit it.

My rule of thumb: no practice in a room that regularly reaches over 85 degrees.

So you can just practice? A note of caution

Now that we've unpacked these myths about practicing yoga while pregnant, it might be easy to conclude that someone who was an avid yoga practitioner before becoming pregnant could simply continue her pre-pregnancy practice with only mild modifications. In fact, I have seen plenty of pregnant students continue with their non-prenatal yoga classes well into their pregnancies. I have even seen students avidly continue practicing deep, advanced yoga postures well into the third trimester. But here's the thing: while the body is not fragile or broken during pregnancy, it is changing. Trying to maintain the same practice one had before they started growing another human ignores this shift. It also runs the risk of creating complications due to the hormonal and weight balance changes inherent to pregnancy.

While most of the yoga practice *can* be done during pregnancy, it *should* not be done by everyone. The postures that are appropriate for a given yogini are very personal. Deciding what to practice requires not only an understanding of how the body is changing throughout the pregnancy but also a recognition of the patterns of muscle and fascial tension or laxity that might have existed before the pregnancy began. Many long-time yoga students become so attached to what they know as "their practice" that they cling to certain postures, even if their bodies indicate that practicing these poses is promoting instability rather than balance (for example, continuing to take a deep asymmetrical posture like Pigeon while dealing with pregnancy-induced sciatica). I have pulled a great number of very flexible yoginis back from deep postures because they told me their hips and back were aching during class check-in .

Our egos are far too attached to showy backbends and inversions. Maybe we think it genuinely feels good, and in fact it may. But if the consequence is pelvic or back pain, the practice needs to be re-evaluated. Yet the internet is filled with pictures of women late into pregnancy performing flashy postures that require a deep range of motion (Just look at the pictures of this author earlier in this chapter!). The honest truth is that I only practiced Wheel five times during my entire pregnancy, and once was for the picture so I could have a great Facebook post. Could I have done it more? Maybe. But my own circumstances (sacral instability from years of ballet; overly tight hip flexors from triathlons) meant that I wanted to exercise caution.

The moral of the story...

The yoga practice has a wide variety of movement options, the pregnant body is often very capable of performing them, and the baby (for the most part) is going to be fine with them. But very few of us are able to tell whether we are moving our bodies too far until it is too late. No, we don't hurt our babies during pregnancy, but our bodies do suffer from the "yogic" focus on range of motion and pushing the edge instead of striving for balance. And this can subsequently affect how labor and birth unfold!

The solution? Recognize that your body both is and isn't the same. Its signals could be different than before. Perhaps the biggest myth around yoga during pregnancy is that we will know exactly what the body is happy or unhappy to do. This would be true if we knew how to hear its calls, but the body sadly doesn't speak in English or even Sanskrit. It speaks in sensation.

I encourage you to let go of what your practice used to be, and move mindfully on a daily basis through the different shapes. Pregnancy is an optimal time to begin tuning into sensation and observing, mindfully and without judgment or ego, how those sensations are changing and guiding you into a deeper connection. This takes a different way of thinking about yoga practice, although I'm sure some of you would argue this is what yoga should be in the first place: a deep inner conversation between our outer and inner selves, between our bodies and our minds, between our bodies and our babies.

I will go over true contraindications in the next chapter, but the bottom line is: go ahead and practice but with awareness. If you already knew how to backbend, do inversions, engage the abdominals and so on, then feel free to continue, as long as you are not striving for a deeper practice and you can be open to the possibility that some days or weeks you may have to let go of certain movements to support your growing pregnancy.

Pranayama should only be free-flowing breath, without any fast or retained breathing. Forward bends simply need to make space for the baby to be there with you, and avoid anything where you might be compressing the little one (twists, prone postures, etc.) since they don't like being squished any more than the rest of us. If lying on your back begins to feel uncomfortable or disturbs your breathing, find a way to take the pressure off your spine, either through lying at an incline or being on one side. Left is slightly preferable, but only slightly. Bring the focus of your practice during pregnancy to finding balance within your body and your mind, not on progressing your postures for the moment. Your body will thank you, your baby will be happy, and you'll probably be back on your mat faster following your baby's birth.

7 — True Prenatal Yoga Contraindications

By now you may have realized that there are few hard and fast contraindications to practicing yoga while pregnant. There are certainly times when we should exercise caution, perhaps working to reduce or relieve our ego around what we thought the posture was supposed to look like or how it used to look or feel. But with a little common sense and some understanding of how the body changes during pregnancy, most pregnant students can discern when a yoga practice is beyond what their body can comfortably manage or adjust for.

Having said that, there are certain yoga postures that should be avoided. These postures have specific negative implications for pregnancy: they can adversely affect the growing baby (without any immediate outward signals); they can adversely affect fetal positioning; and, under certain conditions, they can be dangerous for mom or baby. Some of these proscriptions are self-evident; others are more subtle and thus good to keep in mind.

So, here are the actual things one should not do while pregnant and practicing yoga:

Don't squish the baby!

Obvious, I know! But what does it mean for a yoga practice? It specifically means that the family of prone postures where the belly lies against the floor needs to be removed from regular practice fairly quickly. How quickly? The moment mom is able to feel the expanding uterus while lying on her stomach. The actual gestational age will vary from person to person. Six weeks is probably too early to feel much change. The baby is about the size of a lentil, and the uterus is maybe the size of an apple; both are still well-contained within the protective confines of the pelvic bowl. At 20 weeks, you are definitely showing a bump, so no lying down on top of that bump!

For most students the shift occurs somewhere between 10-14 weeks of pregnancy. In my own case, it was at 13 weeks while I was demonstrating Shalabhasana in a postnatal yoga class. I laid on the floor, raised my legs and upper body, and realized I could feel something the size of a small grapefruit below my navel. That had not been the case two days earlier when I had taught a similar class. Without saying anything, I quietly came out of the posture, got up from the floor, and proceeded to walk around the room, continuing to instruct. (I hadn't yet revealed to anyone that I was pregnant). There were no ill effects from that one-time compression, but from then on I avoided anything that put pressure on my abdomen. I had already been avoiding postures which would have pressed up into the abdomen (such as lying prone over a rolled blanket to relieve lower back stiffness). But with the sensation on the lower abdomen I also began omitting Cobra, Bow, and any other similarly oriented postures.

124

Likewise, I began modifying closed twisting postures. As I mentioned in Chapter 6 on yoga myths, being able to feel the baby is a sign that it's time to stop actively practicing twisting poses, although I had already stopped activating them as soon as I recognized I was pregnant.

Skip the jumping!

Jumping generally comes into play in two places in classic yoga practice. The first is in the Sun Salutation that is commonly used as a base for many Ashtanga and Vinyasa practices. The second is in Iyengar style practices, where students jump the feet wide as they turn to face the side of the mat. Both styles of jumping stress the body in ways that are not optimal during pregnancy.

The Sun Salutation jump usually happens after Uttanasana, with the yogini landing in the low pushup position of Chaturanga. Jumping the feet back in this way creates a sudden force along the abdominal center of the body. It also demands intense control from the transverse abdominals to support the spine and growing uterus. Given the additional stretching that is already occurring on the front side of the body, and given that the connective tissue is more pliable during pregnancy due to relaxin, this forceful movement could overtax the abdominal wall and contribute to abdominal separation (diastasis recti). Additionally, this motion can overstretch the posterior uterine ligaments, changing the position of the uterus within the pelvis. Neither of these conditions are desirable, so this high impact transition should be avoided during pregnancy. Stepping back is just as functional as jumping,

For the Iyengar jumping transition that turns the body to the side of the mat, the problem is not only the strain on the abdominal wall but also the stress on the pelvic floor and pelvic ligaments holding the uterus. These structures need to function well to support the organs and prevent prolapse. They also need to be in good tone to help guide the baby into an optimal position before and during the birth process. Rather than promoting muscle strain and tension by jumping, you could simply step the feet wide without any loss of precision in the yoga practice.

You may have heard that jumping should be skipped because sudden shocks to the body run the risk of dislodging an embryo implanting in the uterine lining and could potentially trigger a miscarriage. Such a shock would have to be fairly intense to actually disrupt a well-established implantation process. There may be a bit of hyperbole in this rationale, and it seems more like yoga myth than actual medical science. That said, I have met many enthusiastic yogis who land their Chaturangas a bit heavily while practicing (one in particular sounded like a Volkswagen had somehow landed in the back of the room). For the sake of your baby, your body, and your own peace of mind, let go of the jumps and step softly through your sequencing.

Stop any practice that disturbs the breathing!

Disturbed breath equals a disturbed mom. The breath is the physical expression of the nervous system. If its rhythm is dramatically interrupted, it signals stress on a deeper level in the body. This is especially true if the disruption was not caused intentionally but resulted from practicing a posture too long or too vigorously. We practice yoga to reduce stress, not increase it, and the stress hormones flooding mom's body have been shown to cross the placenta and affect the baby's nervous system (not to mention their development!). So long as there is another human being relying on the breath, any physical practice that causes mom to breathe in a ragged or shallow manner is worth skipping.

Most significantly, this means removing any *pranayama* practices which might require short, rapid breathing or holding the breath: Kapalabhati, Bhastrika, Breath of Fire, the *kumbhakas*, and breath retention exercises. Fast-paced breathing artificially increases the breath rate and slightly shifts the oxygen level in the bloodstream. Breath retentions obviously reduce the body's oxygenation level. As I mentioned in Chapter 6, it's not that all *pranayama* must be avoided. But any practice which changes the oxygen level going to the baby is out.

The breath can also be disturbed for other reasons. The diaphragm can be temporarily compressed as the growing baby and uterus displace the internal organs, making it difficult to breathe deeply. The maternal heart rate is slightly elevated during pregnancy, which can lead to a lower cardio threshold. A good general guideline is that if you can't carry on a light conversation during practice (or any other physical activity), you're working too hard. If you are gasping for air, it's an indication that the pacing of the class is too rapid. This isn't a time to overstress the body.

Lying on the back if the breath (or mom) becomes disturbed

We discussed in Chapter 6 why restrictions about lying on the back during pregnancy are often too extreme. But the breath is one key way to determine if you can safely remain lying on your back.

Supine hypotension occurs when the uterus compresses the blood vessels in the back of the pelvis. The body responds with a drop in blood pressure to compensate, which can lead to dizziness, shortness of breath, or feeling faint.

This is not a blanket contraindication for every yogini. Some yoginis have supine hypotension right at the 20 week mark, and some will feel fine until well into the third trimester. As with many practices, we must remember to trust in what the body is telling us. Feeling good? Then go ahead and linger in the pose! Short of breath? Then isn't it wonderful that the body can speak to us so clearly and tell you it's time to move?

Also remember that the position of our own body influences how baby positions for labor and birth. During the third trimester, you might want to take postures like Shavasana on the left side so gravity can assist in moving the heavy back of the baby (the spine and back of the head) towards the lower left side of the pelvis. That doesn't mean that back-lying postures are completely forbidden. Rather, there are times when they can be used for relaxation, stability, and function, but they are not the position in which you want to spend the majority of the day.

No hot yoga

Let me reiterate the importance of this contraindication. If pregnant women are told to avoid saunas, hot tubs, and other artificially heated environments, then heated yoga falls under that category as well. I have had students ask whether a room heated to 85 or 90 degrees is allowable—something below body temperature. Keep in mind that the proteins which govern baby's gestation function best at body temperature, and a room initially heated to 90 degrees often becomes much hotter once it is filled with bodies that are actively moving.

Cautions in Malasana (squatting)

We all come to the mat with different aches, pains, and tensions, and each student needs to be considered as their own person and body in their own right. There are truly a multitude of special circumstances that result in contraindicated postures for even non-pregnant bodies; Downward Dog with high blood pressure, for example, or Sirsasana with retinal challenges or a risk of a stroke. But there is one posture which can be contraindicated in specific cases in pregnancy, even though it is useful under many circumstances: our old friend Malasana, the squat.

Malasana can be a wonderful practice to tone the pelvic floor, mobilize the hip joints, and stretch the gluteal muscles. However, it should not be done if mom knows she has, or is showing any signs of, the following:

Placenta previa

Placenta previa is a condition in which the placenta is covering or partially covering the cervix. It can't be seen or felt in a yoga class; mom would have been alerted to this condition by her care provider. If placenta previa is present, Malasana should be avoided because the downward energy (*apana*) of full and even partial squats, combined with the pulling on the lower pelvic fascia in the full position, puts pressure on the organ supporting the baby's life.

Ultimately, there isn't any specific yoga post that will guarantee the placenta moves, but most instances of placenta previa resolve by the beginning of the third trimester. As the uterus grows additional tissue to expand during the pregnancy, new cells develop below the placenta, pushing it up and away from the cervix. Yoginis can try focusing on gentle inversions such as Viparita Karani and gentle breathing to relax the belly, but really this is more to relax the nervous system than to actually move the placenta. If this condition does not resolve, then the baby will require a surgical birth.

Varicose veins

Varicose veins occur when increased blood volume causes vein walls to swell; this condition is most common during the second and third trimesters. A deep squat with fully closed knee and hip joints temporarily constricts the blood return from the legs, placing additional pressure on already weakened blood vessels. If you have varicose veins, you need to practice with support so the back of the knees stay open and the blood flows freely. The same applies for postures such as Janu Sirsasana or Virasana, where the knees are often bent deeply enough to compress the calf muscle into the thigh. Varicose veins can also appear in the groin area during pregnancy. Since the hips are fully flexed when practicing Malasana, this is another reason to avoid full squats. Instead, rest the elbows against the knees in a half squat or "camping squat" variation.

Symphysis pubis dysfunction

Symphysis pubis dysfunction (SPD) is a premature separation of the pubic bones at the front of the pelvis. If SPD is present, mom must fully support her hips on a block during squats. If the condition is severe, she may opt for the camping squat variation or avoid squatting altogether. Symmetrical, supported hip openers, along with strengthening exercises, can help restore pelvic alignment

Baby in breech position

Breech refers to positioning that occurs when the baby's head is still upright rather than turned down into the pelvic bowl. When a baby is in a breech position, avoid strong down-ward energetic postures that would encourage the baby to drop further into the pelvic bones. Once confined in the lower pelvis, there is less room for baby to rotate, making a turn to a vertex (head down) position more challenging. As an alternative to squatting, you might focus on Bridge pose and other inversions to keep the baby floating in the upper uterus where there is more room to turn. Specific variations of inversions can also be used to balance tension in the uterine ligaments, unwinding tension and creating more space for baby to rotate.

Once the baby turns head down, suspend inversions for a few days to give them time to descend towards the lower pelvis, then squat, lunge, and sway away to increase space below the head and encourage further descent. For more information on helping a baby turn from breech to head down (vertex) see SpinningBabies.com.

I should also note that the turn to head down positioning isn't expected until around 28 weeks—when the baby's head becomes significantly heavier than their bum. Prior to this point, a baby isn't technically "breech" but rather hasn't turned yet. Beyond 28 weeks, you want to be proactive in your positioning and avoid postures that would make it harder for baby to turn downward.

In addition to these restrictions, the question of whether or not to practice a certain yoga posture will depend on mom's practice level, her internal sense of what she needs, specifics about her pregnancy, and a recognition of when classic yoga practices might need modification to better support the changing pregnant body. The pregnant yogini is not sick or injured, but her body is changing. If we can remember that things are in a state of flux, we may be able to see more clearly where—and when—adjustments need to be made. By making the practice adaptable to her own unique circumstances, mom arrives on the other side stronger, more balanced, and better prepared to take on the brand new practice of motherhood.

8 — Basic Postures and Essential Movements

"Whatever your reason for practice, yoga is an adventure of self discovery"
—Judith Lasater

Now we come to the yoga *asanas* themselves. This is really where the rubber meets the road—or maybe, we should say, where our feet hit the mat. The movements you make throughout the day impact how the tissues of your body support the changes of pregnancy. Yoga *asana* practice can affect how those tissues continue to function.

Depending on which trimester mom is in, there may be more or fewer adaptations to the classical yoga practice. That said, there are certain conventional yoga alignment and *asana* "rules" which I firmly believe should be removed, or at the very least strongly questioned, during the perinatal period. After all, originally the only people allowed to practice yoga in India were men (specifically teenage boys!). Even after women were permitted to practice, men continued to dominate yoga *asana* thought and instruction for decades. Given that none of these male teachers had ever been pregnant, and given the research in more recent years into connective tissue, fascia, and body structure and balance, it's time to reconsider some of the classic instructions given to female bodies (even in non-prenatal classes!).

Where do we begin? Well, a pelvis born with a uterus was also born with the pathway for the birth process already imprinted within it. The pelvis was already shaped to allow for a baby's passage, and the organs and tissues were built so the body would be able to carry a pregnancy (if the woman so chose). But while we may have begun this way, women often do not enter pregnancy in this same state of harmony and balance. Especially in our modern sedentary culture, our bodies have developed tight spots from whatever movement "diet" we have fed our tissues over the years. As psychologist Bessel Van de Kolk's work so eloquently states, "the body remembers."

Those hours slouching on the couch, that bike accident at 12 years old, those years of ballet training or track and field (or both in my case) leave imprints in the connective tissue that alter how open or closed various parts of the pelvis, and overall body, might be. Through yoga, the challenge and opportunity is to restore the body's original balance and suppleness. Doing so helps a pregnant yogini navigate the changes in the center of gravity, weight, and movement; it also allows the uterus, pelvic floor, and baby to work together harmoniously and maybe facilitate a smoother birth process.

Some basic guidelines for practicing while pregnant

First trimester (0-12 weeks)

During the first trimester there is a great deal of shifting going on inside the body but very little visible from the outside. The result is that you need an increased awareness internally, because while the changes may not be visible, they are nevertheless significant. From the moment of conception, the body shifts its hormonal balance to support and sustain the pregnancy. Both progesterone and estrogen levels increase, along with relaxin. The changes in hormone levels can lead to fatigue or nausea, which often begin around the week six or seven. The progesterone increase slightly elevates the internal body temperature (though most women can't feel it). And relaxin levels peak by the end of the first trimester. This means that mom's joints develop increased mobility and softness long before she needs to modify *asanas* because her belly is getting in the way.

For *asana* practice in the first trimester, the biggest change needed is holding back in postures that inherently call for a deep range of motion—especially asymmetrical ones such as deep lunges and twists. The increase in relaxin affects the body holistically, and key supportive joints such as the internal pelvic joints can easily be overstretched. Practically, this means that a yogini should avoid locking any joints, straining for a pose, and leaning into excessive or sudden increases in range of motion. The body will most likely borrow the movement from a more flexible joint to avoid having to work at the tighter one. These guidelines are generally good in yoga practice anyway—but vital during pregnancy.

Additionally, anything that would create pressure on the growing uterus and abdomen should be reconsidered in the first trimester. Twists which would compress the belly can be done during the first trimester but without "activating" the posture. Don't wring out the baby, especially while the pregnancy is establishing itself. Likewise, jumping in sequences such as the Sun Salutation should be avoided.

Fast *pranayamas* such as Kapalabhati or Bhastrika are also out: too much pumping in the abdominal area, plus someone else is using the oxygen! Gentle *pranayamas* such as Viloma, Ujjayi, or Nadi Shodhanam are fine. These breathing exercises can be of benefit, as the relaxin can also affect how the diaphragm functions, leading to mom feeling slightly winded. And of course, NO HOT YOGA!!! If the baby can't sweat, then we shouldn't be turning up the temperature. Keep the room below body temp, and if you feel nauseous or uncomfortable, leave the room immediately!

Second trimester (12-28 weeks)

Hey! Look, a baby bump! During second trimester, you start to actually see the pregnancy. Both the belly and breasts grow significantly, and the added weight on the front of the body leads to postural shifts in the spine. Blood volume also starts increasing, growing to 150% of the usual amount by full term. This is because mom's body needs to provide fluid and nourishment for the baby as well as herself. The body compensates for the increased volume by dilating blood vessels, which decreases blood pressure. As a result, there can be more dramatic changes when moving from one position to another: those fast swan dives up and down now may make you dizzy.

Second trimester is also when the breasts begin producing colostrum (baby's first food). As the breasts begin to increase in size, they may have a feeling of fullness inside. There is no contraindication to having pressure on the breasts, but it may not be comfortable for some yoginis. Additionally, the uterus can also begin practice contractions during this trimester—even as early as 15 weeks. If mom can sense them, they may feel like gentle tightening or pressure sensations within the abdomen. Uterine contractions may be confused with movements from the baby, which can usually be felt between 18 and 24 weeks, depending on the position of the placenta. During second trimester mom's energy may return as the hormones level off.

For *asana* practice, second trimester is when some of the more obvious pregnancy modifications come into play. Along with everything mentioned for the first trimester, the feet widen in standing postures, both to create a more stable base and to allow for a growing belly. In standing postures such as Warrior poses, the foot placement shifts from a heel to inner heel alignment to a heel to heel alignment, creating more stability and also allowing for less torque on the pelvic joints.

Closed twists and lying on the belly will no longer feel comfortable given the increased size of the uterus. This means usually turning the twist in the opposite direction to create space rather than compression for the belly and baby and using props to create space if continuing prone postures. The ability to practice advanced postures such as deep backbends and inversions will depend on who is doing the practice. If mom was already practicing deep backbends and inversions, she may choose to continue these *asanas* while exercising caution. Evenly distribute backbends along the spine to minimize pressure on any single point of the linea alba, and move inversions to the wall for safety.

Second trimester is also usually when lying fully supine becomes uncomfortable. For those times, incline the body against yoga blocks and bolsters to create a 45 degree angle so as to remove pressure on the blood vessels.

Third trimester (28-40+ weeks)

By this point in pregnancy, the belly is definitely showing, and the uterus will have moved far up into the abdominal cavity. The ribs may begin to expand sideways to make space for the baby and the internal organs, which can lead to heartburn and shortness of breath. Increased fluid can create swelling in the legs and feet, especially if mom is standing or sitting most of the day. Energy reserves may also fade during third trimester. The body is supporting two full lives within one energy field; no wonder mom can't keep going like she used to!

Asana practice should continue with all the modifications made during the first and second trimesters. In addition, take extra care in *asanas* that have a deep range of motion, such as backbends, forward bends, and asymmetrical standing postures. All supine postures are now generally propped up at 45 degrees, and postures such as hip openers and squats are often done with support (promoting symmetry in the body rather than pushing the range of motion). Plank and other postures requiring strong abdominal stabilization may need to be modified if the belly cannot be supported—knees down is a common variation. In general, the modifications during the third trimester are very personalized, as you strive to find a balanced state that will relieve discomfort and support the open channel needed for the birth process. Aches and pains that arise during this trimester can be thought of as invitations from the body to act and restore balance ahead of labor.

Our overall aim with *asana* practice is to release muscles that have tightened during pregnancy and tone those which are being underused. Mom's common postural habits, combined with the postural shifts that occur during pregnancy, usually require releasing muscles such as the psoas and other hip flexors, hamstrings, calves, glutes, and other posterior chain connections. The pelvic floor needs attention, both for tone and for release. Posterior trunk muscles such as the multifidus and paraspinals need stretching, while the abdominals need to both gently stretch and find tone to support the growing uterus. The practice also affects the pelvis, including the support structures of the round and utero-sacral ligaments, the broad ligament, and the tendon of the psoas running into the abdominal diaphragm. There's a lot to look at, but making some specific adjustments can provide global assistance.

Props during pregnancy

Props are an essential component of prenatal yoga, but they do need to be used with awareness. When used, props should promote ease within the poses. But they should teach the student something about the *asana* as well rather than simply serving as a crutch. During pregnancy, props are used frequently. They help create additional space for the belly and baby, stabilize hypermobile joints, and aid in an understanding of how to best support the posture internally.

Here are some of the most popular props, with their common applications, for yoga during pregnancy:

Yoga blocks

Blocks create more space in a posture, by removing the need to be able to touch the floor, and provide physical support for supine and supported postures. While I love yoga blocks, they should not be used simply to bear weight. Rather, think of them as a way to lift the floor up to the hands.

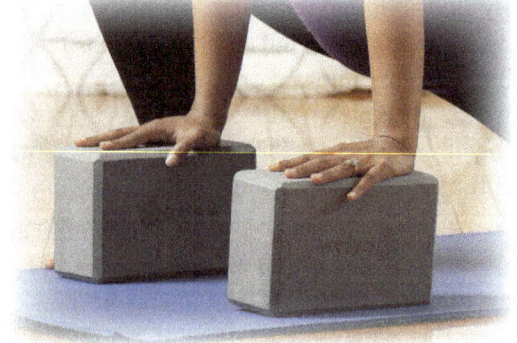

Blocks for hand support

Place blocks beneath the hands in lunges after 28 weeks to accommodate the growing belly and maintain a higher pelvis position. Rather than leaning the weight into the blocks, focus on making the hands light on the blocks. Support the body's weight with the larger muscles of the legs and glutes instead. The goal is to feel as though one could lift off the blocks rather than sinking in.

For Trikonasana and other standing postures, the block is used elevate the height of the floor. In Trikonasana in particular, a block should also provide a solid foundation that a yogini can push off from to create the twist and opening through the upper chest and spine. Make sure the block is high enough that the spine and hips do not collapse when trying to reach for it. The spine should remain elongated as the hand presses the block rather than rounded over due to hip or lower back tension.

For forward bending postures such as Prasarita Padottanasana (or the windmill twisting variation), I recommend placing the blocks on their highest height or even stacking two blocks. The goal is to be able to hinge directly from the hip joint without borrowing movement from the lumbar spine or thrusting the ribs. This helps to focus the action of the pose into the pelvis and pelvic floor. In the windmill variation, the elongated spine and elevated chest helps focus the movement into the lower back and posterior pelvic muscles, rather than dragging on.

Blocks can also be placed under the hands in Downward Dog to promote lifting of the wrists rather than sinking. In this pose, blocks should always be on the lowest height for greater stability. They can also be placed just behind the wrists, which encourages students to lift the forearms rather than sinking into the heels of the hands. This action helps develop internal support from the wrists and shoulders—a good thing to have during early parenthood as well! If a block is too high, a rolled blanket or yoga mat can also be used. The goal is to take the weight off the roll, not rest the wrists against it.

In supine postures, blocks also serve as wonderful supports for freeing the upper spine and supporting the body. (Bear in mind that we limit these poses after 34 weeks of pregnancy to encourage the baby to rotate into a more optimal position for starting labor.)

Yoga strap/sacroiliac support belt

Straps are extremely helpful throughout yoga practice and probably the prop most easily recreated from home implements. In pregnancy I find straps are essential in making space in tight upper back and shoulder muscles, but I also love employing the strap as a stabilizing prop for overly loose pelvic joints.

SI stability belts are tools employed by physical therapists and physicians when the pelvis needs more support than the body can provide on its own. Clinical versions often involve elastic bands which velcro around the pelvis to provide compressive support, but a basic yoga version can be created with a yoga strap. The strap can help awaken students to how much they may need to restrict their movement and provide support to the internal pelvic joints during practice. Students exploring this prop modification are often amazed at how much it restricts their movement—which conversely can illuminate just how often they are over-stretching in their *asana*.

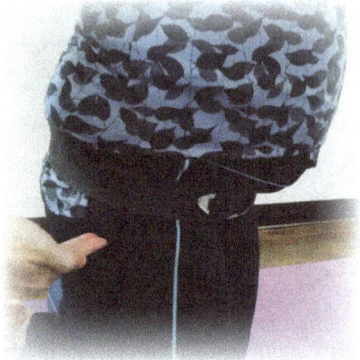
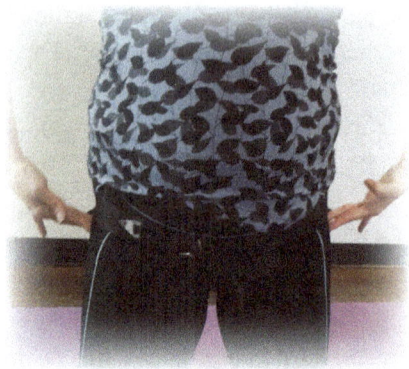

If you are using a yoga strap for stability, you need to put the belt on before beginning the posture, so it creates stability in a neutral pelvis before we add additional twists and stretching into the mix. Begin either standing in Tadasana or lying down in constructive rest (knees bent and the feet flat on the floor). The pelvis wants to be in a neutral position for good initial alignment. Buckle the belt into a loop, and place it around the hips, below the ASIS but above the greater trochanter—that knobby bone on the outside of the thigh. The belt should rest under the belly but just above the pubic bone.

In your current position, tighten the belt as far as possible. Wrap the tail of the belt around the loop you've created, then tuck it in. If you entered the pose lying down, roll to one side and return to standing. Explore your practice, feeling the stability of the bound ring around the pelvis.

When practicing with the stability belt in place, the range of motion will be restricted, which is the whole point. Lunges, side bends, and any posture which pushes against the belt should be done only until the belt begins to compress: no further. Focus on drawing inward, as if pulling away from the belt rather than hanging into it.

Bolsters/Blankets

We would be remiss discussing yoga props for pregnancy without mentioning yoga blankets and bolsters. These of course can be used primarily to help in creating neutral pelvic alignment by raising the hips up so you are not constricted by tight hip and leg muscles in bringing your weight onto the sitz bones.

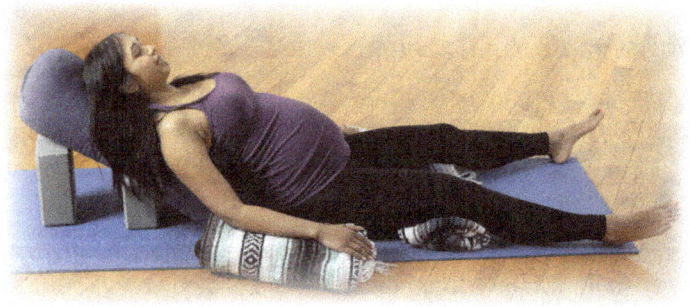

In my experience most students resist using bolsters for seated postures because there is some misconception that using them somehow makes the pose remedial. Far from it! Using a bolster to promote good pelvic alignment not only helps your body stay in good alignment for pregnancy and birth, but also allows the postures to actually affect the areas intended- instead of borrowing movement from other- more supple areas.

Additionally, bolsters create a sense of support and comfort for reclining and restorative postures. Rather than feeling the hard corners of blocks under our back, I have found students far prefer to have a soft, continuous support from head to tail under their spine. If practicing at home, I should note that bed pillows are often not firm enough to provide this support. If you don't have a true yoga bolster in your home prop collection, consider pulling a solid pillow off the back of your couch, or substituting 2 bed pillows for one yoga bolster. The extra firmness allows the props to truly support your body- creating the intended space, rather than simply collapsing under your body's weight.

The foundational postures

The postures described here are what I consider "beginning" yoga *asanas*. This is not to say that they are all beginner level postures, but each of these could be safely included in a level one prenatal yoga class. These *asanas* are not yet in a practice sequence; we will cover possible sequences in Chapter 11.

The instructions provided are what I would give in a general prenatal yoga class, including specific accommodations depending on what trimester mom is in. The aim in most postures is to find an edge of sensation, then explore how to allow the tissues to release unnecessary tension without collapsing. The general rule of thumb is to begin at 50% of the expected range of motion and examine the sensation in the moment, then proceed if things still feel spacious and juicy.

Tadasana

The foundation of all standing postures and the root for our movement! As Cyndi Lee says, "this is the underpants of everything else." The key for Tadasana is to look for both a sense of groundedness and floating within the pelvis.

Stand with the feet hip distance apart to create a strong base. Soften the knees so the bones balance atop one another, drop the pubic bone away from the navel, and draw the hips back. This should bring the navel to point either level or slightly towards the floor.

Placing attention into the feet, lift and spread the toes, activating the arches of the feet, then replace the toes back on the floor. Anchor the ball of the big toe, the ball of the little toe, and the center of the heel into the floor. With active grounding, the arches between these points will subtly lift. This lift, especially in the inner arch, creates an

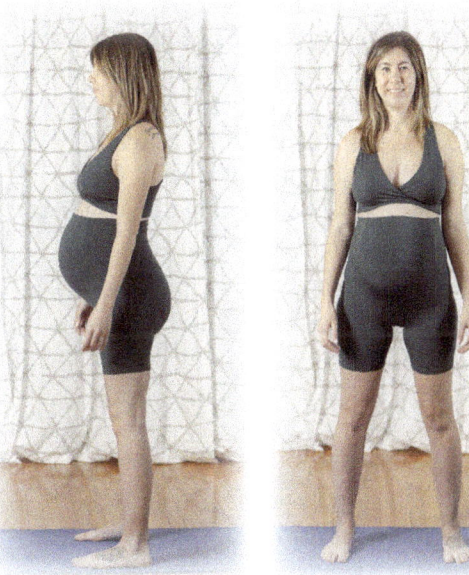

upward lift on the inner leg, drawing the inner knees forward to neutral, and continuing up to lift the pelvic floor.

Feel the pelvis floating on the active legs. The pubic bone dips, as though placing the pelvic bowl onto the heads of the femurs. The tail is likewise heavy but not tucked. Instead, the pubis and tail softly reach towards one another, further activating the pelvic floor.

The belly rests forward and slightly down, cradling the baby. There is a light organization in the deep abdominals as the pelvic floor levels with the earth and responds to the plumb line of gravity. From the pelvis, the spine lifts up, pushed by the feet on the earth. The ribs lift, both in front and in back, so the cathedral dome of the ribcage balances above the bowl of the pelvis. The skull balances lightly on the curves of the spine.

The action has a vibrance to it, energy lifting strongly through the center but then cascading from the crown out and down the sides of the body like a gentle waterfall. The shoulders drop from the column of the spine, with the arms hanging loose but aware and awake. The fingers hang. The outsides of the glutes descend and the outer arches of the feet ground.

Tadasana joins heaven and earth in the same form. This pose is the basis from which all other standing postures flow, and it creates a toned, dynamic action: not too tight and not too loose. In the middle floats the spacious, balanced space where the baby rests, responding to the relative tension and relaxation around them. And although there is a dynamic action through the pose, the body will also continue to subtly sway and shift in a small, never-ending dance to balance within the field of gravity.

Tadasana variation: hip circles

The action of circling and dropping the hip subtly shifts the dimensions within the pelvis, allowing for more space for the baby, and can assist late in pregnancy with engaging into the pelvic inlet. The fluid motion can also help mobilize and balance the SI and lower spinal joints. Look for supple, relaxed movement rather than seeking out a stretch or chasing intense sensation. One note of caution: if mom is experiencing pubic pain, these motions should be done smaller or avoided entirely if they increase discomfort.

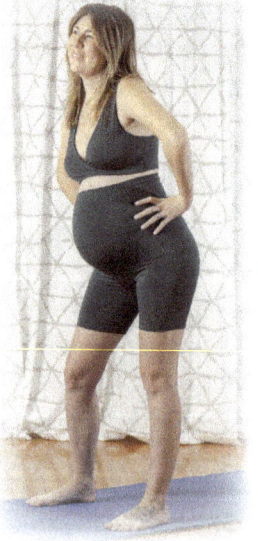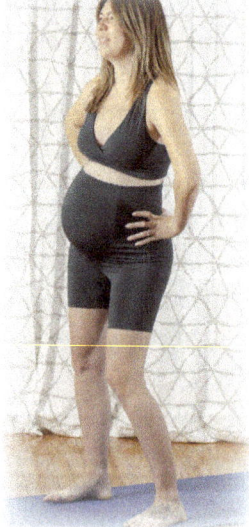

From Tadasana, bend the knees further and begin gently rotating the pelvic bowl in circles, as though swinging a slow-motion hula hoop. Think of the pelvic bowl spiraling around the baby's head as though spinning an egg into a cup. This motion helps lubricate the joints of the pelvis and lower back, and it also can assist in the baby engaging into the lower pelvis.

Practice in both directions (we don't want the baby to get dizzy ;)). When you're ready, begin taking the pelvis in a gentle figure eight motion, focusing on dropping one hip to each side. If you feel creative, you can also try reversing this figure eight motion to see if you can coordinate it in the non-dominant direction.

Calf stretch

Kinesiologist Katy Bowman[45] of Seattle says if there were one stretch she would have everyone do to change how we stand and walk, it would be this one. The calf muscles integrate with a posterior fascial chain up the leg which interlocks with the hamstrings and sacro-tuberous ligaments in the pelvis. Releasing the bottom of the foot and back of the lower leg creates the potential for more movement of the sacrum and thus more space for the baby during the birth process.

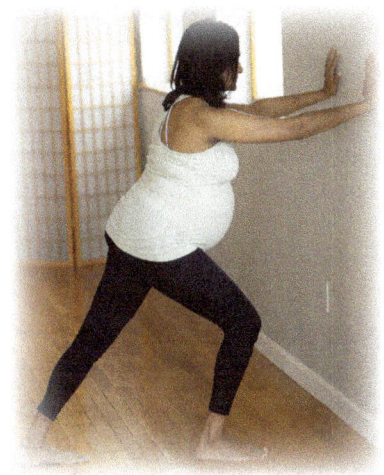

I have found two approaches that are effective for targeting this area. One is to take a gentle lunge facing a wall or chair with the back heel fully contacting the floor. From there, gently bend the front knee, bringing the hips towards the wall and keeping the back heel on the floor to lengthen the calf and Achilles tendon. Hold for five breaths, feeling the calf soften and release, then gently bend the back knee (not very much), bringing the stretch into the slender lower calf muscle, closer to the ankle.

The sensation here only needs to be in the 50% range. Deeper stretching may lead to the fascia binding and tensing rather than releasing. Additionally, be sure to avoid rolling in or out on the back foot if the aim of the stretch is to get the release up to the sacrum. Leaning to the inside or outside of the foot changes the line of the calf stretch and can bypass the back leg line that runs up to the sitting bone. If you are curious to feel the difference, try angling the foot one way, then the other, and feel how the stretch changes. Then return to finding a sustained stretch down the center of the calf and heel, which allows the tissues to gradually lengthen and release into the "sigh" of the fascia. Once released, switch sides and repeat with the other foot.

Alternatively, we could stretch the calf by rolling up a blanket or yoga mat and placing the right toes on the roll with the heel on the floor. Be sure the hips (indicated by the ASIS bones) point straight forward and that the toes and knee face the same direction. Ideally, the feet are close together to make it easier to align the hips forward. Bend the right knee (the one with the foot on the blanket) a few times, feeling the arch of the foot massaging into the roll. If sensation allows, carefully step the left foot in front of the blanket roll, keeping the heel of the right leg still on the floor. Maintain a gentle stretch (around 50% of your capacity) rather than looking for a deep "burn."

---

[45] *www.nutritiousmovement.com*

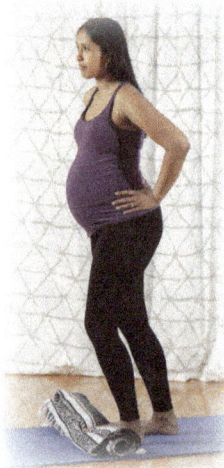
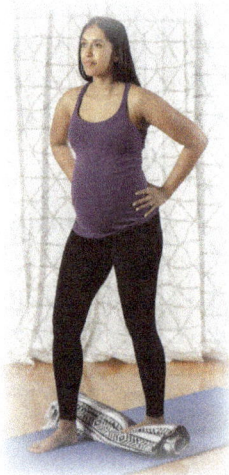
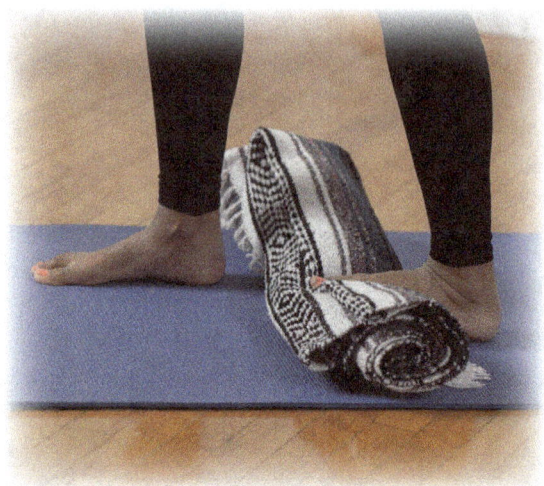

Extend into the right heel while very gently bending the left knee, again feeling for the subtle yawn as the fascia releases. This will move the stretch into the top of the calm muscle closer to the knee as well as into the Achilles tendon. Breathe easily, bending in and out of the stretch. Stay for about 30 seconds. Once you release, stand on two feet for a moment and feel the difference. Then switch sides and repeat with the left foot.

Anjaneyasana/High and Low Lunge

Lunges are a great way to release tight hip flexors, particularly the glorious psoas muscle that runs from the lower back behind the uterus, over the pelvic bowl, and down to the inner thigh. During pregnancy, we want to keep this deep front line balanced, giving the baby enough room to rotate and avoiding lower back compression. When practicing lunges during pregnancy, the first consideration is making enough space so that the belly is not compressed against the front thigh. This can be accomplished by either moving the front leg out to the side or by elevating the hands on blocks.

It is also key to hold back from an intense range of motion in these postures. Increased relax-

in in the body could lead to destabilization of the pelvic bones. Twisting or torquing these bones and their connecting joints not only impacts the internal pelvic space but can also lead to a great deal of pain. Additionally, if the pelvis twists when practicing Anjaneyasana, you lose the opening you are seeking in the psoas and deep front line. Be sure to maintain forward alignment in the ASIS bones when practicing this posture and lift upwards to feel for the lengthening deep within the body.

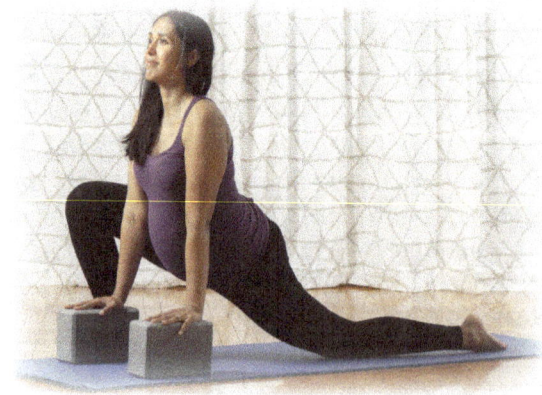

There are two paths to arrive in a lunge: stepping back or stepping forward. If stepping back, begin in Tadasana, bending forward into a half squat with the hands resting on the thighs. Shifting the weight to one leg, engage the abdominals and pelvic floor to support the pelvis and then slowly step the unweighted leg back along the mat. (It can be helpful to have a set of yoga blocks or a chair to place the hands on.) The front leg can be outside the shoulder, with both hands positioned to the inside of the front foot.

Be sure to keep the hip points pointed forward and keep the back heel in the air, with even weight between the big toe and the baby toe. Extend through the back foot to find a stretch through the calf, lifting the chest and belly. Engage the glute of the back leg to suck the femur bone into the hip socket rather than extending it. The groin of the back leg will lift towards the ceiling, creating a slight crease in the front of the hip, as though drawing the pubic bone towards the tail and the tail towards the pubis. This helps to draw the pelvis away from the floor and into stability.

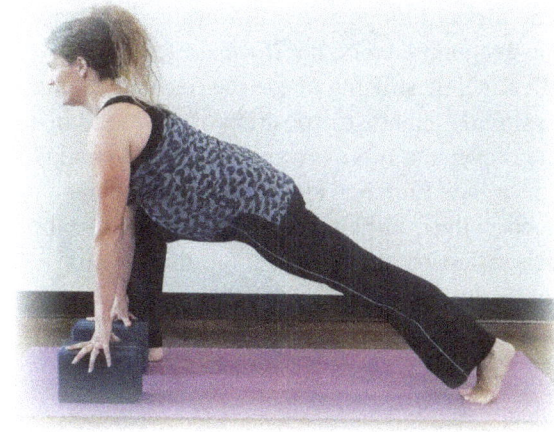

If practicing a low lunge variation with the knee on the mat, maintain this groin lift and pelvic alignment, but lower the back knee to the floor or a blanket. As with the high lunge, the pelvis should remain floating and aligned forward, with the back glute engaged and a feeling that the pubic bone is reaching back and up rather than sinking towards the floor.

If coming into the lunge from the floor, begin in Table pose. Elevate the hands on blocks and step one leg forward to the outside of the hands. The pelvis can lower, but the front

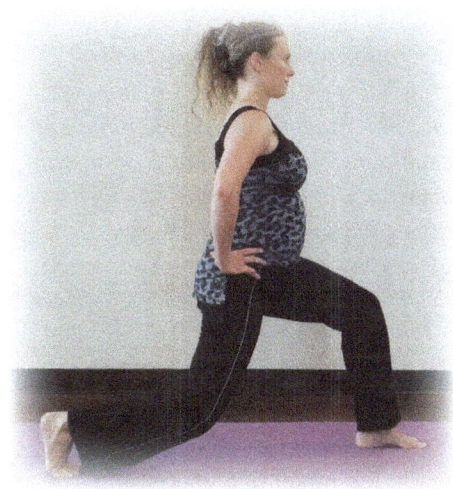

knee should not pass the ankle, and the pelvic bowl should remain aligned forward. Once again, to promote stability and prevent overstretching, the pubic bone draws back and up towards the tail rather than sinking into the floor, and the back glute turns on. If you are experiencing pubic bone tenderness, it is better to do this at 50% range of motion for a while until stability is restored. If lifting to the full lunge and standing pose variations, tuck the back toes and draw the thigh away from the floor to straighten the knee.

To further target the psoas muscle, walk the hands from the blocks up onto the front thigh. This action extends the spine, inviting the psoas to lengthen and gently release. Raising the arms increases this action further, and gently sidebending away from the back leg can invite even more length. Keep the back heel parallel, and keep the hips pointed straight forward. Releasing the psoas can free the lower back and create more room for the uterus and baby. The movement should be gentle, and if balance becomes an issue, either hold a chair or place one under the front hip for stability.

Be sure to repeat the lunge variations on the second side, paying attention to any differences between sides.

Skandasana/Side Lunge

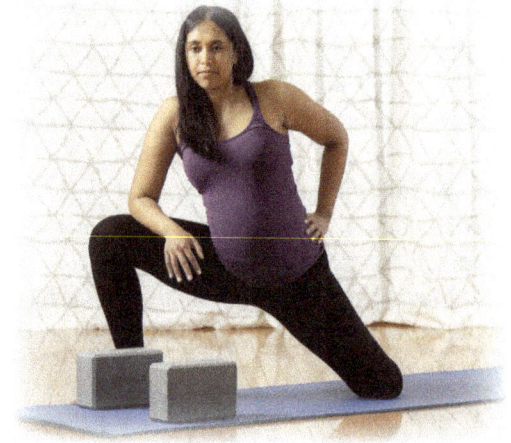

The forward lunge of Anjaneyasana helps ease the deep hip flexors, but if we are looking to affect gentle shifting inside the pelvis, we have to slightly change the position of the leg to bring the movement more towards the side. Skandasana, or Side Lunge, widens the ischial spines deep in the mid-pelvis and can help release the pelvic floor, making more room for baby to rotate during the birth process.

To find the side lunge, begin in a knee down Anjaneyasana and walk the hands onto the knee. From this position, walk the front foot to the side about 45 degrees so the foot points on a diagonal and is probably off the mat. The navel and hips face slightly away from the thigh rather than towards the knee, but the knee tracks with the toes. This creates a subtle external rotation in the femur bone of the active leg. From this position, gently shift the weight into the front leg, bringing the knee out over the front heel. The arms can lean onto the front leg to create a side bend if desired. On an inhale, return to the kneeling position and repeat. This variation can be wonderful for accessing the adductor muscles along the inner thigh as well as spreading the sitz bones and mid-pelvis.

Be mindful that this motion moves laterally and asymmetrically, without a physical stop point. It can be challenging for a vulnerable pubic symphysis. If you are experiencing pelvic pain, it is best to perform this movement gently and in small increments with abdominal support. Omit it entirely if stability is becoming a critical issue. During labor, Skandasana can be one way of releasing and balancing the pelvic floor muscles which guide the baby's head to rotate and align with the birth path. Practicing this movement ahead of labor conditions the body's tissues to be more responsive when labor does begin.

Prasarita Padottanasana/Wide Legged Forward Fold

One of the simplest and yet sometimes overlooked postures for lower back and hip release, Prasarita Padottanasana offers ample room for the growing belly while also opening the backs of the legs and hips. A variation which combines a gentle twist can also be hugely beneficial for the lower back and SI joints. That said, here again, too much of a good thing can

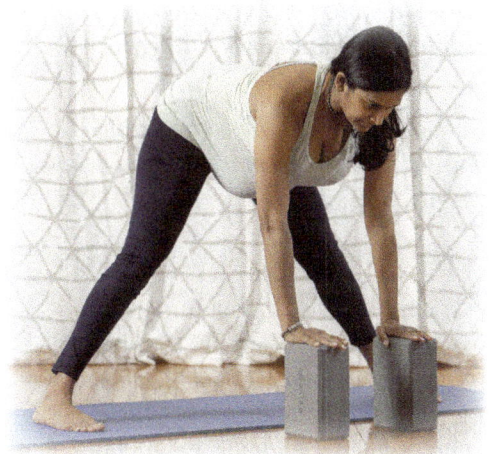

be too much, so the key is to find the middle path where the tissues are gently stretched but the joints remain spacious, especially the hip socket and the junction of the sacrum and lumbar spine.

Begin with the feet positioned 3-4 feet apart. Inhale to lengthen the spine. On an exhale, tilt the pelvis forward to fold from the hips, bringing the hands down onto a chair or a yoga block. Unless you naturally possess a wide range of motion, there's no need to reach for the floor. Doing so can place too much strain on the SI and pelvic joints as the spine flexes forward.

Bring the spine parallel to the floor if possible and lengthen through the crown of the head and tail. Imagine the handle of a broom lying across your back as you fold. Aim to maintain contact with the whole broom as you hinge (rather than allowing the spine to curve like in Child's Pose). Lightly engage the abdominals to "hug" baby up towards the spine to prevent sagging in the lower back. Pause when parallel to the floor and feel the opening in the "back window" where the legs and pelvis meet.

If you're continuing into the deeper forward fold, keep folding from the hip sockets, then walk the hands off the blocks and back towards the feet. The head will move towards the floor, and the belly will drop from the pelvis, gently hanging from the ligaments in the back. Collect the ribcage inward under the belly, as though catching baby to your heart.

Windmill variation

If you want to focus on a deeper release in the lower back and sacrum as well as bring better movement to the ribcage and side body, remain in the initial posture with the spine extended long and flat. If your spine is not parallel to the floor, elevate your blocks or use a chair if the blocks are too low. Press the right hand into the block and raise the left shoulder towards the ceiling. It is ok if the hips shift slightly, but the twist should be focused in the upper spine, not driven from the pelvis. To stabilize the pelvis, push the left leg outwards against the mat.

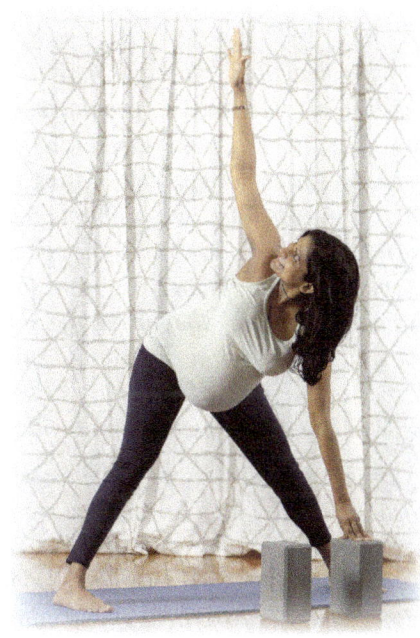

If the shoulders allow, raise the left hand skyward, but watch out for moving your arm past the line of the shoulder. Too often we borrow movement from the shoulder, thinking it is bringing a deeper twist, when in fact it is simply contributing to tension in the

neck. Keep the top arm in line with the shoulder. If you're looking for a neck and upper back release, turn the head opposite to the shoulders. (e.g., if the left shoulder is lifting, turn the head to the right)

On an exhale, return the hand to the floor. The hips should realign towards the ground. Repeat on the second side, and then continue switching sides to gently massage and release the lower back and hips. Aim for around 10 repetitions on each side.

Trikonasana/Triangle

Triangle is one of those postures that seems deceptively simple but is in fact quite complicated. The instructions for practicing Trikonasana have changed considerably throughout the years and can also vary between yoga traditions. Your version may look a bit different than mine, but I encourage you to look at the mechanics rather than the specific shape. This posture can be a wonderful way to access the hamstrings, adductors, glutes, pelvic floor, and even the upper back. The trick is to align the hips and knees in such a way that the SI joints and pubic symphysis aren't pulled into instability. I loved this posture while pregnant, as it gave me a feeling of lightness and space in my chest while allowing me to explore my pelvic alignment.

Beginning with the feet wide and facing the long edge of the mat, turn the right toes to face the front of the mat and the left toes inward about 5-10 degrees. This slight inward rotation allows for more adjustment in the hips, giving them space to float rather than lock.

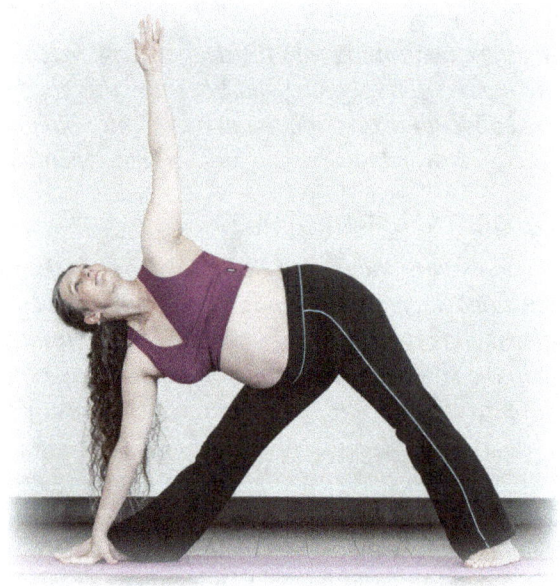

Moving from the right hip, rotate the right thigh so the knee faces the right second toe. Align the feet to stand heel to heel to create a wider base for the shifting center of gravity. The hips will probably need to turn forward to allow this to happen, so let them. During pregnancy we want to avoid trying to "square" the hips to the side of the mat as this creates unwanted shearing forces in the joints. The pelvis is like a crystal bowl to be handled and rotated carefully, not a book to be cracked and opened.

With the right hip, knee, and toes aligned, tip the right hip forward while pressing out through the left foot. Stretch the right hand forward, leaning out over the right leg. Maintain space in the right hip crease. This will feel a bit like doing a forward fold, and in fact, initially it should. When the space in the right hip begins to compress, lower the right hand onto either a block or the floor if you can comfortably reach it. The hand will probably need to come to the INSIDE of the leg, which is fine so long as the hips do not swing further behind you or out to the side. This is a variation from the classic alignment which places the hand outside the ankle, but it promotes more space and freedom in the front hip and focuses the pose into the spine. Engage the glute of the left hip to draw the left sitz bone slightly forward. Look for a neutral pelvic position here, not dumping into the front hip but also not tucked under and thrusting into the front of the groins.

Keeping the right side of the waist long and the right hip drawn back, press into the block or floor with the right hand and lift the chest, rotating the left shoulder towards the ceiling. This twist originates in the shoulders, not the hips. As the chest rotates further, there may come a point where the abdomen lifts, and after that it's possible that the hips will begin to stack. But don't be in a rush to stack the hips. If stacking the hips or moving in that direction causes the right waist or hip to compress or the right knee to roll inward, the body is trying to borrow movement, and it's not time yet. Ultimately the left hip lifting is the final movement of the posture, not the initial one, especially during pregnancy.

Allow the pelvis to float wherever it needs to so that the right knee remains aligned with the right second toe. This may mean that the belly is pointing slightly towards the floor, even in the final expression of this posture, which is good because it preserves the pelvic integrity. A bonus benefit to staying slightly turned towards the legs is that when you want to stand, you can simply exhale to engage the pelvic floor and press the feet into the floor to rise up.

Repeat on the second side for balance, also noting any differences in the body's sensation or range of motion between sides.

Parsvakonasana/Side Angle

A cousin of Trikonasana, Side Angle follows much of the same geometry as Triangle pose, with two exceptions. The front knee is bent rather than straight, and the top arm is often being swept upwards along the cheek. This posture also mimics the space created in Skandasana.

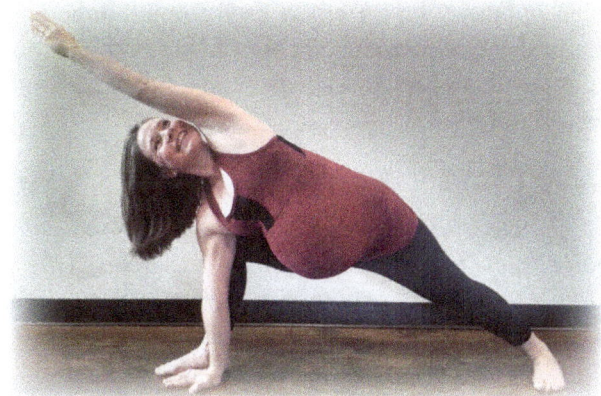

Enter Parsvakonasana the same way you would Trikonasana. Turn the feet, and reach the right hand forward over the right leg. As you reach the end of your limit to maintain space within the right hip, bend the right knee out to around a 90 degree angle. Bring the right elbow to rest on the thigh, or lower the right hand to the inside of the foot or onto a block.

Actively press into the floor, block, or thigh, and rotate the upper chest towards the ceiling. The head should turn fairly easily, following the rotation of the upper back. As in Triangle, the hips remain slightly turned towards the floor, and the left leg presses actively away. Resist the tendency to sag the hips forward and down, and engage the back leg glute.

Stay as long as the breath is steady and comfortable. To exit, press actively into the feet and rise up, straightening the front leg. Alternatively, lower the left hand to the mat, walk both hands to the side of the mat, and roll up to stand.

Repeat on the second side.

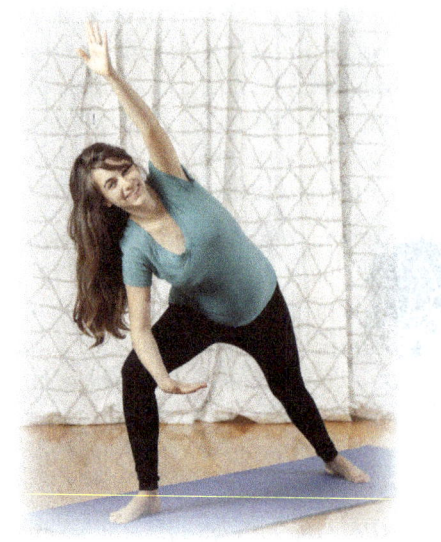

Virabhadrasana 1/2/3: The Warrior Poses

"Wherever we are, we can train as a warrior. The practices of meditation, loving-kindness, compassion, joy, and equanimity are our tools. ... Many of us prefer practices that will not cause discomfort, yet at the same time we want to be healed. Bodhichitta training doesn't work that way. A warrior accepts that we can never know what will happen to us next..." —Pema Chodron

As yogis, we, of course, realize that the warrior this quote refers to is the spiritual warrior archetype rather than an aggressive or violent individual. The Warrior postures usually involve working with physical and mental challenges. Not every variation of Virabhadrasana needs to be uncomfortable, but there is a certain focused strength inherent in these shapes which can be yoked to promote the tools of meditation, loving-kindness, compassion, joy, and equanimity.

Virabhadrasana 1/Warrior 1

Beginning with the feet 3-4 feet apart, turn the right thigh so the toes and knee face the short end of the mat. Adjust the left foot to align the right and left heels on the same line, then rotate the left toes about 45 degrees. Turn the hips towards the right leg, drawing the left hip gently forward and up towards the belly.

The widening of your stance from the classic "foot to inner arch" cue will allow for easier rotation of the pelvis towards the right leg. While easier, it is still key not to wrench the pelvis to fully face the front leg. This "squaring" motion can create a twist within the pubic bone, leading to instability. Instead, draw the back hip

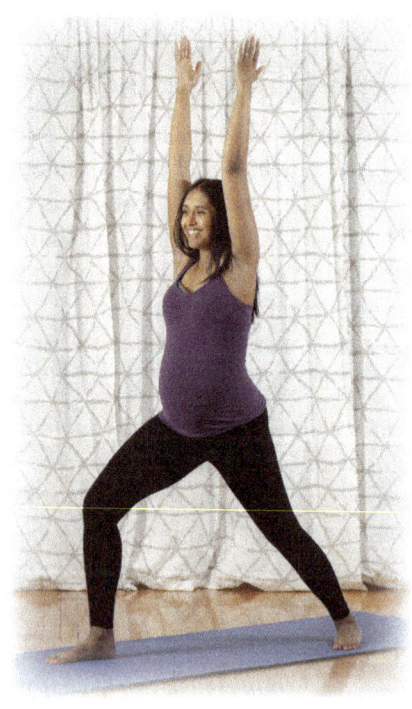

around while lightly engaging the abdominal muscles to support and lift the baby and belly. Maintain a slight downward tilt to the navel as the spine arches up and back. Please note this is a different hip alignment from Anjaneyasana and does not affect the psoas muscle in the same manner.

On an inhale, bend the front knee, sitting down into the lunge until there is either gentle stretch in the pelvis or the front thigh comes level with the ground. Feel the strong connection with the earth and press the legs actively into the ground. If stable, the arms may sweep overhead, creating the warrior's "sword" of awareness. Breathe easily and steadily. If doing this pose in isolation, come out by straightening the front knee and turning to face the side of the mat once again. Repeat on the second side.

Warrior 1 is a pose which is often combined with other postures within a *vinyasa*. If this is the case, this pose is often entered from Downward Dog. This entry involves bringing the front leg forward into a wide lunge, then grounding the back heel before raising the arms off the floor. Due to the increase in upper body weight during pregnancy, it's advisable to walk the hands up the front leg while activating abdominal and pelvic floor support. Doing so avoids the sudden load created by sweeping the hands forward and allows for a more gradual transition to avoid head rushes. If moving from Warrior 1 into Down Dog, allow time to bring the hands inside the front foot and drop the back knee to the floor, moving into Table before continuing on.

Virabhadrasana 2/Warrior 2

One of the most well-known yoga postures, Warrior 2 presents some subtle but profound alignment challenges during pregnancy. Done well, this posture can both strengthen and balance the hips, legs and pelvic floor. Done poorly, however, it can foster significant pelvic and lower back discomfort.

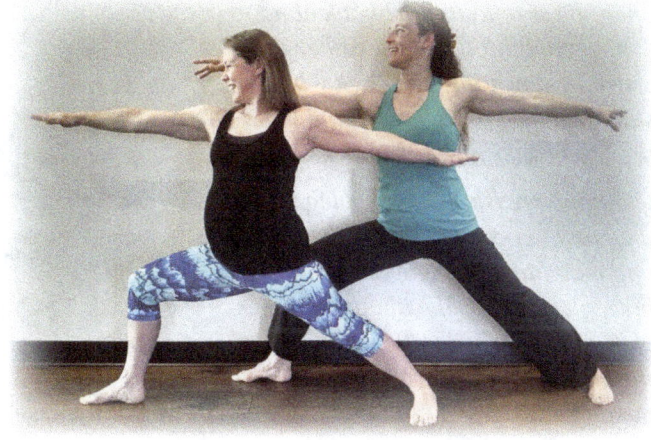

Starting from a wide stance facing the long edge of the mat, turn the right thigh so the toes and knee face the short end of the mat. Turn the left toes in about 10 degrees and allow the pelvis to float at whatever angle makes these two movements easy.

This is the first main difference from the classic Virabhadrasana 2 alignment: the hips are turned! No more squaring the pelvis towards the side of the mat. The pelvis should float, supported in a range where the front hip can rotate the knee towards the toes. The back knee is still able to align with its toes as well. The bowl of the pelvis should also remain as upright as possible. This can often mean lifting the front hip bone and floating the pelvic floor level with the ground. The tail remains long but is NOT TUCKED. Engage the back glute to promote stability without rotating the pelvis past neutral.

With this floating pelvis, inhale to spread the arms from the heart, and exhale to bend the right knee towards the right foot. Press the back leg actively away. The legs can hug inwards, activating the inner thighs and supporting the hips. If you were viewing this pose from the back, you would see that the bowl of your pelvis would remain level with the ground. You might be able to judge this in a mirror via the waistband of your yoga pants.

Press the shoulders down as the head rises up and gaze over the right fingertips. Allow your body to experience the strength required for this posture while still breathing easily. Working and yet releasing at the same time... kind of like in labor!

To come out, straighten the right leg and turn to face the side of the mat. Pause to possibly circle and reset the hips before continuing to the second side.

Parsva Virabhadrasana/Reverse Warrior/Side Warrior

A variation on Warrior 2, and one often performed from Warrior 2 in *vinyasas*, Reverse Warrior combines the lower body placement from Warrior 2 with a half side-bend, half back-bend. The upside is that this pose can be a wonderful stretch for the side ribs and waist. The downside, as usual, is that if done too forcefully or without support, it can overstretch tissues.

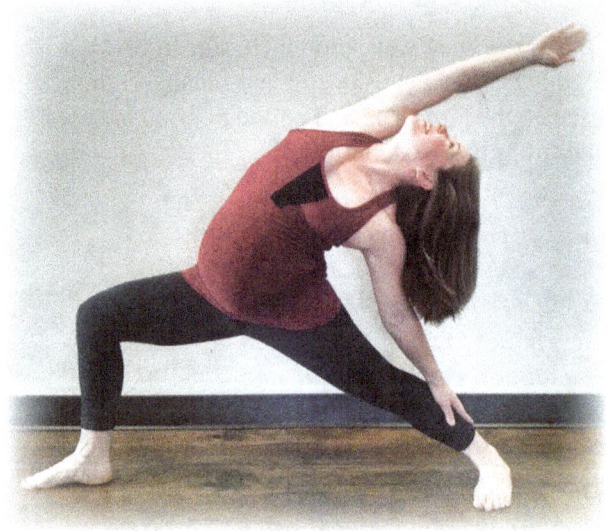

From Warrior 2, place the back hand on the back hip for support. On an inhale, reach the front arm overhead and lean into the back hand and hip while drawing the front waist up and open. Be sure to use the back hand to support and lift the chest rather than crashing down into the back waist. If stable and supported, walk the hand on the hip further down the back leg.

Continue pressing the back leg up into the hand to promote lifting the chest, and maintain the engagement of the back glute. Draw the abdominal muscles gently inward to further support the belly and baby. Done well, this posture should feel light and free rather than compressed or cumbersome.

To return, draw in the pelvic floor and lower abdominals on an exhale, and bring the chest upright again into Warrior 2. Alternatively, you could straighten the front knee, coming into a reverse variation of Trikonasana before returning to stand and continuing on. Repeat on the second side.

Like Warrior 1, Reverse Warrior is a posture which is often done in combination with other asanas in a longer vinyasa sequence. In fact, Reverse warrior, Warrior 2, Trikonasana, and Parsvakonasana share a common hip and leg placement, making them frequent partners, especially in Vinyasa yoga. If being done in sequence, be sure to maintain support through the legs, glutes, and pelvic floor rather than sinking into the hip joints, which can lead to instability.

I'll discuss Warrior 3 in the advanced posture chapter.

Jaiasana/Kaliasana/Goddess Squat

Jaiasana—also known as Goddess Squat or Kaliasana, referring to the images of the goddess Kali giving birth to the universe—is popular in many prenatal yoga classes. Its dynamic leg work is helpful in developing both mental and physical stamina. And the external rotation of the thigh bones helps tone the glute muscles and integrate the pelvic floor. That said, yoginis do need to be mindful when practicing Goddess Squat during pregnancy, especially if hypermobility or lower back pain is an issue.

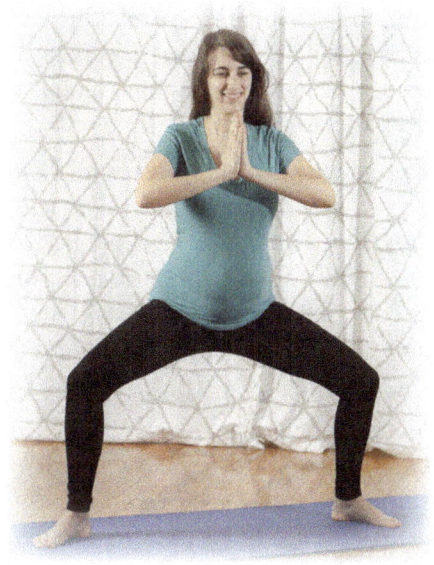

Step the feet a generous distance apart. If you are working with pelvic pain, take a shorter stance, no more than three feet between the heels. Rotate the thighs to turn the toes out approximately 45 degrees. Be sure to drop the pubic bone down to maintain deep groins, even with the external rotation, and anchor the tail to avoid spilling the abdomen forward.

Inhale and raise the arms over head, feeling the spine standing tall as in Tadasana. Exhale, reaching tall. On the next inhale, bend the knees out towards the toes, sitting the hips down into a wide squat. Maintain a neutral pelvis, and bend the elbows to 90 degrees (goalpost arms). Feel the pelvic floor widen as you descend, and actively move the knees apart to activate the glute muscles. You can further activate the glutes by isometrically pressing the heels forward against the mat.

On the exhale, press the feet outward on the mat and rise, drawing the pelvic floor upwards. Repeat several times, gathering the power of the lower body into the heart center.

The key here is to maintain the neutral position of the pelvis and avoid excessively rotating the femur bones outwards. Over-rotation can lead to widening of the pubic symphysis, which can cause instability. Instability in this posture will often manifest quite quickly as an aching or even cramping along the pubic bone and inner thighs on the ascent.

Parsvottanasana/ Half intense forward fold

Often referred to as "intense side stretch" this posture is more accurately thought of as a single leg version of the more common forward fold Uttanasana. For pregnancy this posture can be a great way to release tension in the posterior muscle chain, as well as focusing the action into the muscles of the pelvic floor. Out of consideration for the increased relaxin as well as the expanding uterus in later pregnancy, I recommend raising the hands onto blocks to prevent overstretching.

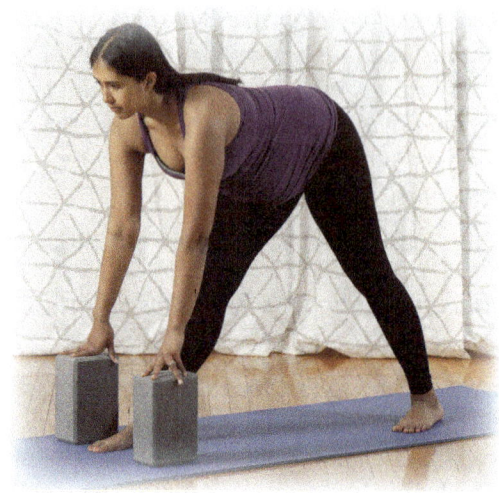

Begin with the feet placed as for Warrior 1, heel to heel about 3-4 feet apart with the back foot turned out about 45 degrees. Ground both feet equally into the earth, and stretch up tall through the spine. On an exhale, hinge from the hips, rotating the pelvis on the femur socket to come forwards over the front leg with a flat back. Later in pregnancy the belly will snuggle alongside the front thigh. Maintain an open chest.

When the hips stop rotating, lower the hands to tall height blocks. Even if you could go lower here, stay with the taller height. Draw the front hip sitting bone towards the back, focusing the action into the back of the leg. Stretch through the top of the head and back through both sitting bones, focusing on the depth in the front hip crease. Breathe smoothly, and actively press the edge of the back foot into the floor to bring the pelvis as level as possible.

To come out, exhale and press both feet actively into the floor to stand up. Turn the feet to the side and pause. Repeat on the second side.

Prone postures on hands and feet or knees

As we discussed in Chapter 7, lying flat down on the belly after the uterus can be felt is not a good idea for practice. You don't want to squish the baby. But there is a whole family of yoga postures which involve the belly facing towards the floor while the body is supported by the arms and legs. These postures can be extremely helpful for lengthening the spine to counter its increased curvature during pregnancy, finding more coordinated movement in the pelvic bowl to relieve back pain, and preparing for labor and birth.

Table

Table might be one of the most overlooked yoga postures in the catalog. More than simply coming onto hands and knees, this prone posture is a great place to practice maintaining an open chest while employing light abdominal engagement. Table is effectively a Plank on hands and knees. Done well, this posture can help build arm and wrist strength and support overall core integration. Done improperly or without attention, however, and Table can lead to wrist compression and sagging into front abdominal connective tissue. Starting with a solid, balanced Table pose sets us up for good movement in the pelvis in Cat/Cow tilts. This posture is also a position for labor and birth, so becoming familiar with its sensations is key during pregnancy.

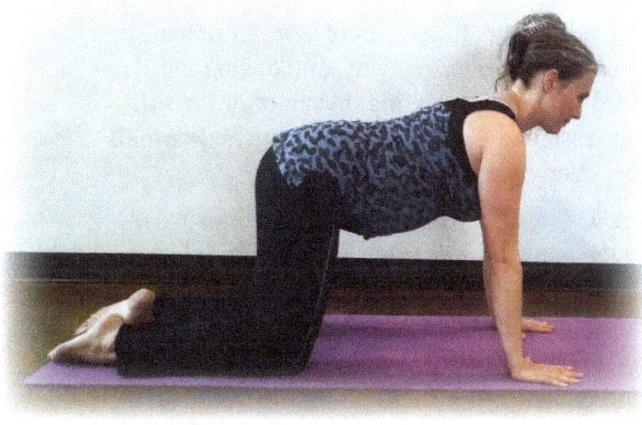

Coming to the mat, bring the hands under the shoulders and the knees under the hips.

Actively press the hands into the mat, spreading the weight throughout the whole palm and fingers rather than sinking into the wrists. Gather the transverse abdominal muscles around the baby and softly lift them towards the spine. This is not a sucking in action but rather a light hugging and support. Be sure the breath can continue smoothly.

From here, move into whatever pelvic tilts or circles you feel called to practice.

Birth ball/ Yoga block Table modification for sore wrists

For some moms, the combination of relaxin and increased fluids in the body can lead to wrist sensitivity or even carpal tunnel syndrome. If placing weight on the palms is too uncomfortable and a prop such as an exercise ball is available, mom can rest her arms and upper chest against the yoga ball to take the weight off the hands and tilt or circle the hips. Alternatively, resting the elbows on two yoga blocks can also remove the weight from the wrists while still allowing for the pelvic and spinal movements.

Cat/Cow variation

Many of us familiar with yoga have experienced the movements known as Cat/Cow. Flexing and extending the pelvis and lower spine can be especially beneficial for freeing the posterior muscles and finding rhythm between the sacrum and the lumbar spine. These movements can also be helpful during the labor process, as the tilting and tucking of the pelvic bowl changes the internal shape of the pelvic inlet and outlet respectively.

The main focus in Cat/Cow is on initiating the movement from the pelvis, then creating a wave-like motion up and down the spine. The tilting motion of Cow allows for easier engagement of the front triangle of the pelvic floor and also helps to widen and release the sitz bones. Conversely, the tucking motion of Cat pose leads to more engagement in the posterior pelvic floor, narrows the sitz bones, and can slightly widen the space between the front and the back of the pelvic inlet (hint hint! useful movements for when a baby is trying to negotiate the twists and turns of our pelvis to be born!).

The movements needed for release do not need to be dramatic. Less is more here. Practice calls for gentle movements, and during the third trimester mom might even omit the full expression of Cow pose if the front abdominals feel overly stretched.

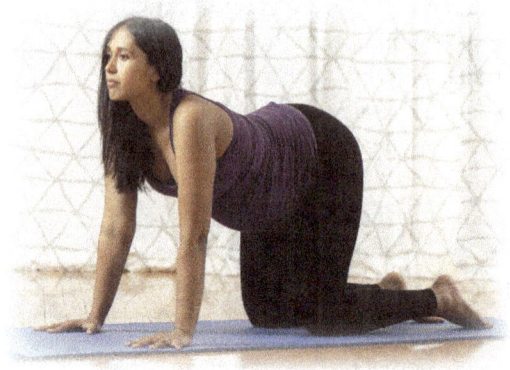

From Table, focus the attention into the bowl of the pelvis. On an inhale, lift the sitting bones and tailbone upwards, allowing the top of the pelvic brim to tilt forwards. Follow this motion up the whole spine, bringing a gentle backbend into the upper back and lifting the head. Be sure to maintain a subtle engagement of the abdominal wall to avoid straining the linea alba, like giving baby a soft hug. This is Cow.

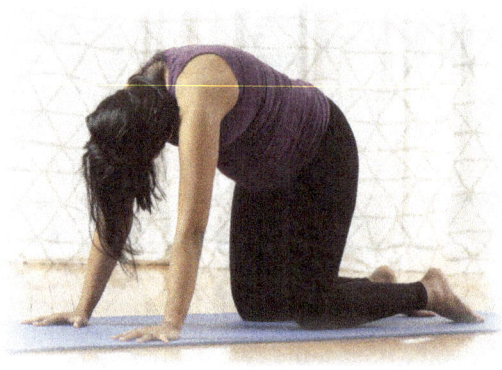

On an exhale, once again focusing on the pelvic bowl, reverse the movement of Cow. Draw the sitz bones and tail downward as the pelvic brim and abdomen lift it. The action creates an opposite wave up the spinal column which eventually drops the head. This is Cat. From the tuck, return to lifting the sitz bones on the inhale, and follow this wave back and forth through the spine.

Repeating this front and back movement helps mobilize the pelvic joints and also builds familiarity with the ways this movement widens or narrows different levels of the pelvis.

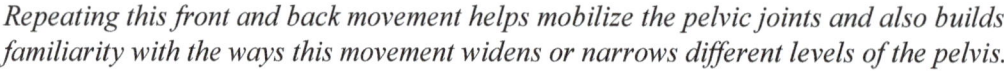

Hip circle variation

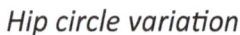

An alternative exploration to the straight tilt and tuck of Cat/Cow is to gently shift the pelvis side to side and begin to explore the movements available, as though drawing a circle in the air with your tailbone. These more instinctive movements can help release gluteal muscles and sometimes even realign

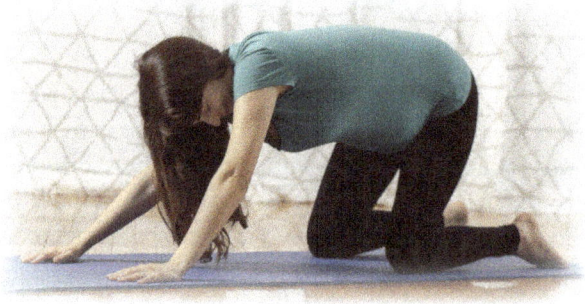

the sacrum and pubic bone. The caution here is around big movements, especially for those coping with pubic bone or SI joint pain. If the pelvic joints are not stable, then shifting side to side without awareness and support can bring further wear and tear rather than stability and freedom. This variation is often a movement women in labor drop into instinctively. The tilting and tucking combined with lateral swaying subtly changes the internal space within the pelvis, sometimes helping to make space for baby to descend and rotate.

Balasana/Child's Pose

Along with the back release found in Cat/Cow, the gentle flexion of Child's Pose can also be

of great benefit for those with lower back pain. This pose not only gently stretches the spinal muscles but also slackens the deep hip flexor, the psoas. Allowing the psoas to shorten can remove pressure on lower back joints being compressed by muscle tension. Balasana can also be a great place to rest and restore the parasympathetic nervous system during a more vigorous practice.

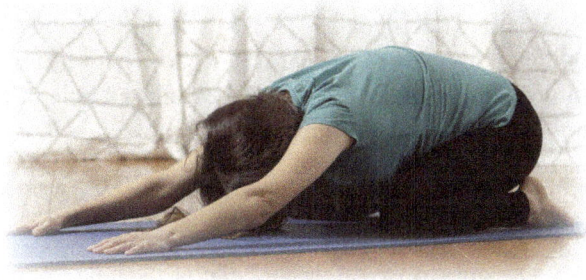

Note: for those with tight abdominal and pelvic fascia who may experience tense round or broad ligaments, the abdominal pressure of Balasana—even with the knees spread wide to accommodate the belly—may feel uncomfortable. If that's the case, focus less on bringing the head to the floor and more on finding space and rest in whatever shape is manageable.

From Table, bring the feet together and widen the knees enough to accommodate the belly. Do not go so wide as to place pressure on the pubic bone. Rather, simply create enough space for the belly to snuggle between the inner thighs without compressing the breath.

Sit the hips back to the heels and allow the spine to drape forward. The arms can either extend forward or rest under the shoulders. The head may come to the floor if that is easy, or it can rest on a bolster or block.

Breathe comfortably and easily, allowing the weight of the body to be supported by the earth. This pose can also be a great place to practice feeling the movement of the pelvic floor, releasing on an inhale and gently drawing inwards on the exhale.

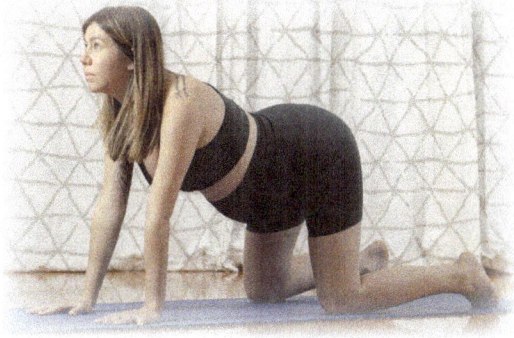

Chakravakasana/Rocking Child's Pose

Chakravakasana, drawn from the Viniyoga tradition, combines Balasana and Cat/Cow in a fluid sequence.

Beginning in a comfortable Balasana, inhale to rock your hips forward into a small variation of Cow. The knees may stay wide or come slightly together if the hips require. On the exhale, reverse the movement, returning to Child's Pose and allowing the spine to

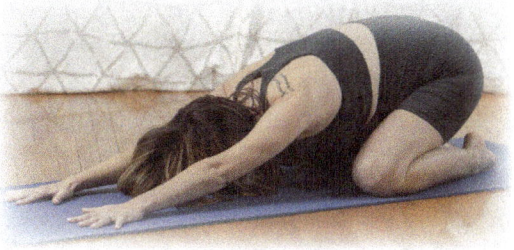

round. The motion gently massages the spine, and also the hips and legs, gently pumping circulation through the whole system.

When timed with the breath, this action also mimics the movements many mothers naturally slide into during labor as they ride the surging sensations of contractions through their bodies. This pose is a great way to both begin to warm the joints and also to quiet down the mind after an active day. It has become a staple in many of my prenatal yoga classes. It also combines nicely with hip circles in Table, which is another natural labor coping technique I have often seen mothers use.

Downward Dog

Ah, Downward Dog. Possibly one of the best known yoga shapes, and of course, one of the key postures in a classic *vinyasa* flow sequence. I have always loved Downward Dog as both a stretch for the hamstrings and as a wonderful way to elongate the spine in dynamic movement. As we discovered in Chapter 6, Downward Dog isn't contraindicated for pregnancy, but there are a few modifications pregnant yoginis may wish to make for safety and ease.

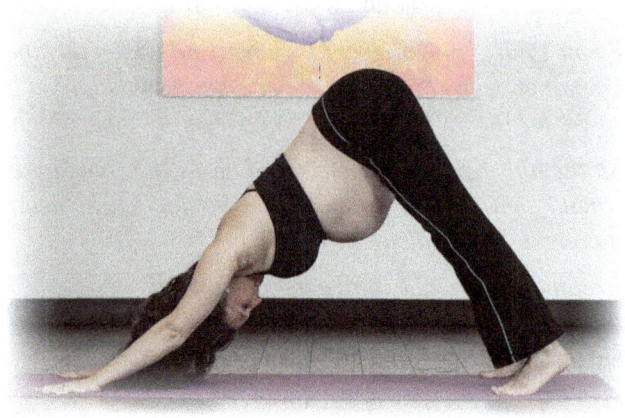

The added weight on the upper body brings extra challenge to Downward Dog, especially if this posture was already strenuous for an expectant mother. So for starters, the duration of this pose may be shorter. If we are not practicing in a flow, we might switch the classic inverted posture for the "L" shape variation described later in this section. If mom has been experiencing heartburn, going upside down may not feel so good either. In this case, either modifying to the "L" shape or keeping the head elevated and looking at the hands can help her maintain an open chest and reduce acid reflux.

Begin in Table posture with the toes tucked under. Inhale to open the chest and lightly raise the sitz bones towards Cow pose. On an exhale, press the hands and feet into the floor, raising the hips up and back, aiming for an upside down "V" shape. Start with the knees bent.

The first aim of this asana is to lengthen the spine. The second is to bring the heels towards the floor. Focus on creating a long line from the head to the tail, paying special attention to creating the curve of the lumbar spine. Avoid thrusting the chest. As the knees do straighten, be sure to keep the front of the ankle open (i.e., skin not wrinkling up) so the joint is not compressed, and maintain the lift of the sitz bones to prevent the tail from tucking. Imagine a broom handle being laid along the spine, with the end of the pole between the hands. Stretch the spine along the line of the broom handle, maintaining contact throughout the whole back and sacrum.

The arms spiral into the shoulders, but the shoulder blades will elevate towards the ears as though reaching for something on a high shelf. Watch that the neck is not compressed or tense. The head hangs easily with the ears resting in between the upper arms, ultimately continuing the lengthening line of the spine. If you're experiencing heartburn, raise the head to gaze at the hands or spend less time in Downward Dog.

Ground evenly through all four corners of the hands, and feel the sitz bones move backwards as though pressing into a wall. Finish either by returning the knees to the floor or by walking the hands and feet together.

Downward Dog "L" Shape Variation

For those with tender wrists, intense heartburn, or severe high blood pressure who should not be inverting, there is also the "half dog" or "L" shape variation of Downward Dog at the wall.

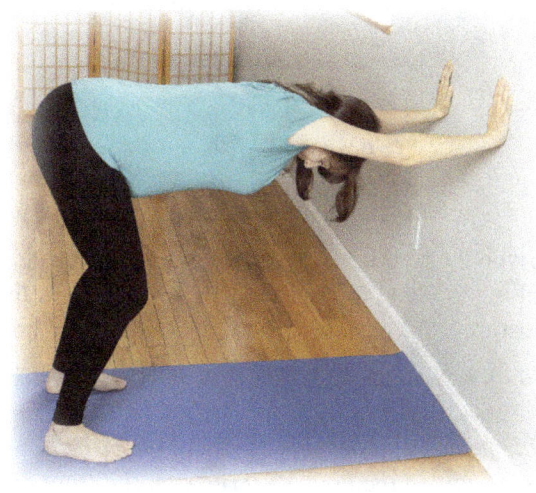

Standing with the feet hip distance apart, press the hands into the wall around hip height, then walk the feet back until the spine comes horizontal and the feet rest under the hips, creating a 90 degree angle.

Work to extend the hips backwards, elongating the spine. Watch for the belly or ribs drooping lower than the hips, and draw them up. The aim is for a long spine, not a backbend. Bend the knees to begin, and press the sitz bones back as though sitting on the opposite wall. Breathe smoothly and evenly.

Seated postures: hip openers and stabilizers

Hip openers are key in birth preparation. Toning the inner and outer hip muscles helps promote stability and suppleness within the pelvis. And since many of the hip rotators also connect into the pelvic floor, balancing their tone can lead to better pelvic floor tone and function.

In any seated posture, just as in the standing ones, it is key to establish a solid, balanced foundation from which the pose can then arise. For seated postures, the foundation is the pelvis. More specifically, it's the triangle created by the sitz bones and the pubis. As we discussed in Chapter 2, when the pelvis is in neutral alignment there is a slight forward tilt to the pelvic bowl. When seated, this means we rest on the front edge of our sitz bones with the pubic symphysis tilted slightly downward. Another way to think of it would be that if a light were shining from the navel, the beam would be pointing across or slightly down towards the ground.

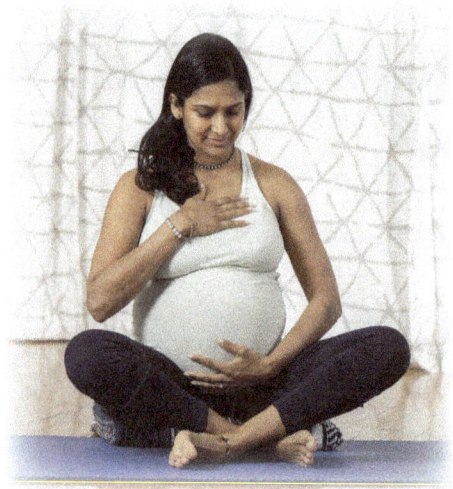

Sukhasana/Easy Pose/Sweet Pose

As the name of this pose suggests, the pelvic alignment here should feel "easy." This is not to say that there is no effort involved but rather that the effort feels pleasant and natural.

For many people, tight glutes, hamstrings, and lower back muscles make finding the sweet spot on the front of the sitz bones challenging. While these imbalances can all eventually be remedied with other yoga postures, in the meantime it is worth elevating the pelvis on props so that it can tilt forward with greater ease. During pregnancy, it's especially important to maintain this forward tilt, as it allows gravity to move the baby's body into the optimal position for birth: head down, facing mom's spine.[46]

Given the frequency with which this posture is used in both yoga and meditation, it is worth taking the time to find good alignment for it. Just as Tadasana is the foundation for standing postures, Sukhasana is the foundation for seated ones.

Sit on a blanket, yoga block, or bolster so the knees are at or slightly lower than the crest of the hips. Cross the legs loosely, either at the ankle or the middle of the shin bone. Shift gently side to side and become aware of your sitz bones buried within the gluteal muscles. Now shift the weight of the body so it rests on the front of those bones.

Allow the spine to stretch up tall but without stiffness or rigidity. Stack the head over the shoulders, the ribs, and the hips. Feel the stable, wide base of the pelvis and legs resting into the floor. Allow the chest to be open and the belly to be soft. Place the hands either on the tops of the thighs or in whatever position feels meaningful for you at the moment. Breathe normally, allowing yourself to simply rest in the dignity of sitting.

Baddha Konasana/Butterfly Pose/Bound Angle/Tailor's Pose

I think almost every pregnant yogini has had her picture taken in this posture! And yet it can also be one of the most challenging *asanas* for those who struggle with tight hips. Baddha Konasana can be fabulous for toning the pelvic floor, releasing inner and outer hip rotators, and developing pelvic balance—but as always, too much of a good thing is still too much!

Seated on a blanket or block as for Sukhasana, bring the pelvis to balance on the front of the sitz bones with the navel tilting slightly downward. From here, bring the soles of the feet together and draw them in towards the pelvis until there is a light stretch on the inner thighs.

---

[46] The heaviest part of the baby is the spine and back of the head. Left to its own devices, this part will naturally move to the lowest point in the pelvic bowl. Since we want the back of the head to rest on the front side of the pelvis, ideal pelvic positioning is to bring the pubic bone towards the lowest point to promote gravity rotating the spine forwards.

The feet should not be so close that the pelvis rocks backwards, so find a middle path, not too close and not too far.

Anchor the pubic bone down while simultaneously grounding the tailbone. This will energetically bring the two points of the pelvis towards one another, activating the pelvic floor. Place the hands behind the hips and stretch up through the spine. At the same time, feel the thighs moving outwards and the sitz bones spreading slightly apart.[47]

If looking for gentle hip opening, lean forward from the hip joints, maintaining a straight spine for the first 1/3 of the distance towards the floor. If you cannot fold further than this anyway, then you have arrived and need not keep bending. Just breathe and observe the stretch. If you stop at this point, you will also be able to maintain an open chest.

If the hips are flexible enough to keep going, then the spine will need to round slightly (as it would in Balasana) so the SI joints in the back of the pelvis aren't strained. This is a very subtle rounding, and if your hips don't yet have the range of motion, the body will borrow movement from other joints. Only fold as far as you can without straining or borrowing movement. Breathe and enjoy the gentle stretch. Inhale to return to sitting.

Pelvic pain variation

If you have been struggling with pelvic pain, actively press the soles of the feet together and draw the thighs into rather than out of the hip sockets. Remain upright. This will cause the knees to lift slightly, but if the pelvis has been uncomfortable this is not a bad thing as it compresses the joints rather than applying further stretching.

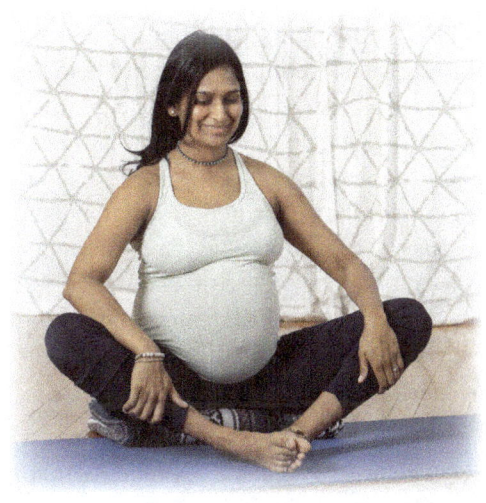

Pelvic stabilizing variation

From an upright Baddha Konasana, place either your hands or elbows on the knees. Breathing smoothly, use the hands to lightly press the knees outwards, but at the same time actively

---

[47] For those struggling with pain at the pubic bone, draw the thighs inward rather than out, as described in the pelvic pain variation.

press the knees into the hands. There won't be any major movement, but you'll feel the muscles of the inner hip and leg working. Press to about 50% activation.

Moving in time with your breathing, switch the hands to hold the outsides of the knees and gently pull up while actively pressing the knees down into the hands. This will fire the outer hip rotators. Continue switching directions back and forth, following the tempo of the breath. Work up to 10 times in each direction. When you are finished, sit up and extend the legs in front to shake them out.

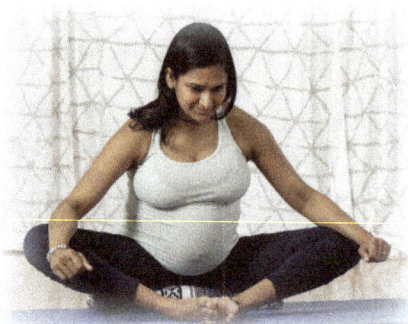
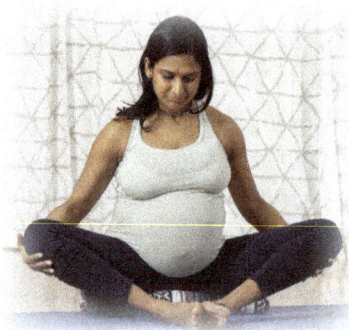

This action is similar to the one described above in the block variation of the wall squat, but externally rotating the knees can bring more activation directly to the internal and external rotators. It is key to maintain a neutral pelvis and only activate to 50% of what you feel you could. This will help prevent overworking and straining the pelvic joints that have already been loosened by pregnancy hormones.

Janu Sirsasana/Head to Knee Pose

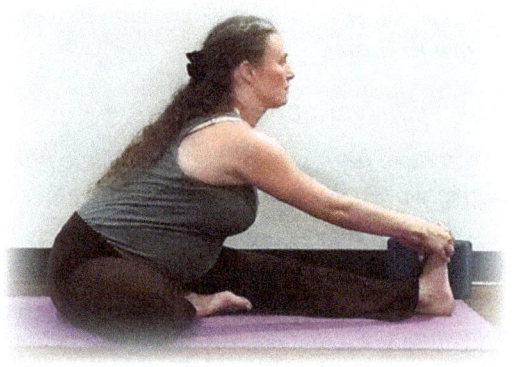

Along with the symmetrical hip openers, there is also the Janu Sirsasana family, which allows for release of the hip rotators and also the hamstrings and adductors. Done gently, these postures can help release the sacrum and lower back with subtle twists and flexion. Done too vigorously, however, and… you may be able to guess where I'm going here. Too much of a good thing is *still* too much, and doing too much here can lead to strain in the SI joints. Apply the law of 50% diligently, progressing further only if it seems easeful.

Begin in Baddha Konasana, with the hips elevated if necessary to come easily to the front of the sitz bones. Extend the right leg forward, bringing the left heel against the right inner thigh. It is not necessary to pull the foot in close to the groin, and this should be avoided if there is a history of hypermobility or hip pain, as extreme ranges of motion can promote pelvic instability.

Inhale to stretch up through the spine. Exhale, turn to face the extended leg, and bend forward, moving from the hip. As in Baddha Konasana, it is critical that you maintain a flat back during the first part of this motion rather than allowing the spine to round.

If it's early in your pregnancy, bring the belly to face towards the extended thigh while maintaining a lengthened spine. Remember, due to the high amount of relaxin in your system, especially during the first trimester, this is not a time to try and force or pull the chest to the leg. If you are further along in pregnancy, the bottom of the abdomen will begin to snuggle into the top of the thigh. Consider this a natural reminder to back off from a deep range of motion.

If able, you can reach out to grab the ankle or toes and draw up against the pull of the leg. If unable to reach (and let's be honest—this is going to be more common during pregnancy), hook the foot with a yoga strap and pull upwards against the press of the foot. The stretch is for both the outer rotators of the bent knee as well as the hamstring of the extended leg. Maintain a long spine.

To release, simply inhale and sit up, letting go of the foot or strap. Bring the extended leg back into Baddha Konasana and reset the sitz bones evenly before repeating on the second side.

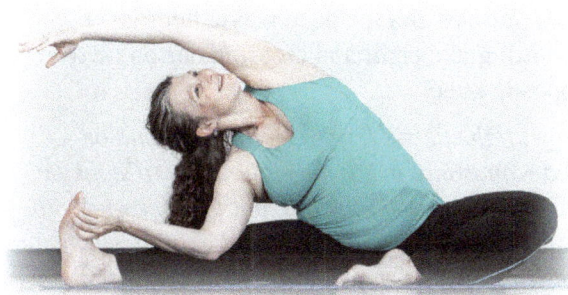

Parivritta Janu Sirsasana/Rotated Head to Knee Pose

Parivritta Janu Sirsasana is a somewhat simpler variation that can be done during pregnancy. It offers a delicious stretch for the side body through rotation. While this rotated side bend can create length through the quadratus lumborum and intercostals (the muscles of the lower back and between the ribs), it is key not to lock the pelvis in place here, since fixing the pelvic bowl can lead to excessive strain at the SI joint. The weight may shift on the sitz bones, but as long as you don't tip over, it is allowable for one hip to lift slightly.

Beginning in Baddha Konasana, with elevated hips if need be, extend the right leg out to the side. The angle will depend on your flexibility, but a good benchmark is that the sitz bones remain grounded and the outer hip does not cramp.

Inhale, stretching the right arm overhead and feeling for length in the right side body. On an exhale, shift the ribs right and reach out over the extended leg, as though you were going to lay the whole right side of the body along the right thigh. This will help maintain the length on the right side body as you stretch the left.

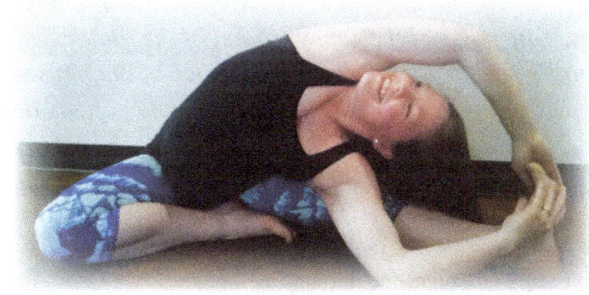

With the chest stretched out towards the thigh, inhale to bring the left arm out at shoulder height. Turn the left palm

towards the floor, and on an exhale sweep the left hand out in front and up across the cheek, as though clearing off a table in front of you. The result will be that the left arm slides into the extended shoulder position without twisting the arm bone. With the arm by the left cheek, rotate the torso to bring the gaze under the arm and look upwards.

Return by inhaling to sit up lowering the arm. Pause to feel the lingering sensation on the left side of the lower back, then return the right foot into Baddha Konasana. Re-center and try the second side.

Agnistambhasana/Ankle to Knee/Fire Logs/Double Pigeon

This more targeted stretch for the glutes and piriformis muscles is effectively a variation of Sukhasana with the ankle stacked on the opposite knee. This variation can be a prep for deeper hip openers (think lotus pose) but the foot further forward than lotus allows for greater contact with the deep hip muscles. A great stretch for those dealing with sciatica, this posture can also be quite challenging. Go gently, and be patient with your body.

The good news is that even minor releases here can be of benefit during the birth process because of the interplay between the piriformis muscles and the deep pelvic floor layer. An alternative and less intense variation involves sitting in a chair and crossing one ankle over the opposite knee.

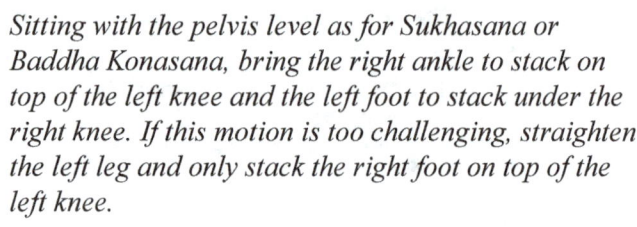

Sitting with the pelvis level as for Sukhasana or Baddha Konasana, bring the right ankle to stack on top of the left knee and the left foot to stack under the right knee. If this motion is too challenging, straighten the left leg and only stack the right foot on top of the left knee.

Actively flex the toes, stretching through the inner ankle to create muscular and energetic support for the knees. Inhale and stretch up through the spine. For many, this will be a sufficient stretch in the outer hip. In that case, simply bring your attention to the sensations and observe how things change.

To further focus the stretch into the piriformis, press the thumbs into the top of the thighs at your hip creases. You may feel the ropey tendon of the quadriceps popping up. Pressing down on this area both grounds the thighs into the back of the hip sockets and helps to activate a reflex in the muscles[48] which relaxes the tendons and softens the hips.

If you can go deeper, gently fold forward, maintaining an open chest and as neutral a spine as possible (the lower back should not round for the first half of the movement). This action

---

[48] This reflex is known as the Golgi Tendon Reflex, which inhibits a muscle from further firing when it perceives excessive tension on the surrounding fascia.

will bring the belly closer to the shins, as though working to snuggle it into the triangle made by the thighs and shins.

The knees should not be involved in this posture. If there is any sensation or pain in the knee joint, either place a yoga block underneath one or both knees for support or back out of the pose (or do both!). Maintain the flexion in the top ankle to engage muscle support around the base of the knee.

Bring your attention to the sensations of the outer hip stretch and observe how things change. To switch sides, sit up and extend the legs out fully for a moment, shaking them in and out to reset before stacking the left shin on top for the second side.

Chair variation

For those with extensive pelvic pain or extremely tight hips (most of the non-yogi population!), the glute and piriformis stretch can also be recreated sitting in a chair, with the sitting bones well balanced and one ankle crossed over the opposite knee.

Sit on a solid chair with the feet placed on the floor and the spine and pelvis upright. Lift the right leg and cross the ankle over the left knee, creating a figure 4 shape with the legs. Maintain an upright pelvis, and flex the working foot to avoid twisting the knee joint. The bottom foot should remain planted on the floor.

To deepen, anchor the hip crease with the thumb and index finger, possibly externally rotating the femur bone. Grounding the femur, rather than leaning forward, will help focus the stretch into the back hip muscles and avoid borrowing from the spine.

A labor preparation practice

Because this posture can bring on strong sensations, it can also be useful in preparing to work with the mind during intense experiences. Try this inner investigation during any of the previous pose variations.

Having found a stretching sensation to focus on within the posture, bring your attention to that space, and become curious about how the feeling unfolds as you gently stay.

Is the sensation a feeling of burning? Pressure? Pulling?

Is there only one sensation or a combination of several?

Do the sensations stay the same, or do they shift as you stay?

What thoughts or feelings arise as you focus on these sensations?

Is there a storyline you are telling yourself? Is it helpful?

Do you feel a desire to push further? To pull back? What is your habitual tendency when you come up against an edge during practice?

Watching our responses to the sensations within our bodies, especially when coupled with steady breathing, can help develop increased mental stamina during challenging situations.

Obviously the analogy here is being willing to feel the strong sensations of contractions during labor, but that isn't the only application for moms-to-be.

The postpartum period has numerous situations which bring up strong emotions (sleep "training" comes to mind). Possessing the ability to not simply react, but to take a moment to pause and observe, can be the difference between feeling overwhelmed and feeling capable. Additionally, while the sensation of hip openers isn't akin to labor contractions—at least to most people—the ability to investigate any strong sensation builds the ability to stay present with other situations. This is one of the hidden benefits to practicing yoga during pregnancy. Even if we ultimately choose pain relief, such as with an epidural, we do so from a more centered and focused place.

Gomukhasana/Cow Face Pose

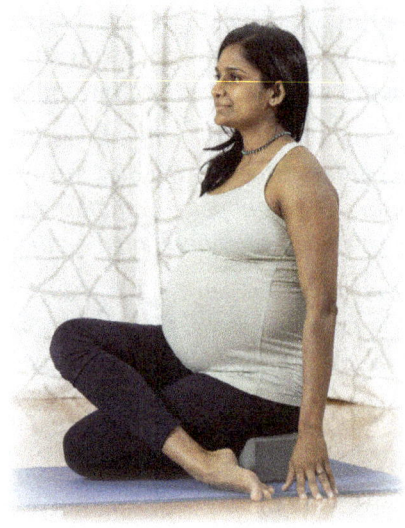

Gomukhasana is a hip opener that many people discount during pregnancy because it requires a deep cross of the thighs at the groin. In its original form, this posture can displace the pubis joint and possibly compress the baby's head as it moves into the lower uterine segment.

Properly modified however, this pose can be one of the only ways to stretch some of the outer hip rotators and medial glutes, which can become extremely tight due to their dual role of movement and stability within the pelvis. And that's not even mentioning the fabulous shoulder stretches which can accompany this posture!

The easiest way to come into this posture during pregnancy is to back into it. Begin in Table pose. Cross the left leg behind the right so that the thighs cross. From here, separate the feet wide enough to make space for the hips and begin to sit the pelvis back, aiming for coming to rest in between the heels.

Allow the thighs to slope down away from the belly, and point the navel forward or slightly down. If you are early on in your pregnancy, and your belly has not yet expanded to where it would press against your thighs, then you may be able to sit fully down onto the floor, but be sure to place the sitz bones solidly onto the earth or a blanket.

If your belly begins to feel compressed or your hips do not have the range to reach the floor, place a yoga block between the heels, high enough that both sitz bones can come to rest on it. If you need the highest height of the block, I recommend using two blocks stacked on their lowest level for greater stability.

Bring the pelvis to rest evenly on the block or floor and sit up tall. The feet can be pulled back almost against the outer hips for one hip stretch, or the shins can gradually be brought forwards until possibly parallel with the front of the mat for a different stretch. Neither stretch is right or wrong, it simply depends on where your body is holding its tension. Since this posture is slightly asymmetrical and also binds the bottom leg in place, be careful of any pulling in the knees or ankles; pain in the knees should be addressed, not ignored.

If combining the hip opener with the shoulder stretch for this posture, bring the opposite arm from the top leg overhead (the left arm in this case), and rotate the arm so the palm spins to face the back of the mat. Rotate from the shoulders, not the elbow or wrist.

Bend the left elbow, reaching the hand down the back, possibly assisting with the right hand. The arm spins so that the left hand moves towards the left shoulder blade rather than across the midline. If this is a sufficient stretch into the triceps and rotator cuff, then remain here. If you wish to add the other shoulder, reach the right arm out to the side, rotating the thumb to point down, and then reach behind to see if

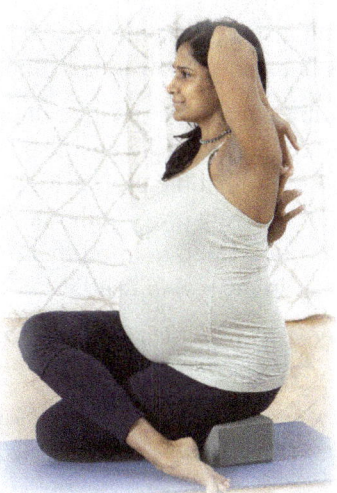 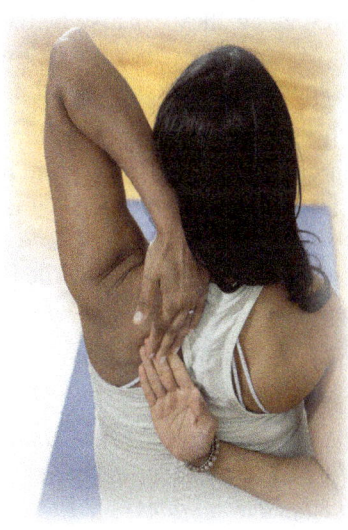

the hands can touch. Gently hold while maintaining the inward spin of the top arm.

If the hands cannot reach, you can use a yoga strap in the top hand to bridge the gap. Be careful not to allow the top shoulder to swing wide as this puts the shoulder integrity at risk.

To release, lower the hands and lean forward onto the palms. Shift the hips forward and uncross the legs, returning to Table pose. Take a couple of Cat/Cow motions to feel the impact on your hips and lower back, and then cross the other leg behind and repeat for the second side.

Eka Pada Rajakapotasana/Pigeon Pose

Ah, the ever-popular Pigeon hip opener. I have always loved this posture for the dual stretch it can bring to the outer hip muscles and the back leg psoas muscle.

We can enter Pigeon in one of two ways—from all fours or from sitting using props.

From Table or Downward Dog, slide the right shin forward to place the knee on the outside of the right wrist, shin on the ground (yes, this is wider than we often use for classic practice, as we must once again make room for baby in this pose). Wiggle the right foot across the mat until it comes to rest directly in front of the pubic bone (this will externally rotate the thigh). From here, scoot the left leg back, working to sit the hips down towards the floor behind the right heel. Anchor the pelvis evenly right to left on the mat or onto props to create a solid base. Inhale to lift the chest, then exhale to walk the hands forward, bringing the chest towards the floor. Feel for space in the right hip, and use the hands to press the sitz bones into the floor.

To come out, either walk the hands back in and slide back to all fours for the second side or sit down onto the right hip and then use the hands to bring the left leg around before returning to Table/Downward Dog for the second side.

Pigeon with a bolster

While hip openers are vital for relieving tension and balancing the pelvic floor during pregnancy, they can also be tricky due to extra hip mobility and the potential to borrow movement from above or below a tight spot. In asymmetrical postures like Pigeon, there is potential to affect not only the hips but also the lower back and knee joints.

Pigeon becomes a more active posture during pregnancy rather than being an opportunity to simply sink into the floor and hang in the hips. When using a bolster or rolled blanket for a hip opener such as Pigeon, it is important that the prop is high enough to remove any torque or strain in the hip joints. In addition, actively press both knees into the floor to activate the pelvic support muscles while in this pose. Keep in mind that injuries frequently occur in the entry and exit to this pose rather than in the *asana* itself.

Begin sitting in Sukhasana on the bolster, with the right leg crossed in front. Moving carefully, swing the right leg over to the side, and internally rotate to sit with the feet tucked to the side.

Placing blocks under the hands if needed, extend the right leg straight behind its hip. Press down on the blocks to lift the chest and open the heart, feeling both hips sit fully down into the bolster support.

Inhale to lift the chest, and then lean forward onto the blocks with an exhale. Rest against the blocks or lower down to the floor. Because of the bolster, the chest will not touch the ground, so be willing to stay elevated as needed. Exit by sitting onto one hip as described in the all fours section. Repeat on the second side.

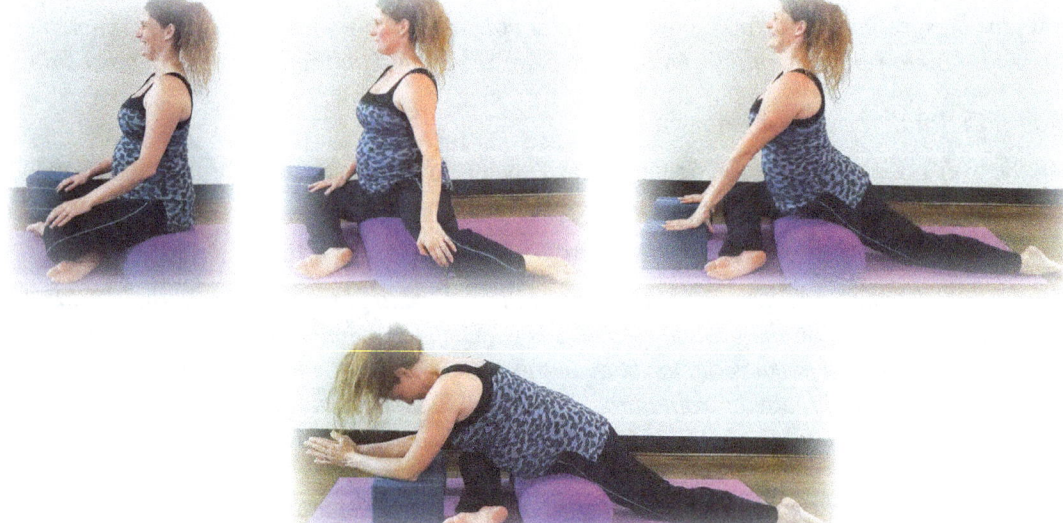

Vajrasana/Thunderbolt

Along with the hip openers focused on external rotation, the seated postures which address the internal hip rotation and extension are also key practices during pregnancy. Releasing and balancing the psoas and hip flexors can have a dramatic impact on the space available in the pelvis for the baby to descend and can also improve lower back and pelvic floor function.

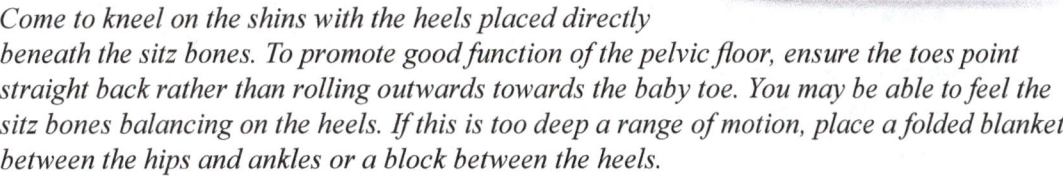

A seemingly simple posture, Vajrasana can be surprisingly effective in balancing the legs, and the position of the ankles and knees can also affect the pelvis and pelvic floor. Like Tadasana, this one posture can have rippling impacts on other seated and standing postures.

Come to kneel on the shins with the heels placed directly beneath the sitz bones. To promote good function of the pelvic floor, ensure the toes point straight back rather than rolling outwards towards the baby toe. You may be able to feel the sitz bones balancing on the heels. If this is too deep a range of motion, place a folded blanket between the hips and ankles or a block between the heels.

Bring the pelvis to rest on the front edge of the sitz bones, allowing the belly to point downward towards the thighs. The spine stretches softly upwards with a quiet dignity, as though resting a crown on the top of the head. As the head stretches upwards, the inner groins softly descend, grounding the pubic bone and inner thighs to match the anchor of the tail.

Breathe smoothly, feeling the pressure of gravity and the body pressing into the earth, and the subtle rebound upwards through the body's center and pelvic floor. The gaze is cast softly downward, with a quiet but steady focus.

If the ankles are uncomfortable, a rolled blanket can be placed beneath the front of the ankle joint to reduce the extension required. Additionally, many people will prefer to have a blanket unfolded beneath the entire shin to soften the surface of the mat.

Virasana/Hero(ine) Pose

While Virasana looks similar to Vajrasana, its function is actually quite different. Virasana incorporates an internal rotation of the femur bone into the leg position and shifts the feet outside rather than beneath the hips. This internal rotation widens the sitz bones and also brings the stretch more fully into the psoas, especially in the reclining variation known as Supta Virasana (described in the restorative posture section of this book).

Begin by kneeling on the mat with the knees and shins together. Lean forwards, and separate the feet slightly wider than the hips, keeping the toes pointed straight back. With your thumbs, grab the calves and draw the muscles away from the backs of the knees, towards the heels.

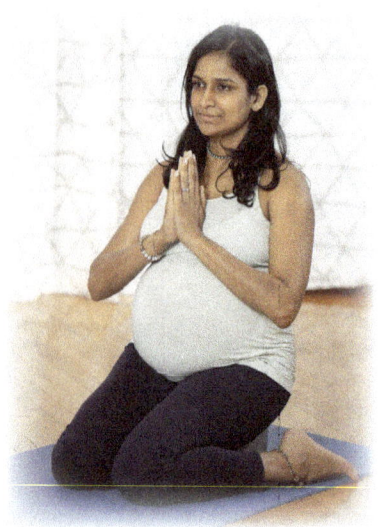

This does not mean roll the calf to the outside of the shin! Rolling outwards can twist the fascia around the knees, leading to injury. Instead, pull the middle of the calf back, creating space behind the knees as you sit back.[49]

With the backs of the knees cleared, sit the hips back, bringing the sitz bones to the floor between the feet. Make sure the tail does not tuck under, as this will round the lower back and disconnect the integration into the pelvic floor. If the pelvis cannot reach the floor, place a block beneath the sitz bones high enough to provide support. For cranky feet, place a rolled blanket beneath the ankles as for Vajrasana.

Draw the sitz bones back so the pelvis rests on the front edge of them once again. While classic yoga keeps the knees drawn together, during pregnancy it may be necessary to widen the legs to make space for the uterus and baby. Regardless, keep the toes pointed straight back and preserve good pelvic alignment.

Stretch the spine gently upwards, and feel the depth of the groins and gentle spreading of the pelvic floor as you breathe. To come out, shift forward into Table and gently extend one leg, then the other, allowing blood flow to return to the lower legs.

Note: because of the deep knee bend, this posture does temporarily compress the veins of the lower legs. If you are experiencing swelling or varicose veins, this is not advisable. Instead, elevate the hips high enough to maintain a soft space behind the knees. This way blood can keep flowing and not stress already strained tissues and blood vessels.

Malasana/Squat

We couldn't talk prenatal yoga without discussing the squat! This is the mythical birthing position supposedly used by all women of ancient times…ok, maybe it was. We can't be fully sure, but we do know they were not birthing lying down on their backs.

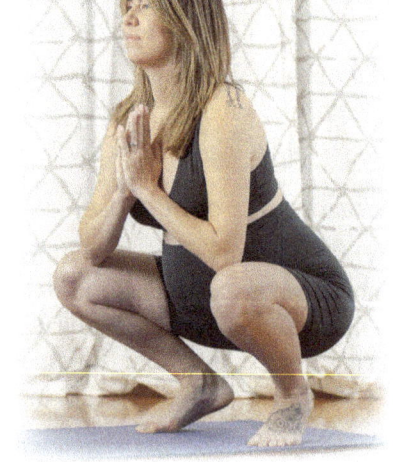

There are certain qualities of the squat which favor the childbirth process. It is an active posture that promotes the natural expulsive reflex built into the body. Depending on the position of the pelvis, squatting can also align the baby's head more directly with the birth path and with the

---

[49]   Also be sure to actually move your thumb out of the way, I have seen a number of students attempt to create space and then leave their thumbs in the back of their knees as they sat down, thereby filling the very space they'd created!

plumb line of gravity—forward tilting helps, while tucking is usually less effective, depending on the baby's pelvic station. Additionally, pressing the thighs into the upper wings of the pelvic bowl, combined with internal femur rotation, can make extra space in the outlet (lower segment) of the pelvis, creating more room for the baby's head to emerge.

If all that wasn't reason enough to practice squats, widening and lengthening the pubic and tail bones promotes toning and better function of the entire pelvic floor. Simply put, squatting can be a key posture to practice throughout pregnancy.

There are several places to be mindful of alignment when squatting during pregnancy. When practicing for birth preparation, the feet should remain as parallel as possible. This promotes the sitz bones spreading and tones the pelvic diaphragm. While a squat with a tucked pelvis may stretch the lower back muscles, it is not helpful if our aim is to prepare the pelvis to bear the weight of pregnancy and be in good balance to give birth. External femur rotation, combined with the spine rounded as in Cat Pose, closes the sitz bones; internal rotation, combined with the spine arched as in Cow Pose, opens them.

When you come into a squat with the knees spread as wide as possible, there is likely to be sensation around the sitz bones and towards the anus. When the thighs are strongly externally rotated, the back pelvic triangle closes. But that back triangle is where the baby begins to emerge… not what we're looking for in birth!

Compare this to a squat where the feet remain parallel and the hips tilt forward. The heels may have to leave the floor, but the sitz bones may spread another inch or more, and the area between the sitz bones and anus widens.

Begin in Tadasana with the feet a comfortable distance apart and the toes pointed forward. Inhale. On an exhale, bend the knees, lowering the hips halfway towards the floor. Rest the arms on the thighs. This half squat position is a perfectly workable variation for those with knee challenges, pelvic instability, low lying placenta/placenta previa, varicose veins, or if the baby is in a breech position.

If you are not in any of these categories and wish to go further, continue bending the knees, lowering the hips down until they are either as low as they will go or until you feel content with the depth. The toes should remain pointed forward, and the pelvis should tilt forward, with the pubic bone moving towards the floor and the sitz bones spreading back. At its full range, the body rests against the thighs and the posture takes very little effort. That said, not many pregnant people are comfortably able to sink into this range.

Squatting with the toes forward often creates difficulty in keeping the heels on the floor: the result of tension in the calves, glutes, and lower back. This tension makes it difficult to lower without shifting the center of gravity too far backwards to remain standing. Rather than tucking the tail as a counterweight, try placing a rolled blanket or towel under the heels to allow the pelvis to maintain its forward tilt while maintaining stability under the feet.

To return to standing, exhale and place the hands on the floor or the knees. Straighten the legs, then inhale to return to Tadasana.

If you are working to tone the pelvic floor, inhale while descending into the squat, feeling the pelvic floor spread. As you exhale, draw the pelvic floor upwards for the return, taking as many breaths as needed in between.

Wall Squat

I have found this squat variation to be helpful during pregnancy in several ways. It tones the legs, inner thighs, and glutes, helping to promote pelvic stability. It also builds physical stamina, helpful in overall body health. But I have found the Wall Squat to be especially useful in birth preparation. It offers the opportunity to work with strong sensations in a controlled way, gradually increasing mental focus and presence while also confronting fear (quite helpful during the birth process).

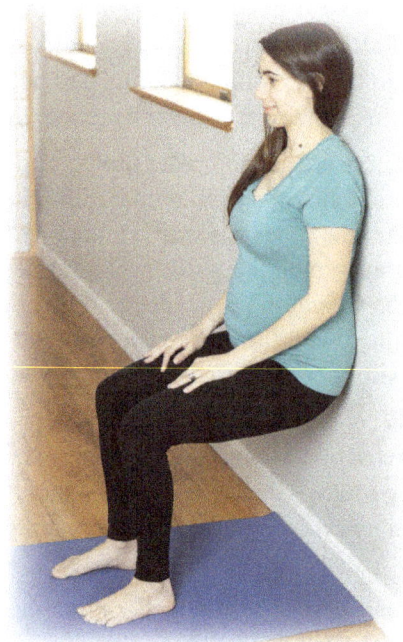

As the length of the hold increases, so does the sensation. In my prenatal yoga classes, we will often use this as a mock contraction simulation, incorporating deep pelvic breathing and mindful awareness of our reactions as we gradually build the hold up to one minute (approximately the length of one contraction during active labor). The sensations of this squat are not what one might feel during labor, but they do offer a chance to observe how the mind may spiral into a "fear-tension-pain" cycle. They also allow for mental training through steady breathing and meditative focus.

Adding a block hold between the knees in the Wall Squat can further increase pelvic floor engagement. Pulsing the inner thighs helps coordinate the connection between the adductors and the first two layers of the pelvic floor. It can be useful for those coping with a hypotonic pelvic floor, but for those with too much tension, the release exercises described in Chapter 3 should be a precursor to any strengthening activities.

Come to stand with your back against the wall. Lean backwards, and walk your feet about two feet away from the wall. On an exhale, bend the knees, sliding the hips down the wall until the thighs come approximately parallel to the floor. The actual angle will depend on individual leg strength and knee function. The knees should be directly over the heels and definitely not in front of the toes.

Press the upper back and tailbone softly into the wall, and rest the palms on the thighs. Begin gradually deepening the breath, observing how the sensation in the thighs begins to build. Watch how the mind may begin to spiral into positive or negative thought patterns. Be gentle with your body, and do not force yourself to stay longer than is workable (if the only thought going through your head is "OW!" and you are suffering, it is time to come out).

Stay with the sensation, and practice keeping the breath steady and deep throughout. At the end of the minute—or whenever your legs demand a break—simply straighten your knees and stand up. Shake out the legs, possibly stretch the quads, and feel the sense of relief within your body.

Block variation

If you have pelvic instability or incontinence from overly loose pelvic floor muscles, place a block between the knees in the Wall Squat. On the inhale, just hold the block, on the exhale, press the block with the legs. Press for the full exhale, then relax on the inhale. Repeat pulsing and releasing for 5 rounds, then take a break. Repeat with the block closer to the groin.

Non-focused awareness variation

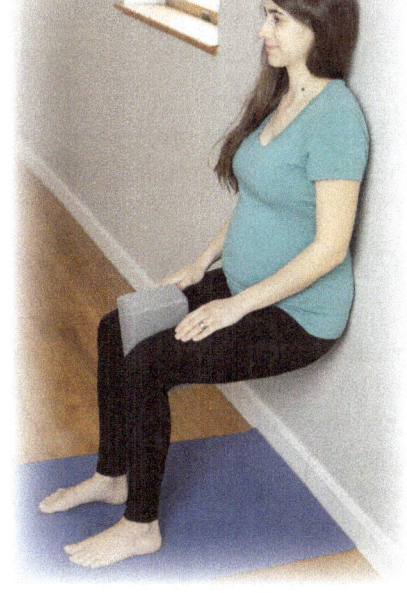

If you are using the Wall Squat to simulate contractions, have a timer you can use to measure one minute. After you complete the exercise with the timer, try this varia-tion to see how your focus affects your experience.

Without looking at the timer, come into the Wall Squat as described earlier. Focus your attention solely on the flow of your breathing. Hear the sound of your breath, and let it anchor the mind. Perhaps expand your aware-ness to take in immediate sounds, smells, or other sensory experiences beyond the sensation in the legs. When your body demands you come out, come out.

Now take a look at the clock. Was that longer or shorter than a minute? Don't beat yourself up if it was not what you expected. This is simply an exercise in awareness. For some, put-ting the focus on an external object helps them stay with a sensation longer. For others, the internal focus on the breath and body is actually what allows for greater mental and physical stamina. The point is to come to know your own mind more clearly.

Shifting perspective

A point I often raise in classes is that the Wall Squat is *not* what labor feels like. Not only do we not feel labor in our thighs (usually), but the sensations in labor are not constant. Even if contractions last up to 60 seconds during active labor, they only occur every four to five minutes. Even at the height of labor it's not unusual for contractions to still be three minutes apart.

That may seem like a short interval, but here's another perspective. If your contractions last one minute, and they come three minutes apart, that means that for every minute you are in a contraction, there are two minutes when you are not.[50] You spend twice as much time

---

[50] Contractions are measured from the start of one to the start of the next.

relaxing as you do in the contraction. As a power yoga teacher I know once said, "You can do anything for one minute."

The key to labor isn't actually what you do during the contraction. That's the easy part! You sway, rock, breathe, and do whatever your body finds most useful to help ease your pelvis open. The real question is: What are you doing between contractions? Are you anxiously worrying about the next one? Or do you take that time to rest, drink, eat, and relax so you are ready for the next contraction—whenever it arrives?

If labor lasts 14 hours (average for a first time mom), the amount of time you are actually contracting might be only 2-3 hours total! What are you doing for the other 11-12 hours? That's the real question. And that's where it's helpful to be able to relax and let go of a contraction once it is over.

Ananda Balasana/Happy Baby

Happy Baby is simply a squat that is rotated on its back, but that shift can have dramatic impacts for the hip rotators and pelvic floor. The change in orientation relative to gravity reduces the pressure on the pelvic floor, allowing for more release and rest. And the pressure from the floor against the sacrum can promote an active reset for the posterior pelvic joints.

To avoid compressing the vena cava in the back of the pelvis, this posture should primarily be done only in the first and second trimester. During the third trimester, it can be approximated from a seated squat or can be done supine for very short intervals, with mom rolling to the left for a rest afterwards.

Rolling to the side, slide to the floor and roll onto the back.[51] Draw the knees in towards the chest, widening them enough to make space for your belly and baby. Reach up between the legs to grab for the outside of either the ankles or the feet. Grabbing the outside of the foot helps to set the femur in the hip socket more securely.

With the head remaining on the floor, gently draw the feet to face the ceiling while pulling the knees towards the armpits. The knees should not splay outwards but rather hug against the arms. At the same time as the legs draw in, arch the tail towards the floor. This anterior pelvic tilt helps reset the sacrum and stretches the pelvic floor muscles that run from pubis to tail.

Breathe smoothly, and feel the groins deepen as the pelvic floor spreads. If it's comfortable, try rocking gently from side to side, pressing alternate sides of the sacrum into the floor. To release, bring the knees in, return the feet to the floor, and roll to the side to sit up.

---

[51] If practicing this posture after another supine posture (such as bridge) check if there are any sensations of supine hypotension (dizziness, nausea, shortness of breath) and shift to the left for a moment before moving into Happy Baby.

Chest opener with strap

Given the weight of the breasts and front body during pregnancy, many of my students come into class asking for shoulder and upper back openers. I always enjoy using a yoga strap to work around the different spaces within the shoulders and help promote gentle opening and release.

Grasping an open strap in each hand, separate your hands wider than your shoulders.

With straight arms—but without hyperextending in the elbows— maintain tension through the strap and raise the arms overhead. Keep the ribs heavy as you do this rather than allowing them to flare forward.

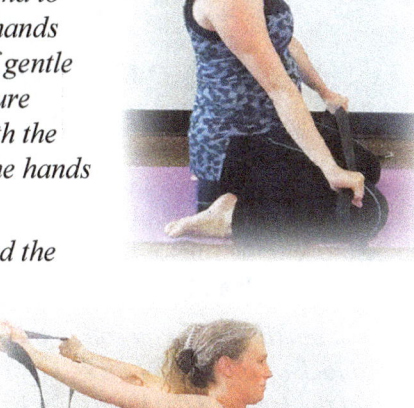

Keeping your arms straight, bring the strap behind the head until you feel resistance through the chest. If the elbows would have to bend to accomplish this, widen the hands a bit instead until a point of gentle stretching is achieved. Be sure to keep the wrists in line with the arms rather than twisting the hands inward.

Lower the arms down behind the back, keeping the elbows straight.

Reverse the movement, bringing the arms up overhead and down in front.

Repeat several times.

This is also a fantastic stretch for new moms who have tight shoulders from carrying and feeding baby.

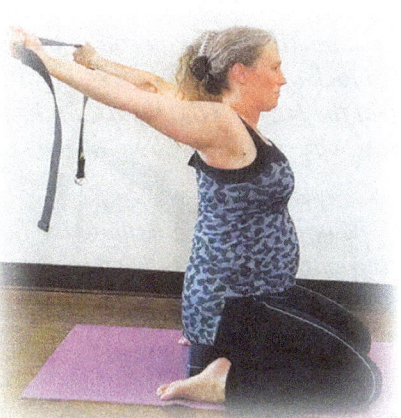

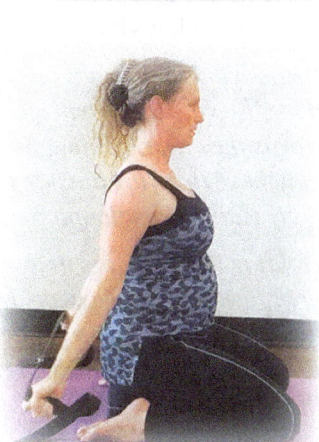

Backbending postures

Backbends during pregnancy are a slightly complicated practice. As discussed in Chapter 6, there has long been a well-founded concern about overstretching the front abdominal line, which could contribute to and possibly exacerbate diastasis recti/abdominal separation. Additionally, pregnancies with an anterior placenta—where the placenta attaches to the front rather than back side of the uterus—can be at risk for complications like placental abruptions if too much strain is placed in the abdominal fascial connections.

At the same time, backbends are an effective way to open the deep psoas muscles, which leads to more space for both the uterus and baby. Gently lifting and spreading the ribs and upper chest can help relieve compression and tension brought on by weight gain in the breasts and counteract the generally rounded posture pregnant women often assume in Western culture. So, as usual, the key to backbending during pregnancy is to find the middle path, one that is neither too aggressive nor too passive.

Begin with the gentle backbends covered in this chapter. Deeper backbends such as Wheel and Camel are covered in Chapter 9.

Psoas stretch

A gentle release of the deep psoas muscles is a great way to free the lower back and make room for the expanding uterus and baby. Before jumping into any backbend practice, I highly recommend addressing the psoas. To do 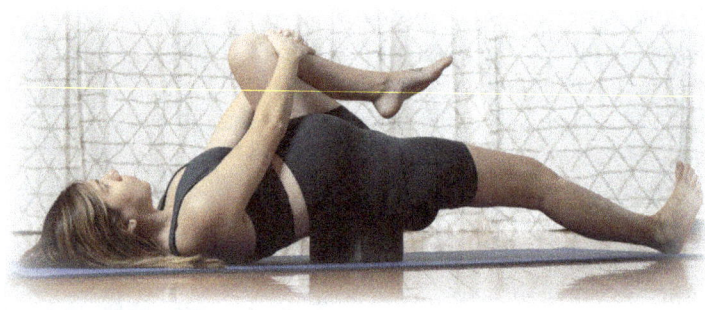 this, we place the spine into a subtle backbend, then allow the weight of one thigh at a time to lengthen towards the floor. The gentle lengthening of the leg combined with a stabilization of the pelvis allows the psoas muscles to stretch and release.

Begin lying on the mat on your back, making sure you roll to the side to come down to the floor. Elevate the pelvis on a yoga block or a rolled blanket. Gently bring one knee in towards the chest, holding the back of the leg with the hands. In the third trimester, the knee may have to swing outside the belly, which is fine as long as the knee is drawn towards the body rather than flopping away.

Holding the knee, begin to extend the opposite leg out along the floor. The foot may want to drift towards the outside edge of the mat, but work to keep the leg in line with the hip. Extend the leg until there is a gentle stretch in the extended hip and thigh. Actively draw the lifted leg into the chest. This will cause the pelvis to rotate back slightly, increasing the stretch for the hip flexors.

Breathe smoothly, and focus on releasing the upper groin, where the thigh meets the pelvis, towards the ground. Hold as long as feels productive—probably about a minute.

To release, bend the extended leg in to place the foot on the floor and lower the lifted leg. Pause to feel the impact on the body and breathing. Roll to the left side if the breath has become disturbed. Repeat on the second side.

Setu Bandha Sarvangasana/Bridge/Shoulderstand

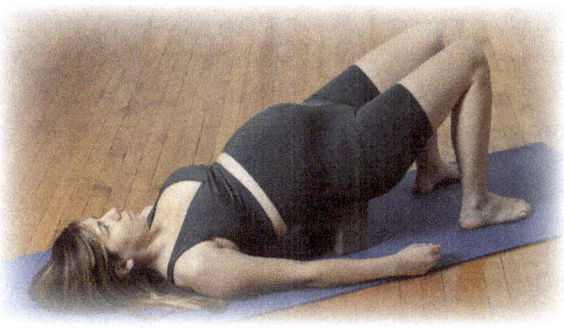

Bridge has an interesting history in pre-natal yoga. Often referred to as "breech tilt" in midwifery circles, this backbend has the ability to both stretch the psoas and, if held for more than 15 minutes with support, may assist in moving a breech baby away from the confines of the lower pelvic bowl. Such movement can create more space for the baby to rotate head down. This rotation usually also requires making space in the lower uterine segment through gentle release of the utero-pelvic ligaments.

In Bridge, it's important to avoid over engaging the gluteal muscles; doing so can lock the sacrum and jam movement into the lower back. The glutes will fire, but they should not become the proverbial "buns of steel" tucking the tail towards the ceiling. Also resist the urge to "walk" the shoulder blades together under the back. This walking together action can feel as though it is opening the chest, but it masks a lack of mobility in the upper spine and ultimately contributes to greater compression in the lumbar vertebrae and overstretching in the shoulders.

Focus instead on pressing the elbows into the floor and lifting the side of the ribs at the armpits, elevating the thoracic spine. The feet may need to step wider than classic yoga usually instructs. Separating the feet slightly wider than the hips allows for more shifting and adjustment within the sacrum and makes the stretch to the hip flexors and psoas more gentle.

Rolling to the side, slide down to the floor and then roll to your back (PLEASE take this pathway to the floor rather than rolling straight down the spine, which can cause abdominal strain). Lying on your back, bend the knees to bring the feet to the floor. Bring the heels in close to the bum, and widen the feet on the mat to hip distance or slightly wider. You may be able to touch the heels, but this should not be the goal for the starting position.

Beginning on an inhale, press the feet into the floor and move the knees out over the toes. This action will draw the hips off the floor with the lower back rounded, as though you were lying in a hammock. You are not yet in the backbend here! The knees will shift beyond the toes for a moment, and the pelvis will hang from the legs, almost able to swing.

Keeping the length in the lower back, use an exhale to press the feet into the floor, opening space behind the knees to raise the pelvis towards the ceiling. Your weight will shift back into the shoulders, creating an arch in the upper back. Let the tail continue to drip down as the pelvis lifts. The gluteals will engage but should fire evenly and not overtake the work of the legs. The arms can press the floor to lift the chest, but keep the shoulder blades open.

If the lower back feels compressed once the pelvis is elevated, use the backs of the legs to pull the hips slightly forward, lengthening the lower back once again. This is different from a pelvic tuck. The feeling is more of trying to bring the hips over the heels than the tail to the sky. The knees can relate to one another, but the common instruction of squeezing a block between the thighs is actually counterproductive here. Instead, allow the knees to widen, but maintain an internal rotation of the thighs as though rolling the inner thighs towards the ground and widening the SI joints. Come out by lowering the hips back to the floor, possibly hugging the legs in, and then rolling to the side to sit up.

To practice with support—as one would if trying to reposition a baby—place a block beneath the sacrum and let the pelvis rest on the block. This can be uncomfortable if the block is very hard, so a rolled blanket or towel may work better for this purpose.

If practicing this posture for pelvic stability or lower back release, try lifting on the inhale and then lowering on the exhale to create a rolling wave through the spine.

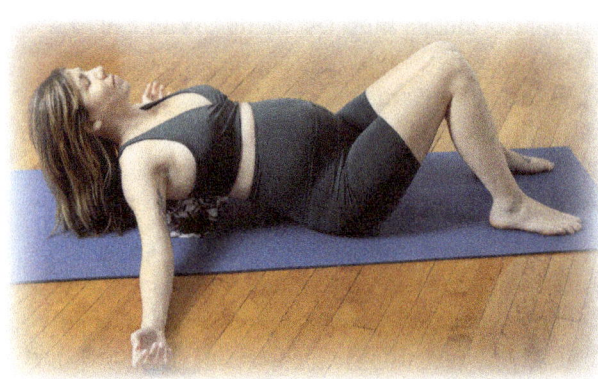

Supported Matsyasana/Upper Back Bolster

One of my favorite practices for relieving upper back tension, and a pose which is helpful both before and after birth, this variation of Matsyasana requires a rolled up surface and either a yoga block or large pillow for head support. You can use a yoga blanket, a towel, a yoga block, or a foam roller if you are feeling ambitious.

Be sure to use your arms to support you when entering this pose because the easiest way to come into it is by rolling straight down the spine. Avoid any straining of the abdominal wall. Since this is a supine (back-lying) posture, roll to the left side if you feel dizziness, shortness of breath, or nausea—or skip it altogether.

Take a yoga blanket or a large beach towel and roll it up into a cylinder approximately the height of one yoga block (about four inches). The roll can be larger if desired but this is a good starting point.

Place the blanket roll horizontally behind you, and put the block or pillow behind the rolled blanket. Place your hands on the roll. Bend the knees and lightly engage the deep abdominals as though hugging baby towards the heart. Inhale to lift the chest. On the exhale, using the hands for support, slowly lower the upper back onto the bolster. The roll should come to rest at the bottom tip of the shoulder blades, or roughly behind the heart. If using a foam roller, aiming for the "bra line" can be a good benchmark.

Once the back is supported, release the hands and let the shoulders and head drop back onto the block or pillow. Be sure the head rests on solid support above the line of the chest. The arms can stretch out from the shoulders in a "T." Depending on the response from the upper back, it may be necessary to shift the bolster slightly up or down the spine to find a workable place. Rest back and let the spine melt over the bolster. If you feel your ribs flaring, place a bolster or large pillow behind the head.

If the lower back complains, keeping the knees bent can help. You can also lift and tuck the tail momentarily to break the contraction of the lower back muscles. Once released, let the pelvis float back down and see if the upper back will let go. This backbend often gets better the longer you stay in it, as long as the breath is able to be smooth and the nervous system can calm. If possible, stay here for several minutes.

To come out, bend the knees and roll to the left side, removing the bolster. Rest on your side for a moment, then sit up and feel the change in the space within the chest.

Parighasana/Gate Pose

One of my favorite things while I was pregnant was stretching my side body. It helped relieve lower back tension and also lifted the ribs off my belly, giving me more space for breath.

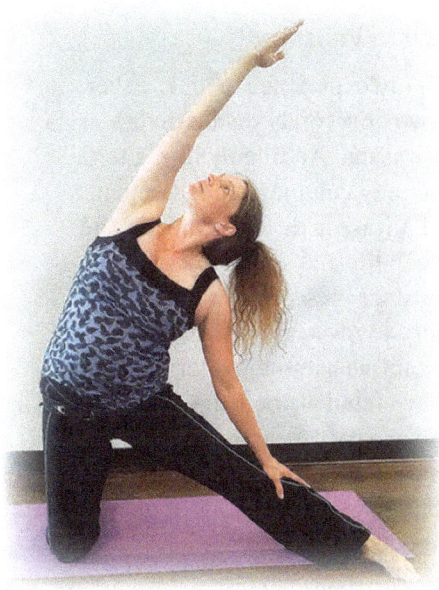

The geometry of Gate Pose can be thought of in two ways. You can focus on the bend of the spine, as one might in a pose like Reverse Warrior, or you can turn the extended knee towards the ceiling and focus on the movement within the hip socket, in which case the structure more resembles Trikonasana with a slight hip rotation. In either case there is also a soft abdominal engagement along with an adductor stretch for the inner thigh.

Begin standing on the knees. If the knees are sensitive, place a folded blanket beneath them for padding. Extend the left leg to the side at a 45 degree angle. If focusing on the side bend, turn the toes and knee forward. If focusing on the hip movement, rotate the thigh so the toes and knee turn skyward.

Inhale to extend the left arm up. Exhale to reach out over the extended left leg, bringing the hand down onto the leg at a comfortable distance. If focused on the side bend, breathe into the upper side ribs and waist, feeling the gentle spinal curve and twist. If focusing on the hip, drop the left hip under to create a pelvic tilt. Keep as much length on the bottom side waist as the top.

On an inhale, raise the right arm and roll the chest open towards the sky. Exhale to reach the arm alongside the cheek. Continue turning the chest to look under the lifted arm. Press the feet and left arm actively against the ground, and breathe into the top ribs.

To return, on an exhale, gather the abdominals and pelvic floor inwards, then raise the chest by pressing the legs into the ground. Return the left leg to kneeling and circle the hips to reset before continuing to the second side.

Restorative postures

We spend so much of our asana practice working on alignment and stretching bones, muscles, and fascia, but the real magic of prenatal yoga comes from cultivating deep rest and a sense of calm during and after the active portion of the practice. This ability conserves stamina during the labor process. And finding time for rest and quiet during pregnancy can be the difference between feeling exhausted and overwhelmed and feeling nurtured and supported. As with most yoga asana, small modifications during pregnancy can dramatically impact the body and mind.

Supta Virasana

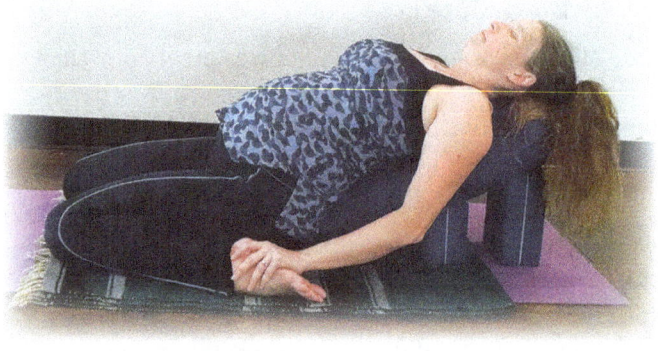

In my experience, people either love or severely dislike Supta Virasana. Adding reclining to the already complex hip movement of Virasana directly impacts the deep hip and spinal muscles. This posture presents a rich opportunity to investigate sensations and examine habitual patterns and can have fabulous benefits during pregnancy. The gentle release in the deep abdomen can help make space around the uterus, relieve the lower back, open the front hip flexors, and create a profound sense of calm and inner quiet. Because it is a reclined posture in which the weight falls towards the back of the body, Supta Virasana does not significantly overtax the front abdominal line.

From Virasana (see Pg 156), *place several pillows or blocks behind you on the mat—you may not need them all, but it is helpful to have them available.*

Bringing the pelvis to the front edge of the sitz bones, lean back onto the hands to bring the spine to rest on the pillows—or floor if you can reach. The head should remain at or above the line of the chest.

It's critical that you do not tuck the pelvis here. While tucking the tail and shifting off the sitz bones may temporarily lengthen the lower back and relieve lumbar discomfort, the movement will drive pressure downward towards your knees and hips. Since the knees are fully closed in this posture, the SI joint will end up taking on the excess movement.

Rather than attempting to lengthen your spine towards the hips, try lengthening it towards the head. Imagine that you could use your back floating ribs and upper back to push the pillows towards the crown of your head. Even better, imagine that a good friend had come along and was gently pulling your ribs back and down into the pillows. The result is a slight upward movement along your spine, which lengthens the lower back without jamming the movement into the SI joints.

You do not need an extreme range of motion in this shape. The psoas needs a gentle but supported stretch that allows things to unwind. Let the hip creases soften and deepen with the breath as you rest back. There should be no discomfort in either the knees or lower back; if there is, put more pillows under the spine and/or elevate the pelvis.

Coming out of this posture can seem complicated, especially if you are farther along in your pregnancy or if you lie back farther than intended. If your knees allow, you can remain reclining on the pillows. Lift one knee to free the leg and step the foot to the floor, then repeat with the second side. For most people, however, this is not possible. In that case, place your hands on the bolsters below the lower back and focus on deepening the groins, as though someone were sitting on your lap. Do NOT crunch the abdominals! With the thighs grounded, press into the hands and allow the spine to arch upwards to sit.

Once you have come out of the posture, extend the knees, either by straightening the legs on the floor or by coming into Table pose, and stretch each leg back.

Supta Baddha Konasana/Supine Bound Angle

Perhaps the queen of the restorative postures, Supta Baddha Konasana supports every joint in the body in a position that allows the muscles to rest in a neutral state and reduces stimulation to the brain and nervous system.

It is possible for the tailbone and sacrum to be uncomfortably compressed during this posture

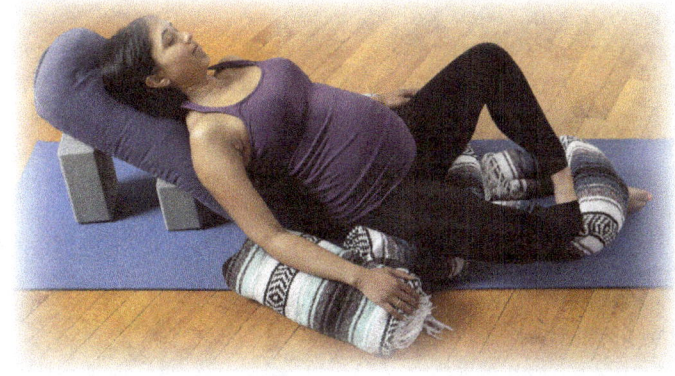

if it isn't properly supported, so if you are experiencing sacral or pelvic pain, make sure that the base of the pelvis is slightly elevated. Place a rolled blanket wrapped around the base of the pelvis, making a "U" shape. The rolled blanket helps lift the tailbone and pelvis off the floor, reducing coccyx and sacral compression. As with any reclining posture, if you begin to feel dizzy or short of breath, roll to the left side to reduce the pressure on the posterior blood vessels.

Set up with two blocks and bolster(s) or pillows, propped to create a 45 degree angle. If you are using a single bolster, place a yoga block on the medium height in the middle of the bolster and a block on the tallest height at the far end of the bolster to support the head. The bolster may not rest on the second block until you lie back, but this is fine.

Sitting against the lowest end of the bolster, bring the feet together in an easy, open Baddha Konasana. Place either rolled blankets or blocks under the knees to support the thighs. It may also be helpful to wrap a rolled blanket around the pelvis to cradle the sacrum and tail. If you're practicing at home, you might even employ a breastfeeding pillow for this role.

Roll a blanket lengthwise, then wrap it over the tops of the feet and around the ankles to support the shins. Place rolled or folded blankets alongside the bolster to support your arms. Have a rolled blanket available for under the neck. Yes, it's a lot of blankets!

To recline, sit directly against the bolster, almost on top of it. Place your hands on the floor behind you directly alongside the bolster. Use the arms to support you as you lie back. The legs should be cradled so that there are no overt stretching sensations. Place the rolled blanket under the neck to gently elevate the head. The elbows should rest against the folded blankets with the hands draping off the ends. You may have to make small adjustments to find total comfort.

The final experience is as though a giant hand scooped you up and supported you from beneath. Once a feeling of full support is achieved, allow the body to sigh into the shape as the breath draws down towards the belly and pelvis, focusing on an easy flow: in and out. Rest in this posture as long as comfortable, feeling the full support from the earth and the sensation of near-floating within the body. 10-30 minutes here is ideal.

To come out, begin by deepening the breath, feeling energy move throughout the body. Notice if you have any awareness of the baby. Bring the hands to the outside of the thighs and help the legs to lift. Then, moving gently, roll onto one side and rest side lying for a moment before pressing the floor away and returning to sit. If you are continuing into Side-lying Shavasana, place supports while you are on your side and continue resting.

Side-lying Shavasana/Side-lying rest

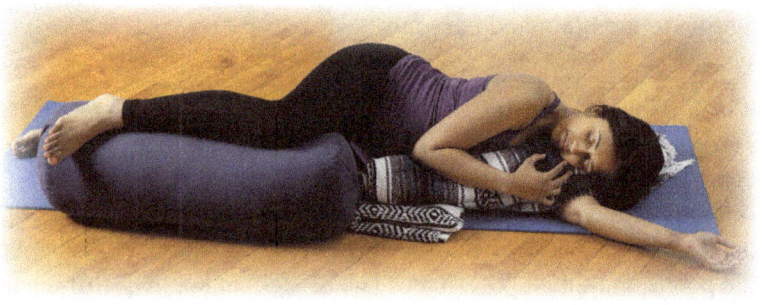

The culmination of the entire practice and the sweet dessert at the end, Shavasana is possibly the most important posture we can practice during pregnancy. With the hectic, busy requirements of our daily lives, taking time for stillness and to allow the nervous system to find quiet is absolutely vital throughout pregnancy—and even more so during motherhood. Simply put, if you are only going to do one *asana*, do Shavasana, and if you are doing a longer practice, don't skip this one…ever!

You're probably quite familiar with the classic Shavasana: lying on your back, legs and arms extended, eyes closed. This position is fine if you are still early in your pregnancy and have no symptoms of supine hypotension (dizziness, nausea, shortness of breath). But after around 25 weeks—and earlier in some cases—many women no longer feel comfortable in this supine position.

While things can be managed for a while by propping the spine up at the 45 degree angle described in Supta Baddha Konasana, at some point it becomes advisable to shift to Side-lying Shavasana. This posture not only avoids compression of the posterior blood vessels but also uses gravity to promote the baby's shift into the optimal position for labor and birth (head down, with the spine curled towards mom's left side). To be comfortable, Side-lying Shavasana requires enough pillows and blankets to fully support the body and allow the mind to let go.

Come to lie on your left side. (If you are sick of lying on the left, you may choose right, but left is slightly preferable for promoting a left-lying baby.)

Place a folded blanket under the waist to support the belly and lower back—this is optional, but most students like it. Place a rolled blanket under the neck at an angle, so it can be hugged by the arms to put light pressure on the chest. Extend the bottom leg straight, and rest the top knee and ankle on a bolster. The bolster can also be placed between the knees and ankles if you prefer. Be sure the top ankle rests supported on the bolster. Allowing the foot to hang creates tension along the side line of the body, eventually pulling on the SI joint—which isn't relaxing.

If you have plenty of props available, place another bolster behind the back to create an additional feeling of security. Every joint should feel supported and at ease, which helps decrease the stimulation to the nervous system.

Once you are fully supported, close the eyes and let the breathing become rhythmic. It's important not to try too hard to relax but rather to simply allow things to be as they are. As you move through thoughts of your body relaxing or place your focus on how comfortable you are, your sense of ease will increase. Shavasana is one posture where we exchange the activity of "doing" with the quality of simply being.

Thoughts will come and go, but you can let them continue rather than getting caught up by them. As though you were under a blue sky dotted with white puffy clouds, let the thoughts simply float by. Remain resting with our body and baby. Stay as long as you like, or as time allows. 10-15 minutes is ideal, but even one minute, done consciously, can be of benefit.

Pranayama: the key breath practices

Breath is the physical expression of the nervous system. Change the breathing, and you change how the mind and thus the body react. This is why every form of childbirth preparation has had some sort of breathing practice associated with it, most famously the technique used by Ferdinand Lamaze in Lamaze Childbirth classes. There are actually several breathing practices involved in Lamaze Childbirth, but the most famous one is the panting, or "hee hee" breathing commonly shown in TV representations of the childbirth process. (Cue the Jennifer Aniston *Friends* sketch or other fast paced breathing scenes from TV!)

What many people do not realize is that this paced, fast breath was actually meant as a sort of "rescue breathing" for someone who was close to a panic state. It was intended to gradually grab hold of the nervous system and slow the breathing down to something much closer to deep abdominal breathing. With this in mind, there are certain fundamental yoga breathing exercises that can be extremely useful for avoiding anxiety and promoting a calm, relaxed, and in-control state.

Calming Breath

This is a breath intended to stimulate the relaxation response in the nervous system. It can be a great way to begin a yoga practice, promote sleep, or re-establish a calm center between contractions during labor, or during pregnancy if you are having trouble falling asleep.

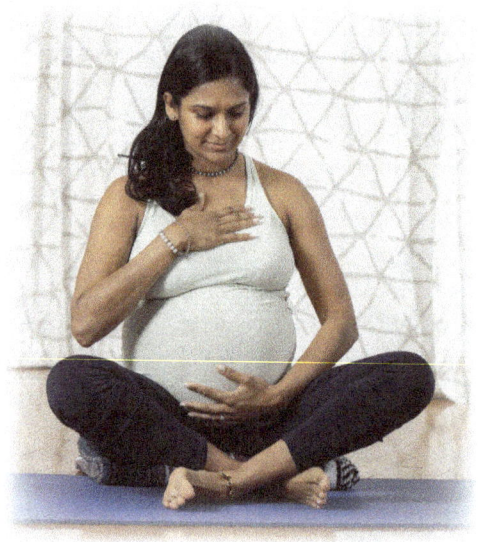

Sitting calmly, tune in to the natural rhythm of inhales and exhales through the body. Begin to count the length of the inhale and exhale. Gradually coax the exhale to become two counts longer than the inhale. There are no set numbers for this exercise, though inhaling for four and exhaling for six seems to be popular when moms are relaxed.

Continue to breathe this way for several minutes, feeling the body and mind relax. When you let go of the breathing and return to normal, notice the impact overall.

Full Body Breathing

This breath promotes reconnecting with your full breath capacity and the instinctual breathing rhythm you had as a baby. It can be especially helpful for maintaining breath capacity in

mid- to late pregnancy, when the organs begin to crowd into the diaphragm. This breath can also be highly effective during contractions.

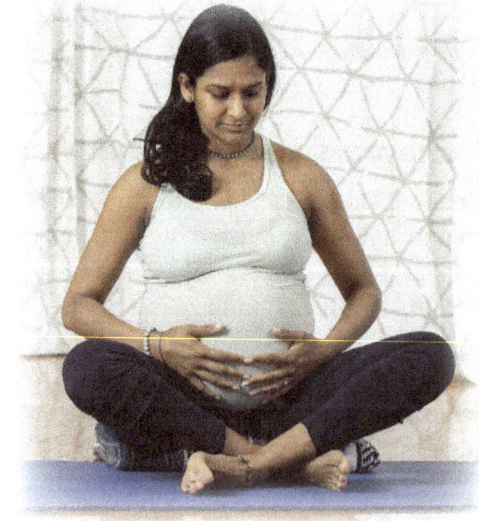

It should be noted that this breath is not solely focused on expanding the abdomen but instead on finding a 360 degree expansion of the whole body. Only breathing into the belly can put additional strain on the front abdominal wall and actually contribute to diastasis recti for those already at risk. Use this breath to expand the front, side, and back body. Breathing in this manner actually increases the available lung capacity and also brings more space during labor, when the uterus surges back and forth as it contracts and releases.

Begin by drawing attention to your abdomen, and

pick up on the motion of the belly, in and out, as you breathe. Late in pregnancy this movement may be smaller, but it is still there. Now notice that it is not just your belly moving but your sides and also the back body. Gradually begin to increase the natural motion of your breathing, as though gently rocking the baby.

Once the belly is moving well, fill the center body as much as you can, and then allow the breath to flow up into the chest, expanding the lungs. Imagine filling your body from the base up, like filling a glass with water. Exhale smoothly and steadily, taking as much time to breathe out as you do to breathe in. Become comfortable with this two-part breath before moving on.

Once you are comfortable with two-part breathing, add the top lobes of the lungs by allowing the breath to flow up under the collar bones after the chest has fully expanded. Feel the entire body full of energy, but do not strain or hold the breath as you inhale. Exhale smoothly and steadily, letting the breath flow out into the space around you. Repeat for a few minutes, pausing if you begin to feel cramped or like you are forcing the breath.

Ujjayi pranayama/Ocean-sounding breath

Like Full Body Breathing, Ujjayi *pranayama* can be extremely useful during labor to help you ride the intensity of each contraction. During pregnancy, avoid contracting the base of the throat and instead open it into as wide a space as possible. This action helps synchronize the neuro-muscular connection between the vocal cords, throat, and soft palette and the pelvic floor, cervix, and vaginal opening. Open throat, open bottom.

Ujjayi *pranayama* can be done first while sitting, then carried through an entire practice if desired.

Beginning with a steady, full body breath, begin to draw your breath towards the back of the throat and into the backs of the lungs. The body should still expand as you inhale, as though filling a balloon just underneath the baby. From the base of the throat there should be a quiet, hissing sound, similar to the sound of waves washing up on the beach or wind rustling through the trees.

Pay attention to the sound of the inhale and exhale. The sound should be steady on each side of the breath, though the tone may be slightly different. The level of sound should be very quiet: almost silent or only loud enough for you to hear it. It is like whispering a secret to yourself. Breathe smoothly and steadily, listening for the sound.

If at any point you realize you no longer hear or feel your breathing, then gently recognize that your mind has wandered. Return your attention to your breath and the movement of your belly, and begin again. Let go of the practice if you begin to feel short of breath, anxious, or dizzy, as these signs may indicate that you have started breathing too deeply too fast and are hyperventilating. If this is the case, let the breath return to normal and sit quietly.

More involved breathing practices are included in the advanced practice section in Chapter 9.

9 — Advanced Postures and Practices

"The true sign of an advanced student is not that they can do the full range of motion. It is that they know when to stop."

—Barbara Benagh

Advanced postures are more than poses that require a deep range of motion, considerable balance, or significant strength. They are postures which, to perform well and safely, need not only flexibility but also an understanding of alignment, balance, and degree of effort. These qualities are usually developed through a regular movement practice (usually but not always yoga). They ask for greater concentration and focus. Advanced postures during pregnancy require even more sensitivity and awareness to avoid overstretching or exacerbating existing imbalances in the body.

The advanced postures included in this chapter need an internal awareness of stability and integration. They often ask yoginis to hold back rather than push into a certain range of motion. In many cases, these *asanas* call for a greater sense of balance, range of motion, or physical ability; with the hormonal and physical changes of pregnancy at play, even postures practiced regularly call for a measure of caution.

When practicing these postures, students ideally should have had a regular practice (once a week) and/or have been practicing the *asana* prior to pregnancy and postpartum. An established practice, however, does not guarantee a sound understanding of alignment. Advanced students often have advanced tricks to work around and avoid tight spots. Therefore, these postures should always be taught and practiced gradually, with a keen awareness of laxity and potential hypermobility. The focus is on feeling for alignment, support, and ease rather than on attaining a certain shape.

Each family of postures has its own specific challenges.

Balancing postures

There are two major concerns for balancing postures. The first is your changing center of gravity and the awareness of where that center is—the shifts lead to an increased risk of falling. We can address the increased risk of falling by always approaching balance postures gradually—and ideally with lots of support options such as a chair, the wall, or possibly a partner. Seasoned students may have enough proprioception (awareness of the body's placement in space) to still attempt balances in the center of the room. If this is the case, practice carefully, without any flinging or "jumping" into the shape.

The second concern around balancing postures is related to the increased relaxin and mobility in the joints. Any standing balance will place asymmetrical force on the pelvis, since you are shifting from two legs (supports) to one. Supporting the pelvis during the weight transfer and throughout the *asana* requires involving the transverse abdominals, pelvic floor, and glutes. Even simpler balances such as Tree or Natarajasana need this support, but it becomes more critical when rotating the pelvis on the standing leg, as in Ardha Chandrasana or the deeper variation of Dancer Pose.

When we are not in an upright position, we need a deeper understanding and awareness of how the core and glutes work to stabilize the pelvis and of where we may be habitually sinking into looser joints such as the knees and SI joints. A general rule is to look for overall space in the joints and a sense of being grounded but floating. Doing so helps avoid compressing the internal joint space and promotes good function for the muscles surrounding the joint.

Beginning balancing postures

Vrksasana/Tree Pose

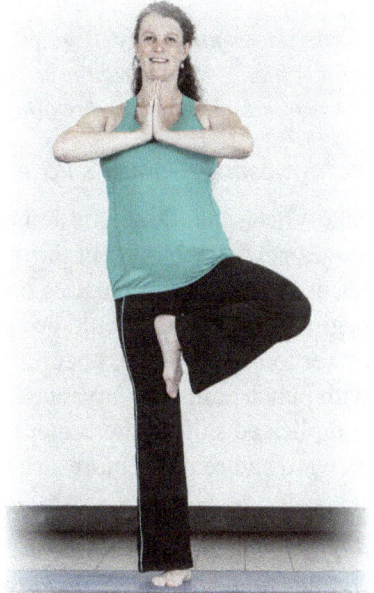

I love this pose—partly because it reminds me of my days in ballet class but also because it brings a dual sense of floating and being grounded at the same time. Done classically, Tree Pose can help open the hips (glutes and adductors) as well as tone the pelvic floor for stability.

However, Vrksasana can be tricky if the pelvis is already hypermobile because the single leg stance creates the possibility of a shearing force through the fixed (supporting) side of the pelvis. What does that mean? It means if there is pain in the pubic symphysis or SI joints, you may have to work a bit harder to keep the pelvis level. Additionally, you may need to engage supporting muscles, such as the glutes, pelvic floor, and transverse abdominals, or be willing to modify the pose—keeping the lifted foot lower or even on the ground.

The standing hip bears the lion's share of the stabilization work and must be engaged as soon as the weight begins to shift. If you feel things collapsing or muscles cramping, then bring the lifted foot to the ground and take a rest.

Out of caution for the shifting center of gravity, start this posture near a wall or chair so you can hold on if you feel unstable. Standing in a strong Tadasana, inhale. On the exhale, shift your weight to the right leg. Engage the standing glute and lightly draw the pelvic floor up, maintaining space within the standing hip socket. Avoid letting the standing hip sink out to the side like a disgruntled teenager.

After shifting your weight, lift the left leg up in front of the body, turn the knee out, and bring the foot to the inner ankle, shin, or thigh. Lift the foot hands-free at first, as it will give you a better sense of your available range of motion. If range and ease allows, the hand can then be used to bring the foot against the standing leg wherever is appropriate. If this movement is challenging or if stability is an issue, it may be worth skipping the hand grab to place the heel.

The foot should not rest against the inner knee, and the hips should remain facing forwards rather than turning open with the lifted leg. Actively press the foot and inner leg against one another, and feel a lift moving up the inseam, as though the pelvic floor was drawing the heel up into the groin. This action may be completely isometric (no visible movement), but it creates stability through the inner leg muscles.

If you are able to release the wall or chair support, stretch the arms out from the shoulders like a tightrope walker. The abdominals may lightly engage but should not suck in. Keep the breath steady and comfortable. If you feel stable enough, either bring the palms to press at the heart center or raise the arms overhead. Notice how the body continues to subtly sway. Bring your gaze to a single point and breathe smoothly.

Come out as mindfully as you came in, maintaining pelvic support. Lower the lifted leg to the floor, placing it once again in Tadasana. Sense the stability provided by having two legs on the ground, and notice any other shifts, mental or physical. Practice on both sides.

Natarajasana/Dancer's Pose

Like Vrksasana, Dancer is a one-legged balance that challenges pelvic stability, but this posture can also be a fabulous release for hip flexor muscles like the quads and psoas. This beginner's variation would be appropriate for anyone who is newer to Natarajasana, uncertain of their balance, or coping with pelvic pain. The advanced variation involves a more complicated shift of the center of gravity as the pelvis rotates forward and requires more strength and stability.

Begin standing in Tadasana, close enough to a chair or wall that it can be used for support. Shift your weight to the left leg, bend the right knee, and grab the ankle with the right hand (same hand as foot). Engage the outer hip and pelvic floor as in Tree Pose to promote stability.

With the free hand on the wall or chair, lift through the chest, drawing the right foot in towards the hip. Do not tuck the tail. Rather, allow the pelvis to float on the standing leg, and actively press the floor away. Lightly engage the abdominal muscles to hug the baby and feel the stretch through the front of the right thigh. Work to bring the knees towards one another to maintain the upright shape of the pose.

For an intermediate variation which increases the deep front line stretch, press the right foot back into the hand, moving the knee and thigh backwards. Maintain an upright chest for this variation, and allow the back to bend slightly. Be sure to maintain a level pelvis rather than swinging the knee and thigh out to the side (no dog at fire hydrant positions here, please).

To return from either variation, draw the knee forward, release the foot, and replace it into Tadasana. Let go of the support and stand for a moment before continuing to the second side.

Advanced balance postures

Natarajasana (advanced variation)

The challenge with the deeper variation of Natarajasana is that it combines a balance with a backbend. This puts additional stress on the expanding abdominal muscles and often requires an anterior tilt to the pelvis, which changes the orientation for stability. That said, going deeper in this pose can be a great way to stretch the quads and psoas muscles. This variation should only be done by students who have practiced it prior to pregnancy and who have good body awareness.

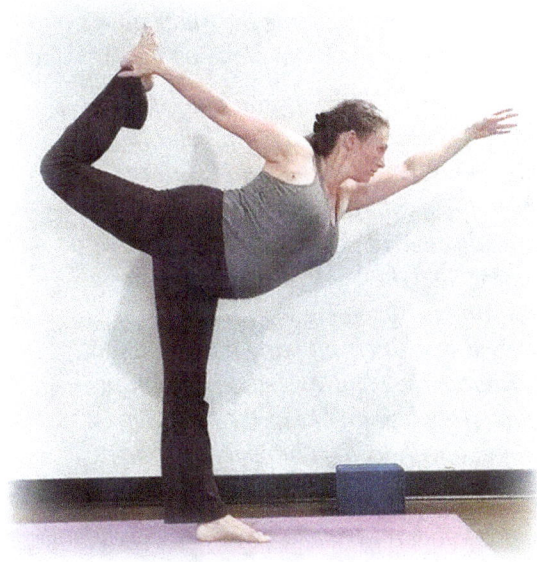

Begin with the basic variation, bending one knee to hold the ankle with the hand. You can hold inside or outside the ankle. If you are holding the inside, be sure the inner elbow faces out so the shoulder is externally rotated. Gently press the foot back into the hand, raising the leg about half of the possible range of motion. Then begin to tip the pelvis forward while drawing the belly gently back and up to support the weight of the baby. Under NO circumstances should the belly be simply hanging forward in this pose, as doing so is risky for the linea alba.

If you can tip to where the navel faces the floor, actively press the standing leg into the floor and feel for a floating sense in the standing hip—as though someone had inflated a cushion in your hip socket. You might begin to press the foot into the hand to raise the back leg higher, focusing on opening the chest. Do not tuck the tail or flatten the lower back, but do maintain the abdominal lift and space in the standing hip.

The free hand can extend forward to a wall or the middle of the room or reach down for a block or chair. Be sure to avoid locking the standing knee, as this will also lock the standing hip joint. To come out, either release the leg into Uttanasana or, engaging the pelvic floor, glutes, and abdominals, slowly raise the pelvis upright again and lower the leg. Rest and then switch sides.

Ardha Chandrasana/Half Moon Pose

Geometrically speaking Ardha Chandrasana is a close cousin to Trikonasana, only rotated on its side. This change in orientation creates some additional challenges and requires extra awareness. Yoginis who are newer to this pose should take it with the back body against the wall for stability.

Begin in Trikonasana, stepping the feet 3-4 feet apart and turning the right (front) foot out towards the short end of the mat and the left (back) foot slightly inward. Inhale, and exhale to tip the pelvis forward over the right foot, bringing the right hand down onto the shin or a block for stability. Press into the right hand to rotate the chest open and stretch up through the left fingers. Your pelvis will be slightly turned towards the floor, but the front hip should still feel spacious. The sitting bone of the front leg moves towards the midline of the posture rather than swinging to the side.

Be sure the belly is engaged and not hanging into the lower back and that the chest is rotated open only as far as can be done without dragging the hips open to the side. The feet actively press apart, engaging the outer glutes and helping to lift out of the front hip. The spine should stay in the same plane as the legs and feet.

To move from Trikonasana into Ardha Chandrasana, lower the top hand to the hip, bend the front knee, and shift the front hand forward about 12 inches to the outside edge of the mat, probably using a block. Step the back foot in, and without rotating the front leg inward, shift the weight into the front hand and front foot. Maintain the same external rotation in your front leg, and keep the lifted leg aligned with its own hip, meaning do not turn the toes towards the ceiling.

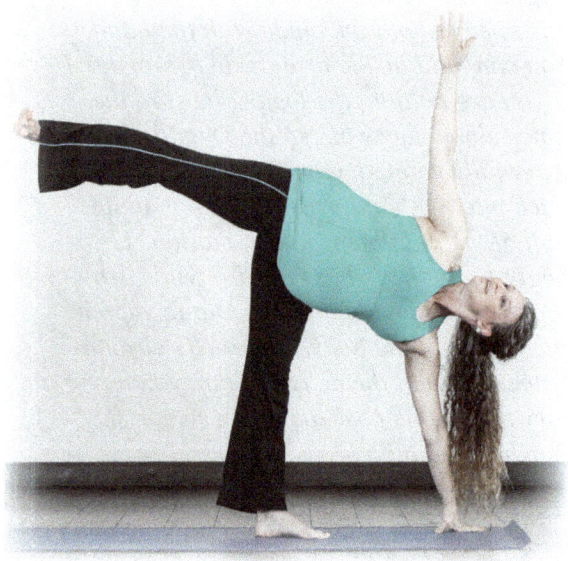

Once you have transferred your weight, engage the abdominals and raise the back leg to hip height or even a bit higher. Keep the standing leg bent to start! Actively flex the raised leg to engage the foot arch and inner thigh line. Press the bottom hand into the floor or block to lift the chest and possibly twist open gently. With the top leg aligned, press the standing foot into the floor to straighten the standing leg, as though taking the whole shape of the pose and floating it upwards in space. Only raise the top arm or look up if it feels easy to do so.

To return, either mindfully drop the top leg next to the standing leg, coming into Uttanasana, or bend the standing leg, carefully step back to the mat, and re-find the Trikonasana shape. Exit fully and repeat on the second side.

Cautions for Ardha Chandrasana: Given the lateral alignment of the pelvis in this posture, the action of actively pressing the standing leg into the floor and finding the floating sensation (rather than sinking into the hip) is key. Maintain the image of the pelvis as a single bowl; moving it as such can help avoid straining the SI or pubic joints during the transitions.

Take care that the top hip does not open faster than the bottom hip can support. Moving too quickly brings the twist into the pubic bone, which leads to a host of aches and pains.

Additionally, because the belly sits off the centerline of this posture, it is worth paying attention to how much stress is being placed on the center abdominal line and how strongly the abdominals have to engage. Strong abdominal engagement can be problematic, as it overly compresses an area which is already expanding. When in doubt, err on the side of caution and apply the law of 50% to this posture. Be willing to back off rather than striving for a hand on the floor, foot high in the air, or chest deeply rotated open.

Virabhadrasana 3/Warrior 3

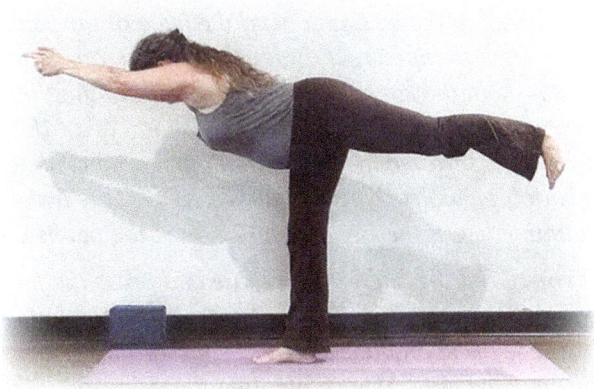

This pose can be done with hands on the wall for stability or in the center of the room with blocks or hands reaching forward if mom is ready. The key points to watch are that the pelvis remains level and that there is no sinking into either the standing hip or the lower back. Practicing this posture, especially later in pregnancy, can be especially challenging for the outer hips and transverse abdominals, as they must support the additional weight of the pregnancy to maintain good alignment.

Entering Warrior 3 can be done in one of two ways. You can step into a short lunge from the back of the mat and then fold forward from the hips to 90 degrees while raising the back leg. Or enter by hinging forward from the hips into Uttanasana, with the hand on tall height blocks, then shift the weight to one leg and raise the other behind and into the air.

While the full pose would have the back leg parallel to the floor, the back foot may initially be just barely off the mat. Seek a sense of floating and lightness rather than aiming to be parallel to the floor. Try to create a straight line from head to heel, even if that line is at a diagonal.

Regardless of how you enter Warrior 3, engage the transverse abdominals to avoid hanging into the lower back, and actively press the standing foot into the floor to float the pelvis to a level position. This is especially true in the third trimester, when the weight of the baby and uterus often cause a sway in the lumbar spine. Keep the knees unlocked and the breath steady and full.

To come out, lower the lifted leg to Uttanasana, or step back into a lunge, landing lightly and with core support. Repeat on the second side.

Utthita Hasta Padangustasana/One-Footed Big Toe Pose

A similarly geometric posture to both Warrior 3 and Ardha Chandrasana, One-Footed Big Toe pose can be a great way to release both the hamstrings and pelvic floor, while also building strength in the standing hip and leg. As ever, be cautious of the (you guessed it) more supple joints of the pregnant pelvis and the potential shifts brought on by the single leg stance.

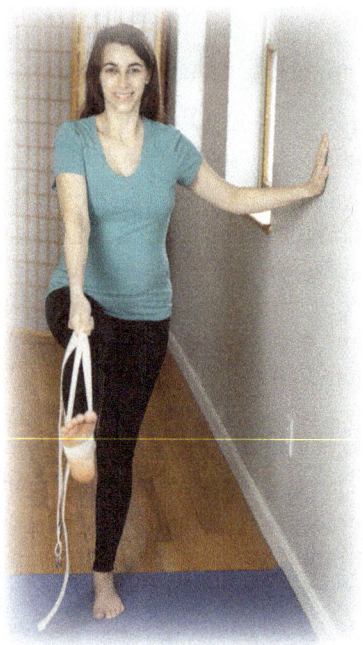

This pose nearly always requires a yoga strap or other way to hold onto the foot. If no strap is available I recommend holding the thigh rather than straining to reach the toes.

Standing in Tadasana by a wall, shift the weight onto the leg closest to the wall and bend the knee of the free leg, bringing it to hip height. Place the yoga strap around the foot or hold the knee. Be sure the outer standing hip engages strongly to maintain a level pelvis, and draw the pubic bone back through the legs to maintain a neutral pelvic position. Avoid tucking the tail. Keep a gentle bend in the standing leg; if the knee is locked, then the pelvis cannot adjust.

If you're ready to move on, exhale and press the foot into the strap to raise the foot forward. Be especially mindful of not tucking the tail or thrusting the hips forward, as this will displace the spinal position and shift the center of gravity. Continue gently drawing back through the inner thighs, planting the pelvis onto the standing leg and setting the lifted femur into the back of the hip. This grounding of the working femur will help draw the breath deeper into the pelvic floor and open the line of the hamstrings further.

The geometry here is akin to that of Warrior 3, simply rotated 90 degrees. If you choose to practice this pose while holding the knee, you may opt not to straighten the lifted leg. Instead, focus the action of the pose into the pelvis and the grounding of the top of the thigh. The movement will have less impact on the hamstrings, but if coping with pelvic instability, that may be preferable to further straining loose joints.

From Utthita Hasta Padangusthasana 1, it's fairly simple to shift to Utthita Hasta 2 where the leg extends to the side rather than the front of the body.

Utthita Hasta Padangusthasana 2

From Utthita Hasta 1, keep pushing the foot into the strap (or holding the knee) and move the leg to the side, opening the inner thigh. The range should only be what the hip socket easily allows, and the movement of the leg definitely should not take the pelvis with it. Keep the hip bones facing forward.

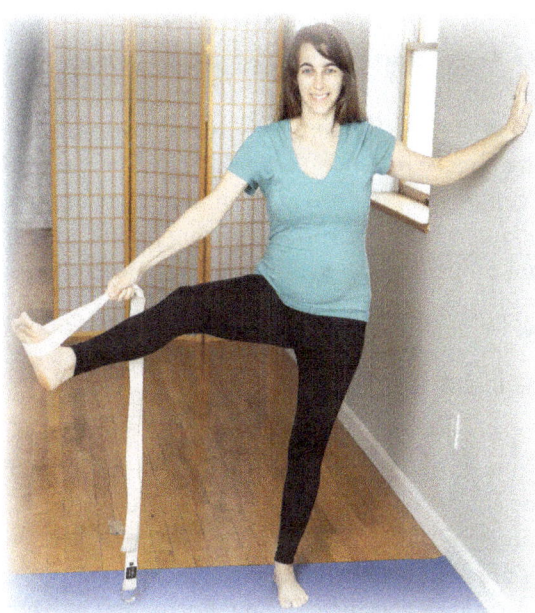

Be sure to anchor the head of the femur into the back of the hip, and gather the sitting bones towards one another without tucking the tail or displacing the pelvis forwards. If keeping the knee bent, this action is effectively the opening movement for Vrksasana.

If you feel stable enough, you can try lifting the hand from the wall to explore the stability required to float the balance on the single leg.

To release either variation, bend the knee in and return the foot to the floor in Tadasana. Stand firmly on two feet, feeling the stability and the internal shift that results from a well-done balance.

Practice both sides.

Utthita Hasta Padangusthasana 3

Given this variation involves not only a single leg balance but also a rotation of the spine, I don't recommend practicing it during pregnancy. While the belly is not usually compressed, the change in the center of gravity and the core strength needed to facilitate this variation safely create too much risk. There are better ways to free the spine and strengthen the pelvis. Try letting this pose go for a while.

Utthita Hasta 1 and 2 (chair variation)

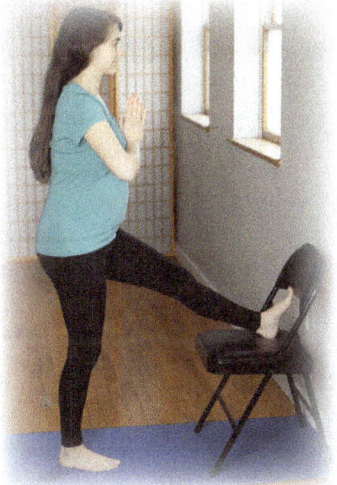
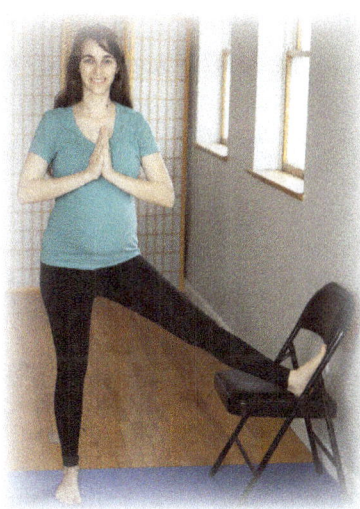

A more stable variation for Utthita Hasta Padangusthasana involves placing the extended leg on top of a chair or bench at the wall rather than holding it out in mid-air. After placing the foot on your chosen prop, lift the spine tall, pressing into the floor to promote stability in the pelvis. The chair or bench allows you to drop the lifted thigh more easily into the hip, as though someone were gently anchoring the hip crease towards the floor.

For the Utthita Hasta 2 variation, return the foot back to the floor and shift the body to face 45 degrees away from the wall. Do not try for 90 degrees unless the chair is placed slightly in front of your hip. Raise the leg closest to the wall, and rest the heel on the top edge of your support with the foot pressing the wall. The pelvis should remain aligned with the top leg. Anchor the lifted thigh down. Feel how the support under your foot allows you to spread the deep layer of the pelvic floor. See if you can feel the breath dropping down into the lower abdomen and between the sitting bones. Inhale, drop and release; exhale, softly gather this area together and up.

To finish, step the feet back to Tadasana and appreciate the changes. Repeat on the other side.

Backbends

Backbends are wonderful stretches for the psoas and quads, and they help to mobilize the spine during pregnancy. But they also pose a risk to the expanding abdominal muscles and the linea alba. Whether this area stretches abnormally will depend on a student's prior fascial integrity and muscle elasticity. Deeper backbends should probably be avoided after 32 weeks of pregnancy unless students have a solid pre-pregnancy practice and know how to free the upper back and hips without borrowing movement from the lumbar region.

Urdhva Dhanurasana/Wheel pose

Urdhva Dhanurasana involves both upper and lower body extension. When done well, it feels like an almost effortless fluid movement undulating along the spine, as though rolling over a large exercise ball. Done incorrectly or overly aggressively, however, and the body will borrow movement from the looser areas to compensate for tighter spots. This means that someone with tight shoulders or tight hips is likely to borrow movement by thrusting into the ribs or sinking into the lumbar curve—both recipes for diastasis recti.

Start exploring Wheel pose by moving into Bridge pose (Setu Bandha Sarvangasana) first. Begin in constructive rest, which is lying on your back with the knees bent, feet on the floor, and the arms resting by the side body. Allow your feet to be slightly wider than hip width. Reach the knees forward over the ankles to lengthen the lower back.

Once the lower back begins to lift, press down into the feet to lift the sacrum and roll back towards the shoulders. The tailbone will feel as though it is hanging rather than tucking (No tucking, folks!). If the lower back compresses, which may happen if the psoas is tight, pull with the hamstrings to isometrically drag the pelvis forward to lengthen your lower back towards the feet again. Press the elbows into the floor, but do not squeeze the shoulder blades together.

To release, roll down through each vertebra. Knees can hug in towards the chest if needed to release the lower back.

... continuing into Urdhva Dhanurasana

From the top of Bridge pose, place the hands alongside the ears on the floor with the fingers facing towards the collar bones or slightly to the side. Draw the elbows towards one another so the forearms are perpendicular to the floor. On an inhale, begin to pull with the legs, drawing the weight into the feet. With an exhale, simultaneously push the arms and legs into the floor lifting the chest into Wheel pose.

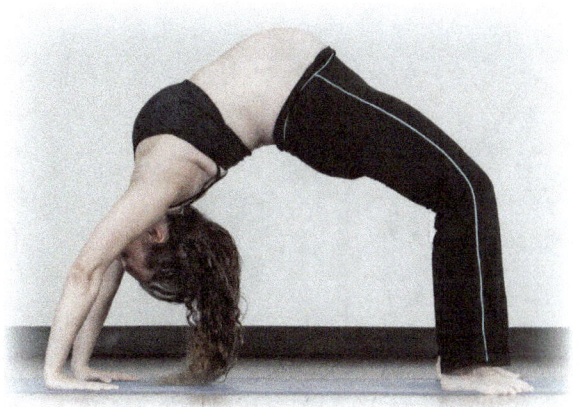

The weight shifts into the feet as the pelvis and spine turn towards the front of the mat, as though standing up into Tadasana. This movement should not be overly muscled. Avoid pausing on the top of the head—this common rest stop places too much weight into the cervical spine and counteracts the fluid movement that comes from a well-integrated entrance. Hug the elbows in towards one another to support the shoulders. Keep the breath steady and full.

I have seen some students pull the head through the arms in this pose, I assume to seek a deeper stretch in the shoulders. This is actually a big no-no, and doubly so during pregnancy! The flexion of the neck right into deep extension in the shoulders asks for too much motion in an already vulnerable joint. Instead of pulling the head through the arms and towards the chest, think of looking back towards the tail to see the hands. This brings the action of the backbend more into the upper spine and helps reduce the load on the lumbar spine.

To come out, bend the elbows towards the back of the mat, keeping them close to one another. As the elbows bend, bring the chin to the chest so the weight lands on the back of the head and neck. Hug the knees in if needed. Wait to repeat until the breath quiets. If the breath is severely disturbed, consider omitting Wheel pose and stick to Bridge.

Ustrasana/Camel

I have always felt Ustrasana was a far more challenging posture than some yoga teachers give it credit for. As an instructor in a workshop once pointed out, "Ustrasana is not a beginner's pose!" This backbend involves not only suppleness in the psoas muscle but also pliability in the quads and mobility in the mid-thoracic spine: all common problem areas for even many seasoned yoginis.

The challenge with Ustrasana during pregnancy is the growing belly adds further abdominal wall stress. There's also the question of how to get in and out of the *asana* safely without asking the abdominals to support weight in an eccentric (muscle lengthening) contraction. I only recommend Ustrasana for yoginis who had a solid practice of this posture beforehand—and who have good body awareness now.

Begin by sitting on the heels in Vajrasana with the feet pointed straight back. Lift up onto the knees. Place the hands, fingers down, on the base of the sacrum. Press the hips back into

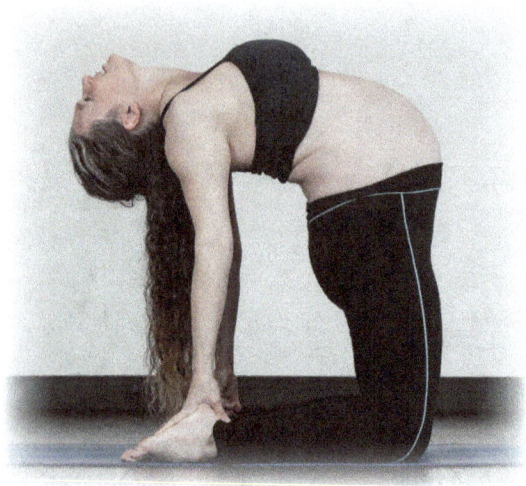

the hands as though beginning a "Cow" tilt of the pelvis. Then draw the pelvic floor and abdominals upward as the chest raises towards the ceiling along with the back ribs. Breathe here. To come out, simply raise the chest back to vertical and sit back down.

To go deeper (and this would have been plenty so far!) from the above variation, tuck the toes or place blocks on either side of the feet. Lifting through the heart, gently reach one hand back to either the block or ankle. It may be advisable to lower the hips a bit to reach the block rather than straining for the grip.

If comfortable, and if there is no undue stretch through the abdominals or strain in the lower back, reach the second hand back and rest it on the other block or ankle. Press the chest towards the ceiling while drawing the inner thighs softly back. Do not thrust the pelvis forward, as this will place pressure on the pubic joint and exacerbate the lengthening of the transverse abdominals. Maintain as even a curve along the spine as possible. The lumbar spine will bend, but it should not be the main focus of the curve.

To come out, sit the hips back to the heels and fold into a wide knee Child's Pose. This "backing out" of the pose reduces the potential for abdominal strain.

Bhujangasana/Cobra and Upward Facing Dog

Cobra and Upward Facing Dog should only be practiced until 28 weeks or so due to the risk of abdominal strain caused by gravity and the expanding uterus pushing into the forward facing abdominal wall. I often find students begin doing this posture only about 50% of the way by around 20 weeks or so, although some may feel comfortable going deeper longer.

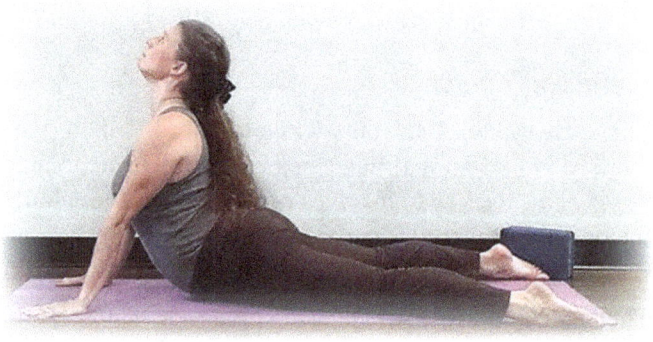

For the first trimester, Cobra can still be done from the floor. Begin lying on the stomach, and place the hands alongside the chest under the shoulders. Rolling the shoulders back and down, start to lift the spine with the upper back muscles.

On an exhale, press the hands into the floor to assist the action of the upper back, raising the chest higher. Be sure to engage the lower abdominal wall upwards to support the weight of *the expanding organs and baby. If this abdominal lift cannot be accomplished, do not proceed further. Focus on opening the chest and grounding the knees into the floor rather than tucking the tail or pressing the pubic bone downward. The feeling is like gently arcing the upper spine onto a beach ball behind your back.*

For Upward Facing Dog, start with Cobra, then press into the tops of the feet to lift the knees and inner thighs while drawing the chest forward. Again, the abdomen should be well integrated, and the pelvic floor will lift upwards.

In second trimester, begin Cobra from Table Pose, and round the lower back as in Cat. Walk the hands a good 6-8 inches further forward. Keeping the lift of the abdomen and pelvic floor, begin to shift the hips forward towards the hands, gradually lowering the thighs closer to the floor. The arch of the spine will gradually unfurl into the backbend as the hips lower. Continue to draw the navel up. If the thighs touch the floor, focus on the knees grounding and the backbend moving evenly throughout the spine.

If attempting Upward Facing Dog, tuck the toes and extend into the heels to lift the knees. Be sure that the belly comes with you and without strain. Bring the knees back down if any pressure drops into the lower back or there is a strong stretch through the abdomen. To come out, pike the hips up into Table and sit back to a wide knee Child's Pose.

Inversions

Inversions are probably the most misunderstood family of postures with regards to pregnancy. Inversions are certainly advanced postures and shouldn't be practiced while pregnant if mom is still learning the basics, but the reasons often provided are significantly off-base—including the claim that the work required for an inversion could deprive the baby of oxygen! Which is flatly untrue. As I mentioned in Chapter 6 on yoga myths, many of the restrictions around inversions are based in superstition and questionable medical understanding.

In reality, caution is necessary during inversions due to the combination of increased relaxin, changing center of gravity, and the hydrostatic blood pressure changes involved with inverting for long periods of time. Essentially, if you don't have a well-established baseline to work from, it will be hard to gauge how far to move and when to draw back in these poses. With that said, even longtime practitioners should be mindful of how they enter and leave these postures and should probably avoid holding them for multiple minutes at a time.

Sirsasana/Headstand

Sirsasana has the benefit of briefly taking the weight off the lower pelvis and also lightly tugging on the network of cervical ligaments supporting the uterus in the lower pelvis. This shift needs to be made gradually however, so I don't recommend holding Sirsasana for more than 30-60 seconds (3-5 breaths) at most. Once you come down, it is critical to give the uterus time to realign before moving on, which is the reason for kneeling up before continuing on to other *asanas*. Again, only consider this pose if you were already strongly practicing Sirsasana before pregnancy and if you have no concerns about inversions in general, such as high

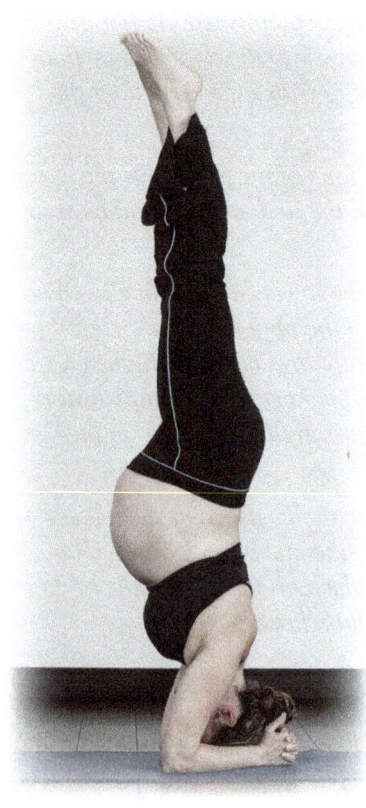

blood pressure, risk of stroke, glaucoma, or any bleeding during pregnancy

Set this posture up so that your back will be facing a wall for stability and as a precaution against falling backwards. Interlace the hands in a basket shape, with enough space between the wrists to hold an egg. Place the elbows on the mat shoulder width apart or ideally a little narrower.

Be sure the outer wrist bone remains connected into the floor rather than allowing the palms to rotate open, as this rotation leads to a more unstable base. Avoid cupping the back of the skull with the palms; rather, connect the back of the skull to the inner wrists. Cross the thumbs to create an "X," and place the crown of the head against that X. Don't press down, as the weight on the hands will deform the basket; just have the crown touching the hands.

Tuck the toes, and with an exhale raise the knees into a variation of Downward Dog. Do not put any extra weight into the head yet. You may choose to simply stay here, feeling the elongation of the spine up and back through the hips.

If going on, walk the feet towards the elbows, widening the feet to make space for the belly if needed. The upper spine should remain straight, without rounding or touching the wall. If you feel either of these sensations occur, work to elongate the spine before continuing. When the hips feel as though they are stacked above the head and shoulders, pause and shift the crown just behind the hands so it can touch down to the floor, with the back of the head in contact with the wrists.

Keep the outer wrist bone on the floor, and do not open the basket of the hands (the "egg" should still be able to be held lightly, not rolling away or crushed.) At this point the body is effectively already in Headstand, and the legs are practically hanging from the pelvis. To raise the legs, focus on rotating the pelvic bowl so the perineum floats towards the ceiling. The lift of the legs should feel almost effortless, with the feet floating off the floor. Bend the knees, and then extend the legs up the wall.

The balance will be subtle and shouldn't be muscled through the arms. Lightly hug the navel back and reach towards the ceiling through the tail and legs. If the feet come to the wall, this is fine, or they may float a few inches from it. In either case, focus on feeling the vertical extension of the spine from head to tail.

To come down, first bend the knees and extend the feet to the ground. The weight of the legs will bring you to the floor. Pause in Child's Pose for a breath, and then sit up in Vajrasana, standing up on the knees to allow baby and the uterus to settle back into position in the pelvis.

Adho Mukha Vrksasana/Handstand and Pincha Mayurasana/Forearm Stand

The setup for Handstand and Forearm Stand is pretty much the same, with the obvious exception that in Handstand we start with the hands on the floor and in Forearm Stand we start with the elbows on the floor. For both poses, set the posture up so the back will be facing a wall. This will prevent toppling over backwards, which could strain the abdominal muscles, not to mention injure shoulders and anything else impacted by a fall (like a baby).

Begin with the back facing a wall and come into Downward Dog on either the hands or the forearms. For Handstand, place the hands shoulder distance apart, and anchor the thumb and index finger into the mat. For Forearm Stand, the elbows should remain shoulder distance apart, and the forearms should remain parallel to one another. If the hands tend to slip together, a block can be placed between them to maintain correct alignment.

I do not recommend binding the arms with a yoga strap, as this can lead to excessive strain on an already loose joint and encourage the body to borrow movement from other places rather

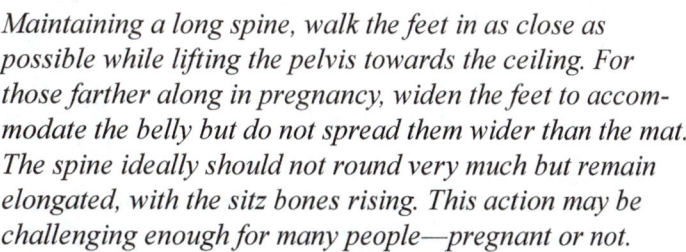

than learning to muscularly support and work with the available range of motion. The shoulders should stay over the elbows to create a stable angle.

Maintaining a long spine, walk the feet in as close as possible while lifting the pelvis towards the ceiling. For those farther along in pregnancy, widen the feet to accommodate the belly but do not spread them wider than the mat. The spine ideally should not round very much but remain elongated, with the sitz bones rising. This action may be challenging enough for many people—pregnant or not.

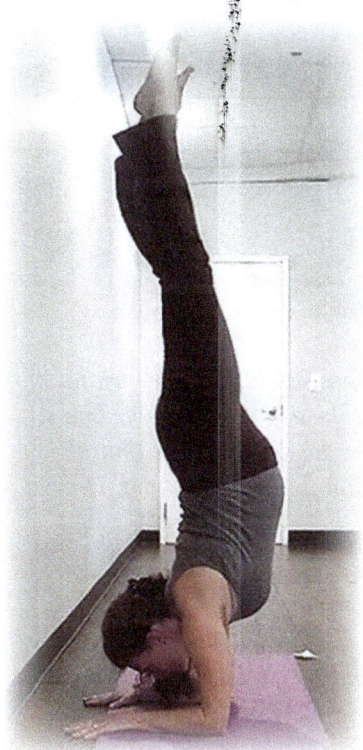

If you want to move on, raise one leg in the air, stretching through the ball of the foot as though placing it on the ceiling. Ideally, one simply steps into this pose without any major exertion from the bottom leg. In reality, you may have to incorporate a slight push from the bottom leg as the top one stretches towards the ceiling, bringing the hips to balance over the shoulders. The effort should be very light, and the landing should be nearly silent. No jarring forces through the body.

With the top foot in contact with the wall, bring the second leg to meet it. Be sure to extend up through the tail and inner thighs to lengthen the lumbar spine, and avoid any swaying in the back. Float the pelvic floor over the crown of the head.

To come down, lightly lower one leg towards the floor while stretching through the upward leg. Allow the weight shift to tip the pelvis, bringing the feet back to the floor. Come to kneeling and take a few breaths, then maybe repeat with the other leg lifting first.

This way of practicing these two inversions removes the "flinging" quality sometimes found when entering these poses. I have found that during pregnancy, flinging is never a good idea, due to both the increased flexibility in the body and the decreased abdominal control over the expanding center. While hopping may be a fun exploration, remember that jumping is one of the true contraindications in the yoga practice. That includes upside-down jumping. Step, don't fling.

Forward Leaning Inversion

A similar-looking but fundamentally different inversion from Headstand and Forearm Stand is the Forward Leaning Inversion. Developed by Dr. Carol Phillips, this posture is used in the Spinning Babies® technique for optimal fetal positioning before and during labor.

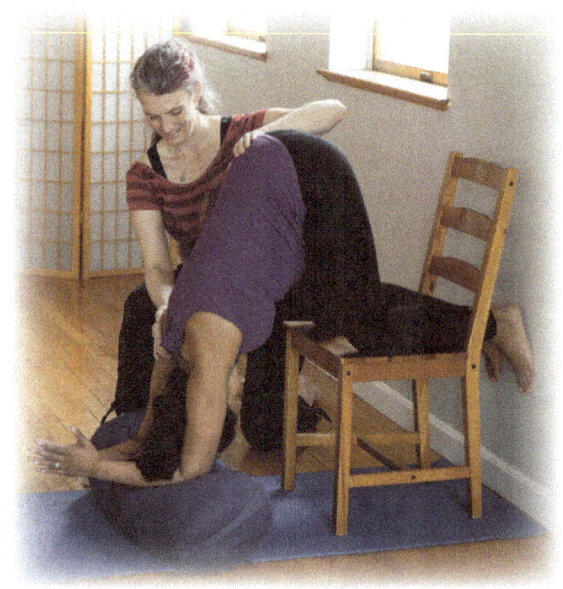

The Forward Leaning Inversion splits the difference between the angles of Downward Dog and a full Sirsasana. It can be extremely helpful for repositioning a breech baby and for balancing the utero-sacral ligaments, allowing more freedom for the uterus to settle into the center of the pelvic bowl.

Forward Leaning Inversion begins with mom kneeling on a chair, couch, or other step unit. The elevation should be appropriate for what comes next. Leaning forward, place the hands against the edge of the chair and sit the hips back onto the heels. From this safe position, walk the hands off the chair onto the floor, then place the elbows down to the floor in the same position as for Headstand. Have a partner spot you in case the body weighs more than you expected.

Place the head between the arms without the head touching the hands or the floor. From here, shift the hips up until the uterus is hanging and pull the chin into the chest to look up towards the belly. Take three deep breaths, maintaining a long spine while the uterus gently hangs down. At the end of three breaths, walk the hands back onto a chair, using a partner for support if you need it. Sit the hips back down, and walk the hands back onto the chair or couch, returning to the safety position.

Pause to allow the blood to drain out of the face. Then lift into a high kneeling position so that the amniotic fluid can wash back over the baby and the uterus can settle back into the pelvis.[52]

Sarvangasana/Shoulderstand

Shoulderstand can be a wonderful release for the neck and upper back, but increased breast and belly size can make it challenging. When practicing, focus on keeping the chest and throat open, even if this means sacrificing the verticality of the legs.

The introductory postures for Shoulderstand are Bridge and freestanding Viparita Karani/Legs Up the Wall pose with the hips resting on a stack of blocks rather than against the wall.

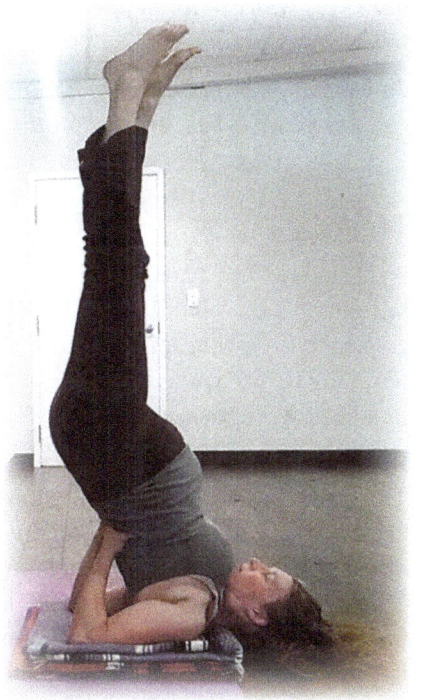

To use Bridge as a preparation, begin on your back. Place a block on the medium height beneath the sacrum. For more flexible practitioners, two blocks can be stacked on the lowest height to create more lift.

To move towards Shoulderstand, press the elbows and the back of the head down into the floor. The pressure should be such that the cervical curve is maintained and the nose feels as though it would lift towards the ceiling rather than tilt towards or away from the chest. The C7 vertebra (the big bone at the base of the neck) will slightly lift away from the floor as the arms and skull actively engage. The tail should be heavy and feel as though it were dropping over the block supports towards the floor.

To explore Shoulderstand further: Leaving the hips resting on the blocks, slowly raise one leg and then the other up over the hips. The sacrum should remain heavy on the block, not tucking upwards. Maintain pressure through the elbows and back of the skull, and feel the chest lifting towards the chin. This effectively brings you into a variation of Viparita Karani in the center of the room.

To move into a fuller Shoulderstand, set up Viparita Karani near a wall, with the feet able to touch the baseboard. Lift the hips, placing the blocks under the sacrum, and then raise the feet to rest the legs on the wall. From this Viparita Karani variation, place the feet against the wall and raise the hips off the blocks. Do not let the chest drop! Move the blocks and replace the support with the palms of the hands. The hips should still tip backwards into the palms, so this can sometimes be challenging for the elbows and wrists.

Maintaining the pelvic tilt, raise one leg and possibly the second off the wall. The verticality

---

[52] For more information on the full Spinning Babies® program see *Spinningbabies.com.*

comes from grounding through the elbows and rooting through the back of the head rather than tucking and thrusting the hips. Breathe and allow the energy to move upwards through the feet. If the breasts are greatly enlarged (honestly, this variation is helpful for those who are naturally well endowed), allow the chest to tilt further into the palms, moving away from pure verticality to allow space for the neck and throat. It is never a good idea to practice without the breath, especially when pregnant.

To come out, bend the knees and place them against the wall. Lower slowly to the floor, then roll to one side. Take a few breaths before sitting up. If done properly, this pose creates a spacious, almost floating feeling in the chest after practicing.

Twists

As discussed in Chapter 6 on yoga myths, the whole restriction on twists during pregnancy has gotten a bit out of hand. The suggestions were probably meant in good faith, but the consequence is that some practitioners have removed an entire family of postures without realizing that twisting is an everyday movement which needs to be fostered and promoted in a healthy, supported fashion. How are you to buckle your seatbelt if you cannot rotate the spine?

The basic rule of no closed twists is accurate, but opinions on what defines a closed twist vary widely. Some teachers say it is anything that reaches across the midline of the body; others say it is anything that compresses the abdomen against the thigh. I fall into the latter camp. I submit that a closed twist means something which would squeeze the belly, either through direct compression or because of the degree of rotation desired. So no cranking into twists or using leverage to get a deeper range of motion, and nothing which squeezes or compresses the expanding abdomen and uterus.

But this doesn't mean that all spinal rotation is out. We can adapt certain postures to allow the belly more space and promote better stability through the hips and legs. In doing so, we return a set of fabulous spinal release movements to pregnant yoginis.

Parivrtta Trikonasana/Revolved Triangle pose

The amount of modification required for Parivrtta Trikonasana depends on the stage of pregnancy and the size of the belly. Some women will feel restricted in the mid-second trimester; others won't need to significantly modify until early third trimester.

Step the feet 3-4 feet apart facing the side of the mat. Rotating from the hip, turn one foot to face the short end of the mat, and turn the back foot inward to about a 45 degree angle. Do not go further than 45 degrees; you'll sacrifice stability and increase the risk of falling. Adjust the feet to stand heel to heel, and rotate the hips to face the front foot. Widen your feet a little more if your hips do not allow for a full rotation in heel to heel alignment. Have a block on hand.

On an inhale, raise the opposite hand from the front foot. On the exhale, begin folding forward from the hips with an extended spine. Pause when you are about halfway down and gently move the belly towards the front leg, trying to shift the belly on top of the leg to the extent possible. Keep pressure in the outer edge of the back foot and create an isometric external rotation of the back thigh to maintain a stable pelvis.

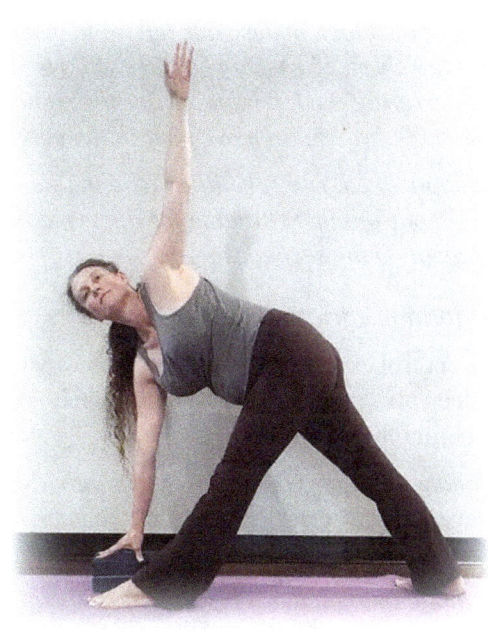

The sacrum should remain level with the floor, and the hips should feel spacious. When the range of motion reaches its limit, place the hand or block to the INSIDE of the front foot and the other hand on the hip. Press down into the block to lift the chest. The top shoulder will lift automatically. Leave the hand on the hip unless it feels easy to raise the arm. The arm should remain in line with the top shoulder rather than drifting behind the plane of the chest.

The head can turn if the hips and belly feel stable, but if not, keep looking towards the floor. Be sure to gently draw the front abdominals in and up to support the expanding abdominal wall. This pose should ultimately feel like it comes from the legs and has a quietness in the belly rather than an active "wringing out" sensation.

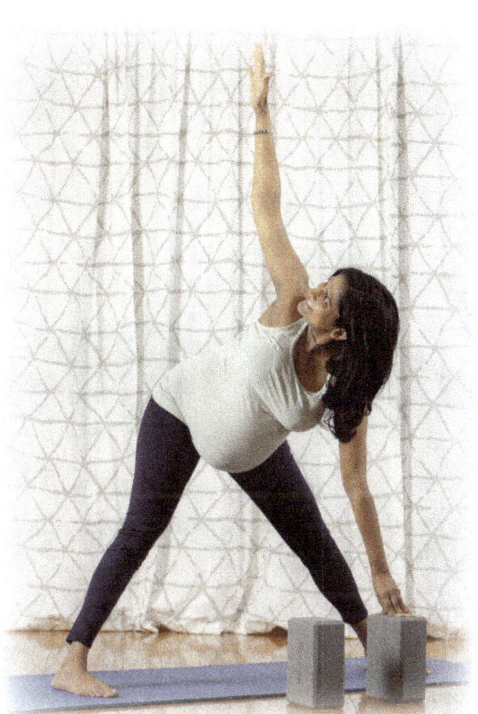

To come out, focus on the back leg and turn it out strongly. On an exhale, engaging pelvic floor and lower abdominals, follow the turn of the back leg to come to standing. Turn to the side of the mat, return the feet to parallel, and take a few breaths before repeating on the second side.

Parivrtta Prasarita Padottanasana/Revolved Wide-Legged Standing Forward Fold

Alternatively, if the forward orientation of Revolved Triangle is too unstable, the spinal rotation can also be achieved from the side-facing position of Parivrtta Prasarita Padottanasana.

Beginning in a wide stance 3-4 ft apart, fold forward to place the hands below the shoulders. Raise the floor by placing your hands on blocks on the highest height. This is helpful even if you are able to reach fully to the floor because the focus is on the spinal rotation rather than hip flexion or hamstring stretching.

Bring the block under your left hand centered beneath the nose. Press the floor away and lift the chest. The right shoulder will rise towards the ceiling, and you might lift onto the fingertips of the left hand. Place the right hand on the sacrum to help maintain a mostly level pelvis. A little bit of movement in the pelvis can feel good at times, but don't exaggerate it.

If so inclined, raise the lifted arm in line with the shoulder and reach the two hands away from one another. Breathe for a few moments, then return the right arm to the block or floor. Repeat on the second side.

Windmill variation

A playful exploration and delicious way to release the lower back, top of the psoas, and the "deep six"[53] rotator muscles of the pelvis is to turn this posture into a *vinyasa* rather than holding the twist.

Inhale to lift into the twist, then gently exhale to lower and switch sides. Go back and forth several times gently mobilizing the back body.

To come out, bring both hands to the knees, bend the knees, and gently roll to stand on an exhale. Bring the feet together.

Parivritta Janu Sirsasana

Janu Sirsasana postures have a great combination of hip flexion, lateral spinal extension, and spinal rotation. I have found there are two variations of this posture which can be helpful during pregnancy, especially for lower back pain.

Parivritta Janu Sirsasana A

Classically referred to as Parivritta Janu Sirsasana, this posture offers a beautiful side bend combined with the spinal rotation and is one of my favorites for students who are complaining of lower back pain, shortness of breath, or rib pain.

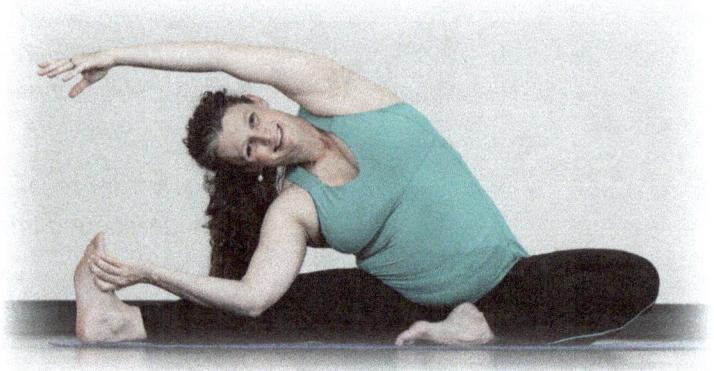

Sitting in Baddha Konasana, with the weight established on the front of the sitting bones, extend one leg to the side and flex the foot. On an inhale, raise the same arm as the extended leg, and with an exhale, reach out towards the foot, maintaining the length on both sides of the body.

The top arm can reach alongside the cheek, possibly grabbing the foot but more likely ex-

---

[53] The lateral rotator muscles of the pelvis are sometimes called the "deep six" muscles and consist of the piriformis, gemellus superior, obturator internus, gemellus inferior, quadratus femoris, and obturator externus. They all affect the sacrum and lumbar spinal stability.

tending over the head. Spin the chest towards the ceiling, and breathe into the stretch in the lower back and side body. Eventually the side body may lie down smoothly along the extended leg. To return, inhale and sit upright. Switch legs for the second side.

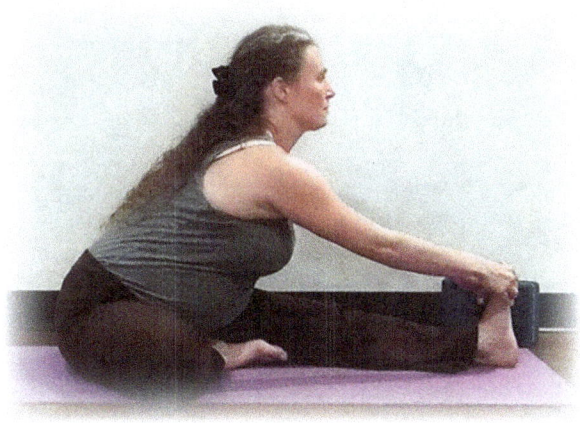

Parivrtta Janu Sirsasana B

Technically this variation more closely resembles the straight Janu Sirsasana, but I find that focusing on the spinal rotation rather than the forward flexion creates more space in the low back and hip rotators.

Set up as for classic Janu Sirsasana, with one leg bent in and the other extended straight forward from the hip. With an inhale, raise the opposite arm as the extended leg. On the exhale, begin to reach forward, gently shifting the belly towards the extended leg. During late second and third trimester you will probably want to use a yoga strap.

Hook the foot with the strap or grab the outer edge of the foot with your hand, and lengthen the chest forwards and up. Focus the rotation into the upper back and snuggle the belly into the extended inner thigh. From here, release the overt twist of the upper back and imagine laying the belly against the extended leg. Maintain a grounded feeling through both sides of the pelvis.

To return, inhale and sit upright. Switch legs for the second side.

Parivrtta Janu Sirsasana C

While there isn't technically a classic version C of this posture, I've included a third variation because for some, turning the pose into an open rather than a "closed" twist provides different sensations and releases within the spine and the adductor pelvic muscles. In my own practice, I like to pair this variation with Janu Sirsasana B to get the counter twist before switching legs.

Begin with the legs set for Janu Sirsasana, then inhale to lengthen the spine and exhale to rotate towards the bent knee. Bring one hand across to hold the knee and the other hand behind you.

Maintain a grounded pelvis and focus the rotation into the shoulders rather than the belly.

The rotation of the shoulders will pull gently into the lower back, and the movement into the bent leg can help to stretch the hip rotators within the groin.

To return, inhale and sit upright. Switch legs for the second side.

Marichyasana

Marichyasana A can easily be performed throughout pregnancy, with the cautions to be gentle with the SI joints at the back of the pelvis and to avoid using force to deepen into the twist.

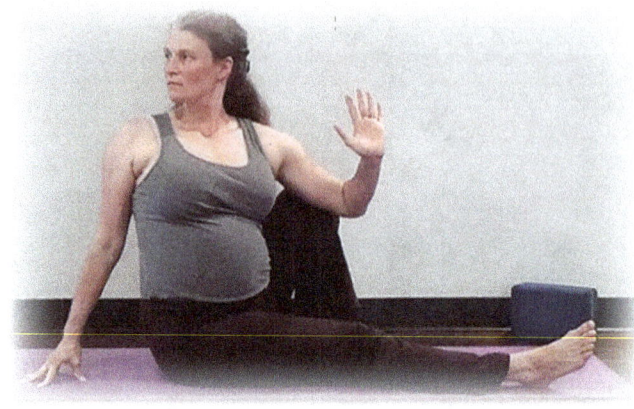

For the variations Marichyasana B, C, and D, I suggest letting them go until the body has returned to its usual hormonal balance. The range of motion required, combined with the cross-body rotation, runs the risk of tweaking the SI joints. Plus, the deep knee bend and hip rotation of the Lotus foot position for Marichyasana B asks for such a big range of motion that the body will likely find a way around existing stiff spots and borrow from pelvic joints. Remember that the pelvic connective tissues interweave with the uterine fascia, and whenever possible, we want to promote balance in this tissue rather than strain.

Begin sitting in Dandasana/Staff Pose, with the hips upright so that the legs and spine form a 90 degree angle. You may need to elevate your sitz bones on a blanket or block to be able to sit tall.

Bend the right knee in so that the foot stands on the floor close to the hip. Move the foot far enough out that there is space for the belly. Do not try and pull the foot back as far as possible as this can affect the SI joint. On an inhale, stretch the right arm towards the ceiling and perhaps lean slightly to the left to make further space for the belly along the right side. Maintaining that space, bring the right upper arm against the inside of the right leg. Actively press the arm and leg against one another to create a dynamic stability. Exhale and rotate the shoulders to the left, feeling the release in the lower back. Maintain the upright pelvis and spine. It may be helpful to place a hand on the floor or a block for greater lift.

Optional increase: To bind, turn the right arm down and reach around the front of the knee placing the back of the hand against the outside of the hip. If it is EASY, the second hand can reach behind to grasp the hands. There should be no straining or wiggling to reach this shape. The hands should simply be able to touch without effort or can reach without touching.

To release, return to center and extend the bent knee back to Dandasana. Take a few breaths before repeating on the second side.

Core Work

Core work in pregnancy is both a needed practice and one which should be done with caution. The expanding abdominal wall does need the support of the transverse abs and pelvic floor. At the same time, these muscles need to be able to release to allow the baby to grow and need to be supple during the birth process. It probably goes without saying, but the focus of abdominal work during pregnancy is not on creating a flat stomach but rather on supporting the weight shift and postural changes that occur as the body grows.

The challenge is to find appropriate engagement of the transverse abdominals (TA) without allowing the lower back to fall and without compensating with secondary muscles such as shoulders or glutes. At the same time, it's important not to overengage the rectus abdominis or obliques; doing so can pull on the already stressed linea alba. Postures such as Plank, Bird Dog, Table, and Cat/Cow are generally preferable to roll-ups or Bicycles, especially in the third trimester. But the back and center need to be fully supported while in any pose or the benefit is lost.

In general, during the first trimester it may be best to back off core work. This is purely my own recommendation, but the compressive force exerted by the TA on an implanting embryo and developing pregnancy seems excessive during the time when that same pregnancy is establishing itself within the body. Certainly abdominal work could be done, but this might not be the best time to start or continue intense core exercises.

Table

I often find that Table is overlooked as a core exercise, yet I also hear yoga teachers describe Table as Plank with the knees down. Done properly, Table can be a great modification for deep core work, allowing for stabilization without the risk of dropping into the lower back or hanging into the front abdominal wall.

Bring the hands under the shoulders and the knees under the hips. Press the hands actively into the floor and lift the chest to open the collar bones. At the same time, gently but firmly draw the abdominals around the expanding belly and lift up, as though gathering the navel up and forwards towards the heart.

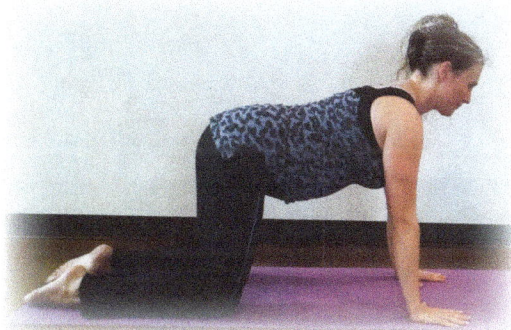

Correct

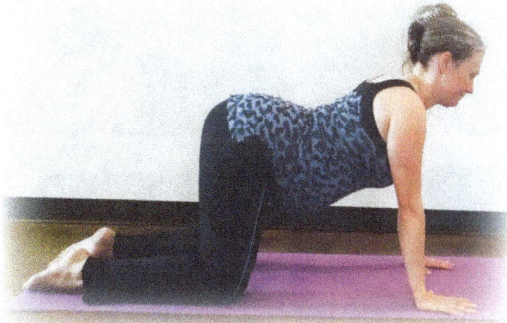

NO! Note the lack of belly support!

The lower back should remain in neutral: no tucking. A student once described this action as trying to do Cow Pose from the waist up and Cat Pose from the waist down, which is an apt description of the sensation created in the mid-body. Maintain a steady breath feeling the deep support from within the abdomen. Release by sitting back to Child's Pose with wide knees.

Bird Dog/Half Plank pose

An increase in challenge from the active Table pose involves extending one leg on the floor as though moving to full Plank. This leg extension shifts the weight support, requiring more engagement from the obliques and lower back stabilizers. After extending the leg, the foot can be lifted off the floor into a variation akin to Warrior 3 on the floor.

This lift further loads the obliques and back muscles as well as recruits the glutes and pelvic stabilizers. As with all core exercises, if the initial stability in the core body can't be maintained, the pose is probably too challenging and shouldn't be practiced at this time.

From an engaged Table pose, tuck the toes of one leg and extend the foot back, pressing into the heel for a calf stretch. Be sure to maintain level hips, and support the abdomen to avoid sinking into the lower back. Breathe smoothly here, feeling the change brought on by the leg extension.

If going further, use an exhale to engage the pelvic floor and transverse abs, then raise the extended leg to hip height. Do not go above the height of the hip, as this will bring a backbend into the spine.

Rotate the toes to face the floor and feel the leg extending back, not just from the hip but from the mid-back as well. This is where the deep hip flexors (psoas muscles) attach, and focusing here helps maintain mid-body stability and coordination. If you feel very stable, the opposite arm can also be raised to shoulder height, but this will require deep control within the abdominal obliques and will make balance more challenging.

Breathe and stretch, long and stable, from the center body to the toes. Then return the knee and hand to the floor and feel the difference in Table. Repeat on the second side.

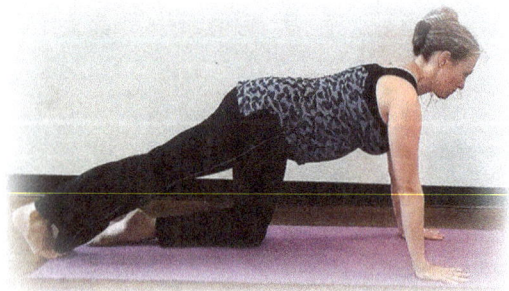 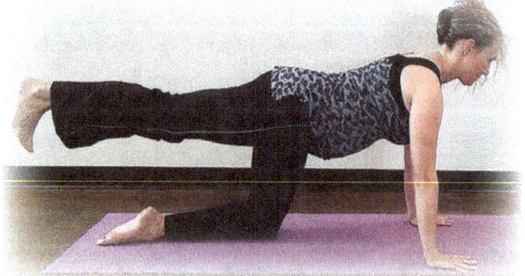

Plank

I don't recommend entering Plank from Table pose in pregnancy. The sudden load of the full weight of the body and baby onto the front abdominal wall is too great of a risk for most pregnant yoginis. Instead, I have students explore a full Plank range coming from Downward Dog, stopping long before they reach the straight line that the fitness world defines as "plank." This gradual entry offers more control over how much weight is being applied to the core body. It also offers the ability to lower the knees back to Table if the support disappears at any point.

I urge students to exercise caution when practicing this pose during both the first and third trimesters. It seems excessive to apply strong abdominal compression during the first trimester while the pregnancy is still establishing itself. And in third trimester, the added weight makes it that much more difficult to maintain the transverse abdominal lift away from the linea alba. That said, if you are a student who can maintain the appropriate support in Plank, explore it to your comfort level.

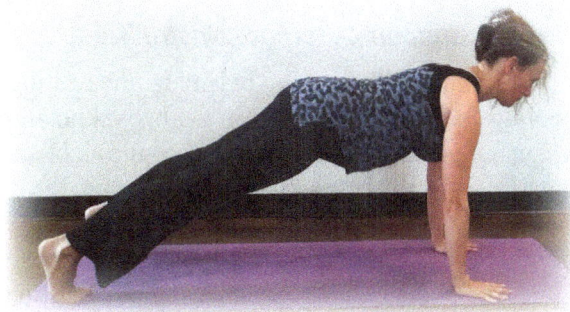

Begin in Downward Dog, with the spine long and the pelvis rotated to a neutral position—which will give the lower back a slight curve. On an exhale, draw the pelvic floor and navel upwards. Begin to shift the shoulders forward towards the hands, as though moving from the feet. Keep an open chest, and only tuck the tail enough to maintain a neutral pelvic position.

Feel for the abdominal muscles engaging. At the moment you feel tightening, pause, and ensure the lower back and belly are still supported. If you can't maintain support here, drop the knees to the floor. If the support is still intact, then slowly begin shifting further forward, maintaining support for your lower back and belly. This posture should not be held for long periods of time during pregnancy. I usually recommend taking 1-2 breaths here and then moving on.

Unlike in a traditional vinyasa flow, moving on from Plank does not mean bending the elbows into Chaturanga. (I have yet to see a yogi in second trimester or beyond who can maintain spinal support through this classic transition.) Instead, drop the knees into an active Table pose, then bend the elbows into a pushup with the knees on the floor. Raise back to Table without backbending, then return to Downward Dog.

Advanced *pranayama* practices

The following are *pranayama* practices which either require more coordination than the basic breath exercises—such as the use of a hand or specific mouth position—or which involve a specific visualization. These practices are all safe to use throughout pregnancy but should be discontinued if they result in dizziness, shortness of breath, or any other feelings of discomfort.

Pelvic floor breathing

Sit in a comfortable seated position with the hips slightly raised and the weight on the font of the sitting bones. The jaw and shoulders are relaxed. Start with visualizing the breath being inhaled from the crown of the head, through the heart center, and down to the center of the pelvic floor at the perineum, like a waterfall. With the exhale, visualize the breath moving upwards from the pubic bone back to the crown of the head.

Do a few cycles of just the visualization of the breath, and then add the movement of the pelvic floor. As you inhale the breath down through the pelvic floor, feel the muscles of the sitz bones spread down and out. As you exhale the breath up and out the crown, feel the pelvic floor gather softly upwards. Repeat for several cycles.

Nadi Shodhanam/Alternate Nostril Breathing

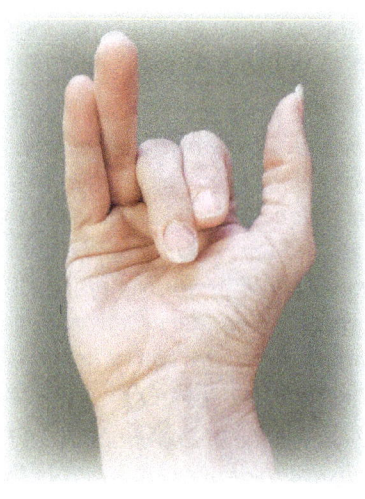

This *pranayama* focuses on balancing the heating and cooling energy channels within the body, known as the *ida* and *pingala*, which correspond to the right and left nostril, respectively. At any one time during the day, the right or the left side of the nose will be dominant, switching roughly every 45 minutes if nothing else is going on. Nadi Shodanam can be used to balance either sluggish or hyper energy states since it brings the solar and lunar energies into balance. It is also said to balance the two hemispheres of the brain.

Traditionally, this *pranayama* is done with the right hand in Vishnu Mudra (first two fingers folded into the palm, thumb resting on the right side of the nose and the ring and pinky finger resting on the left). If this hand position causes the fingers to cramp, it is also fine to rest the first and second fingers on the third eye center between the eyebrows.

Begin by sitting and tuning into the natural rhythm of your inhale and exhale. See if you can tell which nostril is the dominant side. If you are unsure, try blocking one side to check. With the right hand in Vishnu Mudra, rest the thumb and ring fingers just above the flare in the nostrils. Gently press the more closed side so you are breathing only through the open channel.

Exhale and inhale through the open side. Then close that side and open the closed one. Exhale and inhale through the more closed channel, then switch back to the first side. Out and in through each side constitutes one cycle. Continue for several cycles, finishing by inhaling through the second side. Bring the hands down into the lap, and notice any mental or physical changes which have occurred.

An alternate way to practice which can be extremely helpful if the nose is congested, which can often occur during pregnancy, is to omit the hand position altogether and simply practice by focusing the mind on one nostril at a time. While this means the entire *pranayama* is done in the mind, it does not mean nothing is happening. Shifting attention subtly shifts actions within the body, and just paying more attention to the air moving in and out of the right nostril, and then in and out of the left, does have an energetic impact.

Bhramari/Bee Breath

The name of this breath means the humming of the bee, and it can be helpful both in quieting the nervous system and blocking out disquieting sounds in the surrounding environment (hospitals are noisy places!) This breath is very relaxing and can sometimes reduce blood pressure. It also gives the baby a sonic or vibratory massage.

In a comfortable sitting position, close the eyes. Use the thumbs to close the ears, and gently cover the eyes with the hands without pressing on the eyeballs. Keep the arms relaxed so the shoulders do not tire.

Inhale through the nose. On the exhale, quietly hum, listening to the buzzing vibration in the ears and throughout the head. The noise is more internal than external, and anyone around may be only barely aware that you are humming. In a relaxed breathing cycle, keep inhaling through the nose and then exhaling through the nose with a hum.

Practice for about 10 breaths, then sit with your hands in the lap, noticing the lingering effects of the vibratory echo.

Sitali/Cooling Breath

Sitali is great for a hot day or when mom is feeling overheated, as it soothes and cools down the nervous system. The practice is done by sipping the air in through a rolled tongue, as though breathing through a straw. If you are unable to roll your tongue (it is genetic, either you can or can't) then rest the tip of the tongue against the front lower teeth and sip the air in across the surface. The feeling is similar to the cooling effect of sipping a cold glass of water after a hot day's activity.

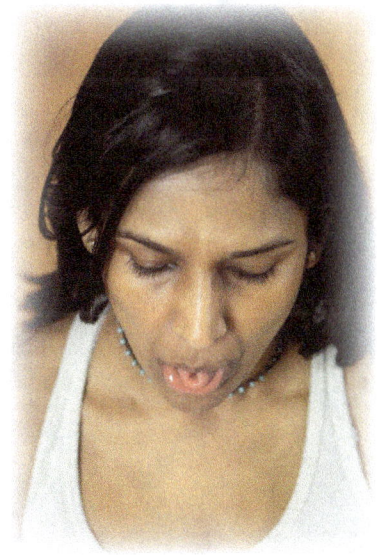

Begin sitting comfortably with a neutral spine and pelvis. Roll the tongue (if possible) and inhale a steady stream of air, expanding the chest and abdomen.

Pause to gently press the tongue to the roof of the month feeling the cool surface. Exhale, holding the tongue to the roof of the mouth. In the pause after the exhale, gently roll the tongue again and repeat the inhalation. Do 5-7 rounds, and then return to calm breathing to check in before continuing.

The pauses mentioned in this exercise should only be held long enough for the breath to change direction. In general, you want to refrain from holding the breath for an extended period of time during pregnancy, as doing so begins to change the oxygen content of the blood going to the baby.

Is this the end of what can be practiced during pregnancy? Certainly not. Yoga *asana* has myriad variations and options depending on the student, their body, their pregnancy, and their experience level. But the basic principles of practicing during pregnancy apply across the board. We must remember how the body is shifting and changing and seek the middle path within our individual practice. Not too restrictive, but not too permissive, either. In this way you can promote your body being not too tight but also not too loose; supple and balanced just right.

10 — Common Discomforts in Pregnancy and Their Yoga Solutions

After nearly 25 years of teaching, I've come to expect certain feedback during the check-in that opens my prenatal yoga classes.

"I'm having a lower backache."

"My SI joint is bothering me."

"I'm having some sciatica down my right/left side."

"I'm having calf cramps at night/in the morning."

"My belly feels itchy/tight/weak."

"My feet are swollen."

The list goes on. There are certain points during pregnancy when the body can get out of balance due to the demands of supporting two full lives. And our modern "movement diet" doesn't particularly help our bodies remain supple and balanced in ordinary times, let alone while coping with the added challenge of gestation.

At the same time, even the most common aches and pains aren't inevitable during pregnancy. Nor is the third trimester fated to be a constant litany of physical discomforts. Each symptom is, in some way, the body offering an invitation to act: to shift something, be it movement, breathing, or even diet, to restore the overall balance to the system.

I've compiled these solutions over years of listening to students, trying out different movements and practices, and conferring with birth workers. Not all of these suggestions are technically yoga *asanas*. But the overall aim of each one is to restore the balance that our bodies are ultimately trying to get back to each day.

Abdominal and/or vaginal pressure

Around the transition into the third trimester (28 weeks), students often mention a sense of heaviness or stretching within the abdominal or pelvic area.

The cause: As the uterus, baby, and placenta grow, there is obviously more weight contained within the body. And once the uterus expands beyond the confines of the bony pelvis, the abdominal organs begin to shift. This shift is what initially leads to the pregnancy "showing." It also creates increased downward pressure that requires the front abdominal wall, pelvic floor, and bony pelvis to bear more weight.

The yoga remedy: Since the feeling of heaviness is related to the gravitational pull on the body, mom may find temporary relief in postures that elevate the pelvis, allowing the weight to drop away from the base for a moment. Try Bridge pose with a block under the hips or Viparita Karani (though avoid this one if baby has turned from breech presentation within the past week). Table and Downward Dog (including at the wall) can also be helpful. Those postures change the spinal orientation to gravity and promote lengthening the spine to make space for the shifting internal organs.

Abdominal weakness

Along with abdominal pressure, students may also express feeling weak or uncoordinated through their core muscles.

The cause: As the belly grows, the abdominal muscles do have to stretch and expand to make room for the growing baby and uterus. Additionally, the shifting center of gravity can lead to a lack of coordinated support from the transverse abdominals (TA).

The yoga remedy: TA toning exercises. These exercises are not contraindicated for pregnancy and can be helpful in preventing abdominal muscle separation (diastasis recti). They may assist in the second stage of labor as well. Try hugging the baby with the abdominals while in Table or Cat/Cow movements from Table, Sukhasana, or standing. These exercises should be done gently and mindfully, as the goal is not to recreate any sort of "flat stomach" but to develop support around the entire abdominal container.

Diastasis recti

As discussed in Chapter 2, diastasis recti refers to a separation of the rectus abdominis muscle along the linea alba. Usually described as a pulling or tender sensation along the abdominal midline, students may or may not realize they have this condition. For some, a bulge or gap can be seen and felt at the center of the abdomen around the navel. This condition is more common in subsequent pregnancies and in women who had rigidly taut abdominals before becoming pregnant.

The cause: Excessive pressure and stretching on the fascial sheath at the center of the rectus abdominis muscle can lead to the fascia splitting along the linea alba as the baby grows. There are no nerve endings in this fascia, so mom may not be aware of the split. Though diastasis recti can occur in response to weak abdominals, hormonal softening, and extra strain, it can also be the result of years of unbalanced posture. A tucked tail posture with the hips shifted forward (see the common posture described on pgs 36-37) places consistent strain on the front line of the body, making it thinner and more prone to separating.

The yoga remedy: The best way to treat diastasis recti is to prevent it if possible. Ways to soften the pressure against the linea alba include standing with good posture that distributes the body's weight through the bones, avoiding tucking or thrusting the pelvis, and gently activating the TA muscles. Think of moving the weight back from the front line of the body so it stacks up over the bones, and we take the pressure off the front abdominal fascia.

Additionally, be gentle in postures which could strain the front body, such as backbends like Cobra, Camel, or Wheel. While these postures aren't completely contraindicated during pregnancy, they should always be done with caution and awareness to avoid placing excessive strain on the tissues. If the strain is severe, mom can employ gentle belly wrapping techniques with a Rebozo or even Kinesio tape to help support the fascia.

Postpartum, many cultures employ belly wrapping techniques, such as *bengkung* from Malaysia, to support the stretched out tissues as they return to greater tone and strength. Core exercises should initially focus on developing the internal "corset" of the TA along with toning the pelvic floor. For an abdominal separation wider than 1-2 fingers (diastasis recti is usually measured by feel), a yoga strap can be wrapped around the back and crossed in front over the widest section of the separation. Mom can then splint the waist and surface layer of the abdominals layer by pulling the strap tight as she engages in core exercises such as lifting one or both legs.

If the abdomen "tents" or bulges upwards away from the spine during core work, or if the spine or pelvis feel unstable, the exercise should be discontinued until more stability is developed. Prone core postures such as Plank require mom to maintain a lift to the abdominal wall; otherwise, the pressure of the organs falling forward could push the separation wider. If the abdominal lift can't be maintained, then the exercise should be discontinued or modified.

Backache

Backache is probably the most common complaint during pregnancy—and the one moms assume is the most inevitable, especially in the third trimester. But I always take the complaint of a backache as an invitation to look at the overall balance of the body and find the places that need release and relaxation.

The cause: Poor posture. This can be from old habits or from changes to the body's center of gravity due to the growing uterus, baby, and breasts as well as the hormonal softening of the ligaments.

The yoga remedy: Releasing back pain can, and should, be a gentle process. Soft twists and circling of the spine can help release tense paraspinal and lower back muscles. Back pain nearly always involves some psoas contraction which leads to compression of the lumbar region. Poses which bring gentle length to the spine such as Downward Dog (including the wall variation) can bring some relief. Then, consider moving into postures targeted for the hip flexors, such as Virasana or Bridge, to lengthen the deep front muscle lines. Side-bending poses such as Parivrtta Janu Sirsasana can also help lengthen tight quadratus lumborum muscles.

Once the tense muscles have been loosened, work to find and maintain an aligned, balanced posture that avoids tucking the pelvis and distributes the weight through the bones rather than into muscles or connective tissue.

Shoulder tension

Neck and shoulder tension is a variant of back pain. Given our cultural tendency to stand and sit with the head jutting forward or to constantly look down (as when looking at a cell phone), shoulder tension is extremely common throughout pregnancy. When we add the extra weight of the growing breasts to the mix, the upper back muscles can wind up in a chronically long and tight state, leading to discomfort.

The cause: Incorrect sitting or standing posture combined with increased weight in the breasts.

The yoga remedy: The solution is the same as what a non-pregnant student would receive. Any and all gentle shoulder openers can feel wonderful during pregnancy. Especially popular are Garudasana/Eagle arms and clasping the hands behind the back.

Breathlessness

About once every two weeks, I hear a student say that she feels like she cannot take a deep breath in. This condition usually occurs in early or mid-third trimester, but occasionally someone in their first trimester mentions feeling easily winded as well.

The cause: In the third trimester, the cause is decreased space for the abdominal diaphragm, the result of the uterus and baby pushing internal organs up towards the chest cavity. In the first trimester, breathlessness is usually more of a hormonal response to the increased progesterone and relaxin, which slow down smooth muscle function.

The yoga remedy: Working with the breath is always a gradual process, as it is inherently tied to the nervous system. Slow abdominal and full body breathing that also allows the ribs to spread can be helpful during the third trimester. Side bends, which stretch the muscles between the ribs, can create more space for the lungs to expand. So can supported supine backbends such as Supta Baddha Konasana, which temporarily lifts the rib cage off the expanding abdomen. Lifting the arms overhead can also raise the ribcage for a moment, allowing for deeper inhalation.

Ultimately, however, the ability to inhale depends on how well the previous breath has been released. Focusing on creating a full exhalation before inhaling again can bring a sense of greater space within the lungs.

Rib pain

If the abdominal organs are moving upward and compressing the abdominal diaphragm, it is also possible that the rib cage itself may need to spread outward to accommodate this movement. This is especially true if mom was naturally short-waisted before pregnancy.

The cause: The growing baby and uterus cause the internal organs to press up against the diaphragm, which causes the ribs to spread outwards. The intercostal muscles between the ribs, as well as the fascia, can become strained and uncomfortable, especially if those muscles were tight before pregnancy.

The yoga remedy: Side stretches to lengthen the intercostal muscles. Prenatal massage and Rebozo manteada (an abdominal sifting technique that involves gentle jiggling of the tissue) to help soften the belly and connective tissue in the ribs.[54]

---

[54] For more information on this technique, see: *https://www.spinningbabies.com/pregnancy-birth/techniques/other-techniques/rebozo-manteada-4/*

Wrist pain, including carpal tunnel and De Quervain's Syndrome

The increase in blood volume during pregnancy can make tissues swollen or inflamed. For some women, swelling around the wrist (which may not be outwardly evident) can compress the carpal nerve at the base of the hand, causing carpal tunnel syndrome.

Another nerve bundle sometimes affected is the nerve running up the base of the thumb into the wrist. Called De Quervain's syndrome, this condition can be especially tricky. Most pressure will aggravate it, and in extreme cases it can become chronic if left untreated. Both of these conditions are also common in new moms, the result of holding babies in awkward positions for long periods of time.

The cause: Swelling of tissues in the wrist, leading to compressed nerves, or allowing the weight to fall into the wrist in quadruped poses like Table. Overuse can also be a cause, especially for those working at a computer.

The yoga remedy: Get off the wrists for a time. Do poses on the forearms or blocks, or make fists with the wrists straight to relieve compression. Some women wear wrist braces at night and even occasionally during the day to keep the wrists neutral. Stretches for the wrists can help, but keep them gentle so as not to increase inflammation. Stretching overhead can reduce swelling, and avoiding prolonged periods of flexing and extending the wrists can also help. If symptoms worsen or are severe, seek medical advice.

Constipation

Often not discussed, constipation affects many women during the first trimester because the increase of progesterone and relaxin slows all smooth muscles in the lower abdomen.

The cause: Increased progesterone and relaxin, which relax the soft muscles of the digestive tract and cause food to move through the system more slowly.

The yoga remedy: Part posture, part diet. Try Happy Baby Pose, rocking side to side, and rocking Child's Pose to gently move the belly and assist the digestive tract in moving food through. I also encourage students to eat a high fiber diet. This is a great time to up your salad game!

Leg and foot cramping

I've taken to calling it my prenatal check-in magic trick: A student says she's waking up in the middle of the night with charley horses in her calves, and I immediately ask, "Are you about 25 weeks along?" Right around the end of the second trimester some pregnant women experience sudden and severe cramping in their feet, calves, or legs. I have heard moms report that their legs cramped so tightly they could still feel the contraction days later.

The cause: The exact cause for calf and leg cramping isn't completely understood, but it may relate to an imbalance of electrolytes in the body. Around week 25, some babies begin calcifying their bones, pulling the needed minerals from their mother's body. Muscle fibers need three of these minerals in order to break a muscle contraction: calcium, potassium, and magnesium. Without these minerals, the muscle fiber continues to contract because it cannot release back to a relaxed state. Dehydration can further contribute to muscle cramping since water is the liquid which carries the electrolytes to the muscles.

The yoga remedy: The first course of action is to stretch the affected muscle group, since gentle tugging can help release the fascia and loosen the muscle fibers around the contracted area. Calf stretches, such as treading feet while in Downward Dog or standing with the ball of the foot on a rolled blanket and leaning into the foot, can be helpful. Remember to pull the toes back towards the knees during stretching. The fastest remedy to relieve calf cramps is often to stand up and put pressure on the foot—though it can be hard to remember this if they occur in the middle of the night.

Dizziness/light-headedness

Another consequence of the shifts in blood volume and blood pressure during pregnancy can be feelings of dizziness or light-headednes. It should be noticed that prolonged dizziness, or dizziness accompanied by headache, severe swelling in the hands, feet or face, or vision changes may be a sign of preeclampsia or unregulated high blood pressure. If you experience these symptoms, seek medical care immediately. Absent other symptoms, however, dizziness or lightheadedness may be the result of mom's body having nearly 150% blood volume by full term, along with a compensatory drop in resting blood pressure. This feeling can be especially profound when coming up to stand, as you would at the end of a Sun Salutation.

The cause: Decreased blood pressure causes the blood to circulate to the brain more slowly and, during standing postures, pool in the feet and legs.

The yoga remedy: When exiting forward bends, come up slowly and in stages. Remember to exhale strongly once you're fully upright to ground the body's energy through increased *apana*. Drink lots of water.

Groin pain/round ligament pain

Sudden, sharp pains in the groin or belly can be extremely uncomfortable and startling. Students usually describe groin or round ligament pain as sudden cramping or stabbing sensations, especially those associated with baby's movements ("It hurts when the baby kicks"). However, it is difficult to determine if you are specifically having round ligament pain, especially because you may be unaware of this ligament's existence until it contracts.

Groin or round ligament pains can often indicate excessive tension in the fascia surrounding the uterus. Tense fascia can have an impact on the amount of space available inside the uterus for baby to turn as well as on the positioning of the lower uterine segment and cervix.

While round ligament pain is not usually a cause for concern, check with a care provider if the pains are persistent or severe. A chronic, sharp pain near the groin that feels like a pulled muscle or a sharp pain under the right ribcage should be evaluated immediately. These pains could indicate appendicitis or a serious liver condition called HELLP syndrome.[55]

---

[55] Hemolysis Elevated Liver Enzymes, Low Platelets is a rare but severe condition which can be life threatening to mom. Providers understand how to work with and treat this condition if it arises during pregnancy, but it should never be ignored. americanpregnancy.org/healthy-pregnancy/pregnancy-complications/hellp-syndrome/

The cause: Excessive tension in the round ligaments connecting the uterus to the pelvis. Overstretching the round ligaments during brisk walking or sudden twisting can cause these ligaments to contract to protect themselves from damage. These are some of the only ligaments in the body which contain muscle tissue. Sudden twisting motions or poor posture can increase their tension and thus their reactivity.

The yoga remedy: Use gentle, symmetrical pelvic movements such as Cat/Cow to stretch the round ligaments evenly. Avoid fast twisting motions. Leaning towards the side that the pain is felt, or gently holding the area with the hands until the sensation subsides, can help the ligaments relax. Rebozo manteada (belly sifting) can be helpful as well.

Sciatica

The sciatic nerve is a huge nerve bundle, almost the thickness of your pinky finger. It runs from the inside of the sacrum, through the greater sciatic notch just under the SI joint, and down the outside of the thigh. The sciatic nerve sits just below the piriformis muscle or in some cases interweaves with the piriformis. If the fascial connections in this area become sticky, it can cause a literal pain in the butt—experienced as shooting pains up and down the hip and thigh.

There are so many nerves in this area of the body that we can't usually say with certainty that the condition is sciatica as opposed to compression of another nerve. Nevertheless, the outer hip seems to be one of the crankiest spots for pregnant students.

The cause: If the condition is truly sciatica, it's caused by pressure on the sciatic nerve from either tight hip muscles or a shifting SI joint. If the pain is caused by compression from a different nerve, the cause is similar: some type of muscular or joint impingement.

The yoga remedy: Loosen the external hip rotators with poses like Ankle to Knee or Gomukhasana which stretch the outer hip rotators. Once released, be sure to then stabilize the SI joints with postures that strengthen the glutes and piriformis muscles, such as Baddha Konasana. Baddha Konasana can be especially effective done at the wall with a block behind the hips, activating the external rotators while pressing the heels together. Another glute strengthener could be side-lying Clamshells—lifting the top knee while keeping the feet together.

Tailbone pain

Adjacent to sciatic pain, but with quite a different cause, is tailbone pain. Especially common in pregnant students who sit a lot, tailbone pain occurs when the tailbone becomes a mobile joint due to the hormonal changes softening the body's connective tissue. When combined with poor or unbalanced posture, the coccyx can become compressed or strained where it joins with the sacrum.

The cause: Relaxin in the body softens the ligaments holding the coccyx to the sacrum, exacerbated by postures which bear weight into the lower end of the sacrum at the joint with the tailbone. Tailbone pain also often indicates tension in the pelvic floor muscles which attach in the back to the coccyx.

The yoga remedy: Sit upright, with weight resting on the sitz bones instead of the coccyx. If the pain is really bad, place a rolled blanket under each sitz bone but nothing under the tailbone, to allow the coccyx to hang freely and relieve pressure. Practice releasing the pelvic floor with gentle self massage around the inside of the sitz bones and towards the tail to encourage tone and elasticity.

Pubic symphysis pain

More challenging than the tailbone pain is discomfort in the front of the pelvis at the pubic symphysis. Sometimes called pelvic girdle pain, it can result from an excessive looseness in the connective tissue between the front two pubic bones of the pelvis. These bones are meant to join together to complete the stable pelvic ring, but they can shift during pregnancy, especially in bodies which were loose to begin with or in cases where yoginis have pushed their range of motion rather than maintaining joint integrity. In severe cases this pain may prevent pregnant students from walking, as any lateral weight shift can exacerbate the discomfort.

The cause: A separation or misalignment of the pubic bones at the pubic joint due to softening tissues from hormonal changes, specifically the introduction of relaxin during the first trimester.

The yoga remedy: This one is tricky, as any split stance pose (Virabhadrasana 1, Anjaneyasana, Pigeon) can put strain on the pubic symphysis. Balancing hip openers such as Baddha Konasana (without the forward bend) allow gravity to realign the pelvic bones and can be helpful. So can engaging muscular support in all standing and asymmetrical postures and using props wherever possible.

It may be helpful to work on engaging the pelvic floor, but be cautious, since excessive laxity can often lead to increased muscle tension as the body tries to hold the joints together. This may be a case where mom would want to sit on a chair for some standing postures to provide extra support which the muscles are not providing. Any pose which aggravates or causes pain at the pubic bone should be avoided, and hip opening postures such as squats will need lots of support.

Weak pelvic floor muscles

Saying one has weak pelvic floor muscles really demands further investigation, because a muscle can be weak from either too much or too little tension, and knowing which will intrinsically affect what the yoga solution will be. As we talked about in Chapter 3, the pelvic floor forms the foundation of the abdominal core. It bears significantly more weight during the latter half of pregnancy, when it must hold up not only the regular internal organs but the growing uterus, baby, and placenta as well.

This increased pressure can lead to muscles either lacking strength and sagging under the weight, or—more commonly in my experience with yogis—becoming overly tense as they try to constantly hold up the additional weight. Tense pelvic floor muscles can pose as many, if not more, challenges as muscles that are too loose. These challenges can range from incontinence—leaking urine, either when laughing or coughing or from a full bladder—to pelvic pain, to—in extreme cases—chronic vaginal inflammation and discomfort (vulvodynia). If I have a student who complains of weak pelvic floor muscles, I ask follow-up questions that revolve around whether there is pain or tension when doing a self-massage (this can be done over clothing—no need to get too personal in yoga class) or if the tissue feels soft and lacking in tone. For many, differentiating between the two may be the first challenge.

The cause: A "weak" pelvic floor is caused by either too much or too little tension in the muscles of the pelvic floor. This is due to extra weight from the baby and uterus pressing against the pelvic floor. Pre-existing tension or weakness, trauma, or poor posture may also be possible causes.

The yoga remedy: We're looking for tone, not tension. In many cases, the first action may be to develop the ability to release and stretch the pelvic floor before working to engage it through pelvic floor toning exercises (Kegels or Mula Bandha). Squats with an anterior pelvic tilt can be helpful. See Chapter 3 for additional exercises to help release and then tone the pelvic floor.

Swollen hands and feet

By the end of pregnancy, the body will have increased its blood volume to 150% to accommodate the fluid needed for the baby as well. While the baby's blood does not mix with mom's, the fluid exchange between the two—which carries nutrients and resources needed for growth—requires enough volume to cover both bodies.

Whenever we are standing, nearly 1/3 of our blood does not fully circulate due to hydrostatic pressure within the body. The result is that the tissues of the lower leg and sometimes the lower arm absorb this extra fluid for a time, leading to swelling. While minor swelling, especially after 28 weeks, is normal, extreme swelling can be a sign of high blood pressure. If you experience extreme swelling, contact your care provider immediately.

The cause: Swelling is caused by increased fluid in the body, combined with spending long amounts of time in seated or standing positions that cause blood to pool in the lower portions of the body instead of circulating fully.

The yoga remedy: Stimulate circulation to the legs through active movement such as rocking Child's Pose and active standing *vinyasas* which pump the muscles of the legs. Change the orientation to gravity with postures such as Viparita Karani or simply side-lying with the feet slightly elevated. Self-massage techniques such as patting and stroking can also help mobilize lymph and blood for better circulation. Drink plenty of water, as dehydration causes the body to hold onto fluid rather than flush it out. If seated or standing for long hours, prop up one foot at a time on a box or small stool to help with drainage.

Varicose veins

A more dramatic and sometimes uncomfortable impact of increased fluid volume is a distention of the vein walls in the legs and sometimes the groin. These varicose veins can usually be seen externally (though obviously you won't see the groin ones during a yoga class). For some, they are uncomfortable; for others, the visual may be the most disturbing part. If you have varicose veins, you want to be careful to avoid increasing intravenous pressure, which can further damage the vein walls.

The cause: Varicose veins are caused by stretched vein walls, the result of increased fluid volume and possibly lax connective tissue.

The yoga remedy: There isn't anything that can be done to consistently relieve the stretched blood vessel walls, so the focus in yoga is two-fold: avoid increasing the pressure for long periods of time and keep blood flowing to maintain good vein function.

For varicosities in the legs, elevate the feet in Viparita Karani, and rotate the ankles frequently to use the pumping of the calf muscles to move the fluid. In other *asana*, make sure to keep the back of the knees open so as not to cut off the blood return from the lower leg back to the heart. This means postures like full squats, full Virasana, and other poses which fully close the back of the knee must be modified. Maintain enough space to easily slide a pencil into the back of the knee crease.

For varicose veins in the groin or vagina, focus on horizontal or even slightly inverted postures which take pressure off the base of the pelvis. Child's Pose with the hips over the knees (so the hip creases don't fully compress) or Bridge can be helpful. I have also known students to find some relief from gentle perineal massage to promote blood flow (again, this was done at home, not in yoga class!). For others, applying ice packs to the affected area gave some relief (10 minutes on, 20 minutes off) Incidentally, these postures can also be helpful for hemorrhoids, both before and after birth. Drink lots of water!

Nausea/vomiting/"morning" sickness

Anyone who has been pregnant knows that instead of morning sickness, it really should be called morning-noon-and-night sickness, because it certainly doesn't affect everyone the same way. The exact reason for morning sickness isn't completely known, though it does seem to be correlated with the growth hormones the body puts out to help establish and maintain the pregnancy. This can be cold comfort for the mom who finds it uncomfortable to eat even saltines.

The cause: Hormonal changes within the body which affect appetite as well as overall balance are thought to be the root cause of morning sickness. Common in the beginning of the first trimester, it can return late in the pregnancy as well. Symptoms can range from feeling ravenously hungry (as with hypoglycemia) to frequent vomiting (hyperemesis gravidarum). The latter may require medical attention.

The yoga remedy: For mild cases of nausea, lying on the left side may help to quiet the abdomen, since the stomach lies on the left side of the body and the esophagus enters it from the right-hand side. Ayurvedic practices encourage lying on the left side to promote better stomach and digestive function following meals, so we can employ this energetic support for the upset pregnant stomach as well.

Nutritionally, mom can also try eating smaller meals, avoiding spicy and oily foods, drinking liquids separately from solids, and sipping ginger or peppermint tea. Reduce or eliminate coffee intake, as this increases acidity in the stomach. Personally, I also found it vital to take any prenatal vitamins with food rather than on an empty stomach. (The only times I actually threw up were when I forgot this rule, and I was reminded of it within minutes—but I had a very mild case of nausea.)

Heartburn

Along with morning sickness, some women may experience acid reflux, especially in the latter half of pregnancy. The combination of shifting internal organs and hormonal softening of internal connective tissue can lead to the esophageal sphincter not fully sealing off the lower segment of the esophagus. Students have reported everything from slight chest discomfort all the way to burning in their throat, depending on the pregnancy.

The cause: The abdominal cavity becomes crowded as the baby grows, leading to less room for the stomach. This crowding, combined with relaxin and other hormones softening the opening to the stomach, makes reflux more common.

The yoga remedy: Avoid inversions such as Downward Dog or Uttanasana or keep the head up with the gaze forward in these poses. Keep the head elevated in supine positions by bringing the body up to around a 45 degree angle with blocks and bolsters.

Anti-heartburn pose

Face a wall and kneel close to it. Stretch your arms up the wall, and allow the chest and head to sink forward until your head touches the wall.

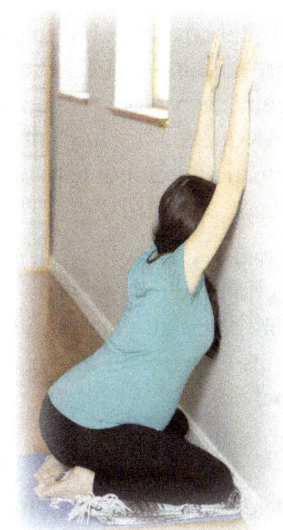

Practicing Urdhva Hastasana (Upward Facing Hands Pose) can also be helpful, actively pressing the hands to the ceiling on the inhale and maintaining the lift through the exhale.

Herbal and medical remedies often suggested are papaya, taking Tums or other heartburn tablets, possibly taking magnesium, or eating almonds chewed to a paste before swallowing. As always, consult with our care provider about any supplements or dietary changes.

Breech presentation

By around 28 weeks, the baby's head has grown to be heavier than their body. Around this time, gravity will usually begin to move the baby into a head- down position, assuming the body is balanced with its muscles, organs and connective tissue. I am always frustrated when I hear students in their second trimester refer to their baby's position as "breech." I feel this term should not be used until at least 30 weeks because prior to that time we might not expect the baby to have turned, and describing it in these terms only creates stress and anxiety in mom's mind, when in reality nothing may need to be done.

The cause: There are numerous factors which might affect a baby's ability to turn head down, but in many cases, it may be due to an imbalance of tension within mom's body. That tension can create a tight spot that baby has difficulty moving around. In some cases there are more involved circumstances, such as the umbilical cord being wrapped in an odd manner or the placenta being in the way, but in many instances, it is a combination of baby having more space upright and fascial connections creating subtle but profound twists within the uterine tissue.

Sometimes these issues can be resolved, and sometimes not. If they cannot be resolved enough for baby to turn, it is still possible to birth vaginally with the breech baby, though this option is rapidly diminishing for many women as providers often are not trained in this manner of birthing.

The yoga remedy: From the yoga perspective, we can try postures to help open and balance the space around the uterus and also practice postures which would encourage baby to stay up in the abdomen where there is more room to rotate as opposed to sinking down into the bony pelvis where things are more confined. Gail Tully of Spinning Babies® has developed a series of positions for creating space for babies to move (for more information visit *spinning-babies.com*).

For our yoga practice, gentle lunges can release and open the psoas muscle which, if tight, would compress the space behind the uterus. Bridge pose on blocks—also sometimes called breech tilt—can also be helpful, both for releasing the psoas and for using gravity to move baby away from the lower pelvis. Additionally, you can try Child's Pose with the hips elevated, allowing the belly to hang, or Table while circling the hips and abdomen. If baby's position does not resolve, the Webster chiropractic technique and acupuncture treatments may be helpful.

Postures to avoid while baby is breech are squats and big hip circles while standing, as these actions help move baby downward into the pelvis. Once baby has flipped head down, squat and circle all you want, but keep doing the exercises to release the psoas and mobilize the hips to maintain the space created for baby to drop lower and more fully engage into the pelvic bowl.

Placenta previa and low-lying placenta

The placenta can attach anywhere inside the uterus, depending on where the baby first implanted at the beginning of pregnancy. For most pregnancies, the placenta grows on the upper half of the uterus and is of little concern (the occasional caution around back bending and belly sifting when the placenta is on the front of the body notwithstanding).

The main concern for the yoga practice occurs when the placenta is close to or covering the cervix: called full or partial placenta previa when the placenta covers the cervix and low-lying placenta when it is close. This position can impact which postures you can safely practice and, if it does not resolve, may dictate a surgical rather than vaginal birth for the baby.

Most cases of low-lying placenta and placenta previa are detected during an ultrasound early in pregnancy and are then monitored as the pregnancy continues. Of the pregnancies with a full or partial previa, the vast majority (around 90%) resolve by the beginning of the third trimester. This is because the uterus grows at an accelerated rate during pregnancy and the placenta usually moves upwards with the expanding uterus. If the placenta moves outside of the radius where the cervix will open during labor, then there is no further concern. If it does not, however, it will almost always lead to a scheduled cesarean birth.

The cause: The exact cause of low-lying placenta and placenta previa is unknown, but it is at least partly due to where the fertilized egg happens to have implanted on the uterine wall.

The yoga remedy: There isn't anything in the yoga canon which can resolve a low lying placenta or placenta previa. Some birth practitioners suggest that practicing Viparita Karani and breathing deeply into the lower abdomen may help relieve fascial tension, allowing for greater movement as the uterus grows, but this is not scientifically proven.

The bigger impact on the yoga practice is in indicating certain postures that should be avoided. No squatting or other postures which would direct energy downward, such as Goddess Pose, as downward energy moves things in the wrong direction for the moment. If you have had or experience bleeding during the pregnancy, check with your care provider about the possibility of more serious complications.

Again, the vast majority of previas will resolve on their own, but if you are dealing with this condition, exercise caution. You will likely have been told by your care provider if you are dealing with this; if it hasn't been mentioned, you can assume that all is well. It should also be noted that one practice with squatting will not cause harm—it is the cumulative effect we want to watch out for and potentially avoid.

11 — Home Practice Guide

"Yogas chitta vritti nirodhah.
Yoga is the stilling of the fluctuations of the mind"

—Patanjali Yoga Sutras 1:2

I will admit that practicing at home was always something I struggled with. Faced with the chance to explore the intricacies of Trikonasana in my own living room or go bend and move in the company of other yogis at the studio, I chose the studio practice almost every time. Even during my multiple teacher trainings, I often chafed at practicing alone at home. It was lonely, and sometimes quite boring, and I much preferred the company of my fellow yogis to the silent echoes of my own yoga space.

Then the pandemic of 2020 hit, and most avid yogis were forced to move their practice into the virtual world or struggle through on their own. For some this meant livestream classes, but for many others it meant pre-recorded classes, practiced without the supportive guide and camaraderie of the in-person or even virtual space. I certainly heard many colleagues bemoan the missing personal connection of the in-person practice. But there were also those who relished being able to practice when they wanted, in the same space where they lived their lives. As I made time for virtual practice, or noticed when I didn't, I came to a deeper understanding of the place for home practice along with the benefit of group classes—in person or virtual.

Yoga is a spiritual practice as well as physical exercise; it inherently incorporates philosophy and possibly even mystical experience. I began to realize that in the same way that a religious practice might involve going to church/temple/meditation center to be in community and hear inspiring teachings, it also involves the day to day faith that supports the larger connection with life. I'm not suggesting that we start a debate about whether yoga class equates to church (though I know some yogis who would say so). Rather, I'm suggesting that we recognize that we need both sides of the practice for a full experience. Buddhists have the three jewels of *buddha*, *dharma*, and *sangha*; in the same way, we yogis have their group class, which might be as much socializing as it is physical exercise, but also our day to day awareness in our bodies. Ultimately, all yoga practice moves off the mat and into the world, and it is in our home practice that this transition begins to take place.

If you are practicing yoga during pregnancy, the practice is eventually brought off the mat in its own way. As the body begins to physically shift, daily movements require more awareness and have a greater impact on our physiology. Plus, your very sense of identity may begin to change as you consider welcoming another human being into your life—with all the uncertainty that entails.

Developing a home practice is more than simply stepping onto the yoga mat at home. Home practice during pregnancy involves cultivating a sense of coming home to your body, finding ways to feel comfortable living in this space and form. It would be so easy if we could say there was one yoga practice that every pregnant person could do which would ensure no aches and pains, a balanced body and pelvis, a smooth birth, and a quick postpartum recovery. But if that were true, then birth would not be the individual process that it is. Just as each pregnancy has its own unique characteristics, each pregnant body has its own unique tensions.

The aim of this chapter is to provide a framework for cultivating a purposeful space for finding comfort in the body during pregnancy. The good news is that the work you do to find better comfort and ease during pregnancy actually has a positive impact on the body's preparedness for birth. And those same actions that create space and ease in pregnancy can help restore balance and function postpartum. There are some daily motions which I recommend students explore, since they can reveal where the body holds certain tensions and sometimes relieve discomforts which, if unaddressed, might lead to more serious challenges.

A little movement each day truly is enough to unwind the lingering echoes of our movement diet from the rest of our lives. Ultimately, the point is to take a moment and explore. Just doing that nurtures our inner awareness and attention. As a good friend and yoga colleague of mine once said, "80% of practicing at home is getting your backside on the yoga mat. The rest is gravy."

Creating a practice at home

Setting a space

For practicing at home, begin by clearing a space where your body has room to move. This need not be a full room; it could simply be an area to the side of your bed or in your living room. Wherever you set down your mat, be sure it is fairly clean and clear of objects which might get in your way. Move the coffee table over, or shift the pile of laundry onto the bed for a moment.

Dropping in

Take a pause to drop into the moment you are in. You can do this sitting, standing, or even lying down. Bring your focus to where you have placed your physical body. Feel the contact you are making with the earth. Notice where you become aware of the sensations of your breathing. There isn't any specific place you should be feeling the breath, this is simply the act of taking note of where it actually is.

Maybe at this moment you also note any sensations coming from the baby: physical pressure, feelings of fullness, or other subtle or overt movements. If your pregnancy is still early on, you might tap into the more subtle layers of the body—energetic or emotional shifts. You might notice if you feel aware of someone else with you on your mat at this moment. You don't have to do anything with this information. Just sit with it.

Setting an intention

As you drop your awareness into the present moment and feel whatever it feels like to rest in your body here and now, you may check to see if there is a specific intention you have for practice. Maybe this is part of a larger practice of balancing and strengthening your body in preparation for birth. Or maybe you carved this time out for rest and introspection. Maybe there's a specific area of your body which is beginning to ask for some attention, either through discomfort or just a feeling of tension and compression. Whatever your reason, give a moment to acknowledge why you are choosing to be here, and also thank yourself for taking an active role in your health and your baby's health. The simple act of getting on the mat is the first step in this process, and this intention may guide you into the specific movements and postures you wind up practicing. Even if just pausing is all you can do today, it is still a valuable practice.

Free movement

Once you have set your intention for practice, you may already know where you need to begin. But if not, start by moving your body in any way that feels opening and explorative. This could be done standing, sitting, on hands and knees, or even lying down. My first trimester, my home practice started almost entirely on the floor, then gradually moved onto the hands and knees. There were days I never went beyond there. The idea isn't to jump straight into a formal *asana* but rather to discover more fully what the body might be saying. If, during this exploration, you find a particularly delicious stretch, feel free to linger there, allowing the body to speak to you in its own language: sensation

Common areas of tension during pregnancy could be:
- Shoulders and neck
- Hip flexors
- Lower back and back muscles in general
- Hip rotators (inner and outer)
- Hamstrings and calves
- Side body and ribs
- Pelvic floor

Common areas which need support and strengthening:
- Hip rotators (inner and outer)
- Pelvic Floor
- Core body (but gently)
- Back muscles
- Arms and shoulders
- Hamstrings and calves

You can probably notice that there is some overlap between what might need to be released and what needs to be strengthened. The needed movements to create overall balance and comfort will vary from person to person, depending on where your body normally carries tension.

Suggested basic movements

The following movements are a basic list of daily ways to help bring overall balance to a developing pregnant body. Pick one of the suggested postures and explore how it can bring space and fluidity to certain areas of the body or overall. The poses suggested are meant as places from which to begin. They can be incorporated into free movement or worked into a more formal *asana*.

- Calf stretch
- Hamstring stretches (Parsvottanasana, Prasarita Padotanasana, Downward Dog)
- Hip movements (hip circles standing, sitting, from Table, or supine if in early pregnancy, Cat/Cow)
- Pelvic floor toning (strengthening active Malasana, stretching Prasarita Padotanasana, Pelvic Floor Breathing)
- Psoas release (Bridge Pose, Anjaneyasana, direct psoas release on block)
- Side bending and release (Parivrtta Janu Sirsasana, Windmill, Reverse Warrior)
- Hip strengthening and stretching (Ankle to Knee, Baddha Konasana (active and passive), wall squat with blocks)

These movements can all be achieved in a fairly brief yoga practice, but given the body tends to tighten after even 30 minutes of sitting, I often recommend students work short yoga practices throughout their day. These "yoga snacks" can relieve general body tension and also help maintain awareness and good posture. From any yoga snack, you might move into a fuller exploration and practice depending on the time, curiosity, and energy available. Which *asana* you practice is up to you, but here are some suggestions for ways to access these parts of the body and find more balance overall.

Basic yoga movements to prepare for labor

(These are ideally practiced each day)

Calf stretch

The calf muscles integrate with a posterior fascial chain up the leg which interlocks with the hamstrings and sacro-tuberous ligaments in the pelvis. Releasing the bottom of the foot and back of the lower leg creates the potential for more movement of the sacrum and thus more space for the baby during the birth process. Since the calf muscles are working most

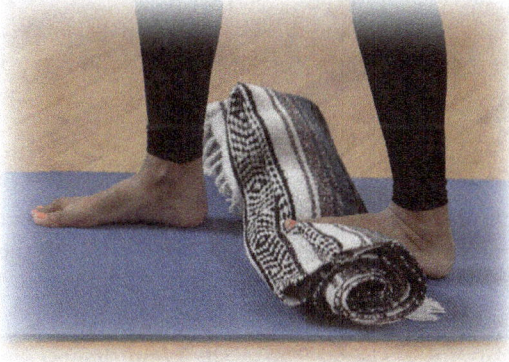

of the time when simply walking or moving around, for birth preparation the main focus here is stretching.

Begin either facing the wall in a gentle lunge with the back heel on the floor, or standing with the toes of one foot placed on a rolled blanket or yoga mat. Be sure to align the foot and knee directly forward rather than rolling in or out on the ankle. Inhale to reach into the heel, and exhale to softly bend the stretching knee, feeling for about a 50% stretch level in the calf and ankle. (For more detailed instruction see page 137.)

Hamstring stretches and strengtheners (Parsvottanasana, Prasarita Padotanasana, or Downward Dog)

The hamstrings are the continuation of the calf muscle line up the back of the leg. While most pregnant people need to release these muscles, there are some who either from lack of movement, pre-existing yoga practice, or simple genetics may have overly lengthened hamstring muscles. In these cases, strengthening actions along with lengthening may be appropriate. An easy way to tell if your hamstrings fall into the looser camp is to explore your forward bend alignment. If you are able to fold easily from the sitting bone, maintaining a flat back more than 50% of the way to your thighs, or if you have previously been plagued by hamstring pulls

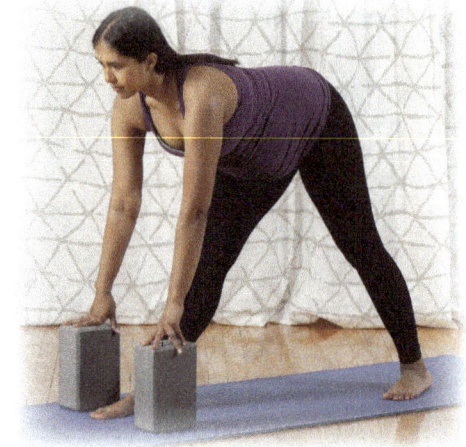

or aching at the sitting bone, this may be an indication of needing strength as well as release. (When assessing the forward flexion, do not be fooled by movement from the back masking tension in the hamstrings: loose hamstrings will allow the sitz bones to lift dramatically, almost bringing the tailbone towards the sky. Tight hamstrings will, by contrast, keep the sitz ones drawn downward, leading to a rounding in the lumbar spine—not what we want in forward flexion.)

To focus the stretch into the hamstrings, being in either Parsvottanasana (pg 148), Prasarita Padottanasana (pgs 140-141), or Downward Dog (pg 152), and imagine a good friend placing their hands on the back of your buttocks. Without moving the femur bones back, energetically press the sitz bones into the imaginary hands, focusing on deepening the crease in the hip flexion. The sensation should focus into the belly of the muscle, not shift into the attachment at the bone itself.

To strengthen the hamstrings (or to prevent overstretching if the sensation seems to be zeroing into the sitz bone attachment), instead of pressing the sitz bones up, imagine a rubber band stretched from the sitz bone down to the back of the knee—and possibly even extending to the heel. This is the deep back fascial line of the hamstring. While in the hamstring stretching postures, imagine gently pulling down on the rubber band line, activating the muscles to stabilize instead of lengthen. It should also be noted that this action will help create space in the hip socket if the joint is collapsing and, if fully engaged, would stand the pelvis upright. This same action of drawing down on the sitz bones (not tucking but rather engaging) can also be employed in any standing posture, such as Goddess Squat, Warrior 2, or High Lunge. (For more specific instruction on these postures see the basic postures chapter. pgs 138-139, 145-147.)

Hip movements

Along with providing support and stability, the tissues around the pelvis also need to be pliable, which in this case means well hydrated by motion. This allows the pelvis to shift and open throughout pregnancy as well as during labor. Pregnancy is a time when the body is going through daily changes. So forget trying to match what it felt like yesterday because that body is already gone.

Cat/Cow

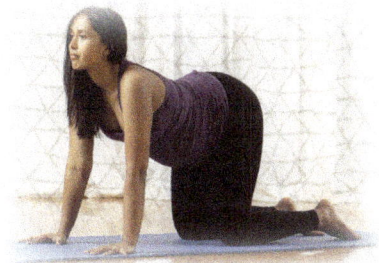 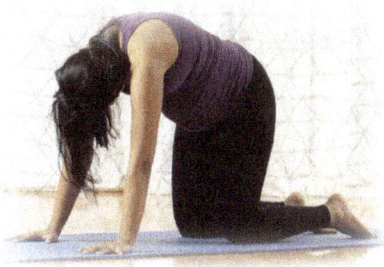

Begin on the hands and knees or, if the wrists are sensitive, rest the upper body on a chair or birthing ball. Focusing the action into the base of the pelvis, inhale, lifting the sitz bones upwards towards the ceiling. This will tip the pelvic bowl forwards and arch the lower back (it is also important to maintain some engagement through the front abdominal wall so as not to overly stretch the linea alba). On an exhale, actively tuck the tail and sitting bones, tilting the pelvis backwards and rounding the lower back towards the sky. Repeating this front and back movement both helps mobilize the pelvic joints and builds familiarity with the ways this movement widens or narrows different levels of the pelvis. (For more instruction on Cat/Cow see pgs 149-150.)

Hip circles

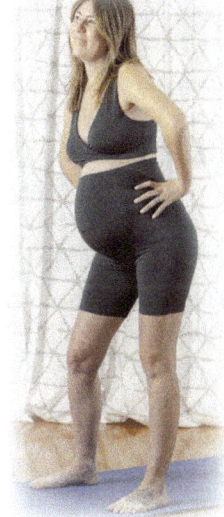

A fun further exploration (and a nice release from lower back pain) is to begin making circles in the air with the tailbone. This can be done horizontally or vertically to the floor. The circling and rocking of the pelvis can help open diagonal planes through the pelvis to access different muscle groups and is also a useful motion for labor preparation. (For more instruction on hip circles see pgs 136 and 150.)

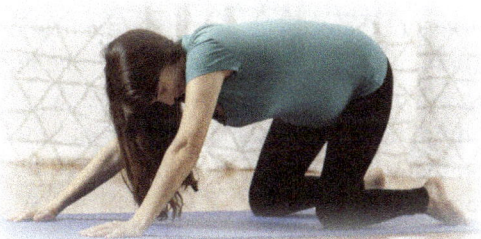

Pelvic floor exercises

As mentioned, the pelvic floor is responsible for the direct support of the uterus and pelvic organs during pregnancy, but the relative tone of the different muscles therein not only controls things like peeing (or not peeing), but also guides the baby's head through the mid-pelvis. Toning exercises are described more fully in Chapter 3. Some basic exercises to begin birth preparation are:

Pelvic floor breathing

This is the breath where the abdominal and pelvic diaphragms mirror one another to promote gentle stretching and toning. Sitting so the pelvis is upright, or lying down with the head supported and the lower back in neutral, let the breath drop into the lower abdomen as though filling the pelvic bowl. Feel the muscles between the sitting bones spread softly downward as the pelvis fills. On the exhale, feel the same muscles gently draw inwards and up. This upwards movement can be done actively if looking for more strength but should be avoided if the muscles are currently overly contracted. (For more instruction on pelvic floor breathing see pg 58.)

Pelvic floor toning

For strengthening as well as stretching the pelvic floor, practice a variation of the yoga squat Malasana. Begin standing, holding onto a solid prop (like the kitchen sink or a doorknob). Inhale to sit the pelvis back and down, focusing on an anterior tilt which will spread the sitting bones. Sit down about halfway to the floor. (Note the reason for holding the support is the weight shifts far enough back that you need to hold the support to stay upright.) The thighs may work a bit, but the focus is on the glutes and pelvic floor. On the

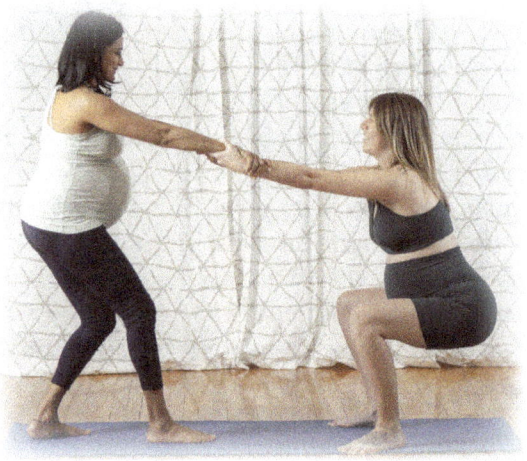

exhale, press the feet into the floor and stand back upright (no tucking!). Repeat this action several times. (For more instruction on pelvic floor toning see pg 70.)

Pelvic floor stretching

There are numerous stories out there about stretching the pelvic floor muscles manually. I find myself constantly reminding my students in childbirth education classes that the vagina is made of folds of tissue which it is not necessary to stretch in order to make room. Do you have to stretch an accordion to make it expand? But for those with hypertonic pelvic floor muscles (chronically contracted), breathing and widening can be a useful practice to add into any strengthening exercises.

Begin in Prasarita Padotanasana with the hands elevated on a chair or two stacked blocks. The spine should be at most parallel to the floor. Bending the knees and internally rotating the thigh bones to turn the toes in, press the sitz bones back as when focusing the stretch into the hamstrings. From here, deepen the inhalation, focusing on the sensation of the vaginal and pelvic muscles spreading and opening. The stretch here is done with the breath, not the bones. If no movement is felt, check if the ribcage is hanging towards the floor or overly rounded—both of which would misalign the abdominal and pelvic diaphragms. (For more instruction on pelvic floor stretching see pg 63.)

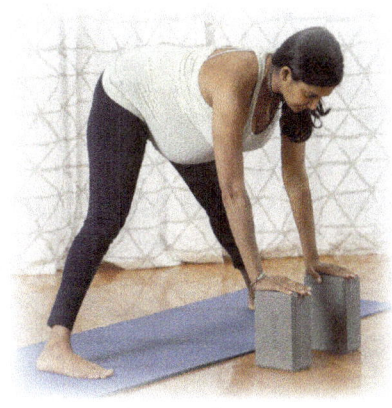

Hip strengthening and stretching

The internal and external hip rotators serve both to move the pelvis and to support the pelvic bowl. Along with the calves and hamstrings, strengthening and stretching these muscles each day can assist in creating overall muscle and pelvic balance.

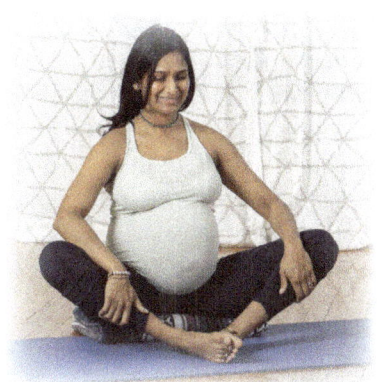

Stretching hip rotators

Come to sit on the floor or a chair with the sitting bones planted and the weight shifted towards the front edge so the pubic bone angles downward. If on the floor, bring either the soles of the feet together in Baddha Konasana (pgs 154-155) or stack the shins over one another for Ankle to Knee (pg 158). If seated in a chair, crossing one ankle over the opposite knee and flexing the foot will achieve the same stretch as Ankle to Knee. Be sure to maintain an upright pelvis and ground the thigh bones down to focus the action into the glutes and outer hip rotators.

To stretch the internal hip rotators sit in Virasana (pgs 163-164) with the hips elevated far enough to both relieve any pressure on the knees and allow the pelvis to tip to neutral. Gentle pelvic tilt actions here can help move the stretch around the different internal rotators contacted here.

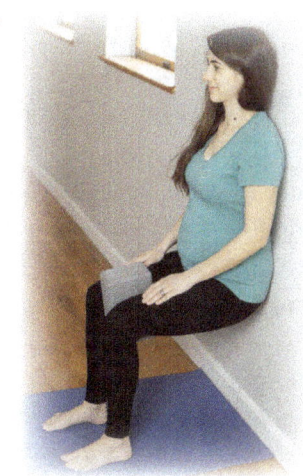

Strengthening hip rotators

Begin either leaning against the wall in a Wall Squat with a block between the knees or sitting against the wall in Baddha Konasana. Alternatively, you could also sit on a chair with the feet planted and a block between the knees. If using the block, gently pulse the inner thighs and knees against the block for the full exhale, releasing on the inhalation. This helps activate the adductor group and engages into the second layer of the pelvic floor which runs between the sitz bones. (For more instructions see pg 166.)

If sitting in Baddha Konasana, gently place the elbows or palms against the inner knees, maintaining an upright pelvis. Gently press down against the knees while resisting upwards (the knees won't actually move). Then switch to pull up with the hands but press down with the knees. Switch back and forth feeling the different sets of muscles engage and release. (For more instructions see pgs 155-156.)

Core toning

While we are certainly not attempting to maintain a flat stomach during pregnancy (this can lead to problems for the growing baby) maintaining light abdominal tone can help both with back support and preserving abdominal integrity postpartum.

To strengthen the abdominals daily during pregnancy we can use a variation of the Cat/Cow/Table pose, but rather than focusing on the movement of the pelvis, we can bring attention to the engagement of the transverse abdominal muscles which wrap around and support the growing uterus and baby.

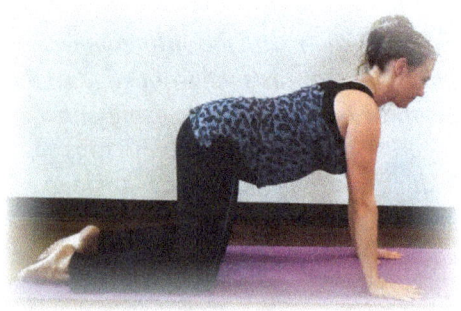

To tone abdominals gently during pregnancy, begin on hands and knees with a neutral spine. Inhale to release the abdomen, but for this variation do not allow the lower back to arch. On the exhale, gently draw the abdominal muscles up and forwards, as though trying to softly lift and hug the baby towards the heart. Again, the spine should not move much, as this is not the Cat/Cow variation. Repeat, alternating release and engagement with the breath. Finish in a middle ground position, not released or engaged. (For further instruction see Table pose on pg 201.)

Psoas release

Releasing the psoas helps free compression in the lower back and makes space around the uterus within the pelvic bowl so the baby is more easily able to move and rotate. As a deep hip flexor, and also a muscle deeply connected with self-preservation, the psoas is best accessed through gentle, more passive stretches than huge backbend movements.

For a direct psoas release, come down to the floor (roll to the side, then onto the back) and place a yoga block on low height beneath the sacrum. Bringing one knee in towards the chest, hold the back of the leg with one or both hands. With the knee drawn in, extend the opposite leg out along the floor until the tissue begins to lengthen at the hip socket. Roll the extended leg inward to drop the inseam towards the floor, and maintain the foot in line with

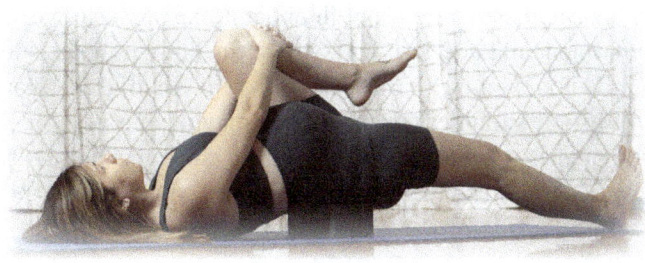

the hip (i.e., do not let the leg drift out to the side). Breathe deeply, as the psoas originates at the abdominal diaphragm. Allow the leg to hang towards the floor for a minute or more, actively drawing the bent knee in to slightly tuck the pelvis. Switch sides.

Other options for accessing the Psoas could be a supported Bridge pose resting on a yoga block (pg #), or the high lunge of Anjaneyasana. To focus the action of Anjaneyasana into the psoas, stabilize the pelvic bowl and then raise the same arm as the back leg overhead, leaning slightly away from the extended hip. This side bending action lengthens the working leg side of the spine, elongating the psoas further. (For more instructions see pg 170.)

Side bending and release

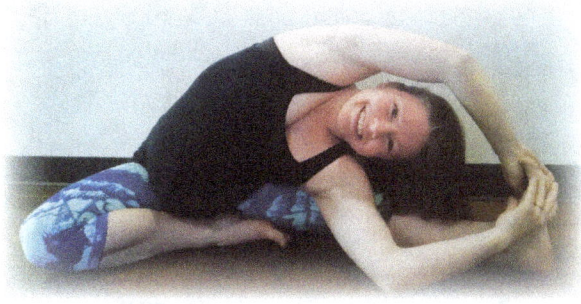

The increase of weight on the front body and postural shifts can often mean compression and tension develop in the side body muscles. Additionally, for those with short waisted torsos, the ribs can become overly compressed as the abdominal organs shift later in pregnancy to accommodate the baby. Lengthening the side body can be helpful to release the lower back and to make space within the pelvis and abdominal muscles on one side while simultaneously engaging the opposite side.

To lengthen and engage the side body, begin either in Prasarita Padottanasana, Warrior 2, or seated in Janu Sirsasana. From Warrior 2 or Janu Sirsasana, inhale to reach one arm up and exhale to lengthen either back over the back leg (from Warrior 2 pgs 145-146) or forward over the extended leg (from Janu Sirsasana pg 157). In both cases focus on the subtle rotation spiraling along the spine to stretch one side and strengthen the other. From Prasarita Padotanasana, place the hands on tall height yoga blocks, and then gently twist the spine by pressing down into one hand while raising the opposite shoulder. Repeat on both sides. (For more instructions see pgs 197-198.)

Classic sequences modified for pregnancy

Along with the basic movements, you may wish to explore further yoga *asana* in a safe and playful manner. I've included a few classic yoga sequences adapted for pregnancy which can serve as good overall movement breaks while addressing several basic movements. In each of these sequences, keep in mind the core definition of *vinyasa*, which is "to place with awareness." The goal is an overall body stretch that promotes the fascia, muscles, and joints arriving at a place of "not too tight and not too loose."

The order listed here is not intended to be prescriptive. Upon completing one sequence, take a moment and check in with where the body now feels tense or loose. Then practice accordingly. For example, if after warming up you find that your shoulders are stiff, you might start with some shoulder releases. Then maybe your body feels stiff in the hips, so you shift to hip openers. Then you feel a need for some grounding, so you get up and practice a standing series. And then, because you only have time for one more posture, you shift to Shavasana or resting meditation.

Let go of the conventional yoga class sequence when practicing on your own, and discover for yourself what feels useful.

The Prenatal Sun Salutation

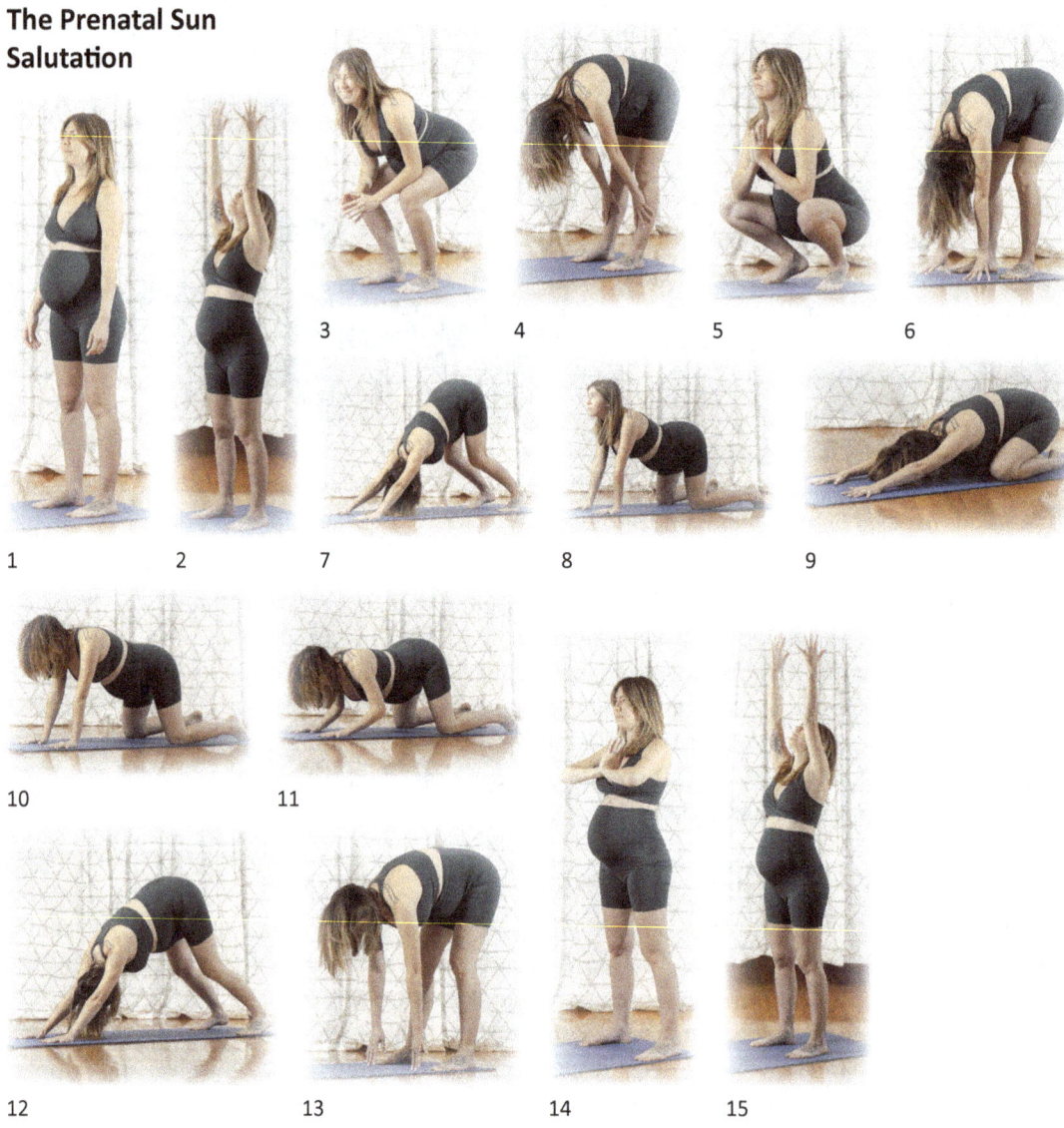

The Earth Salutation

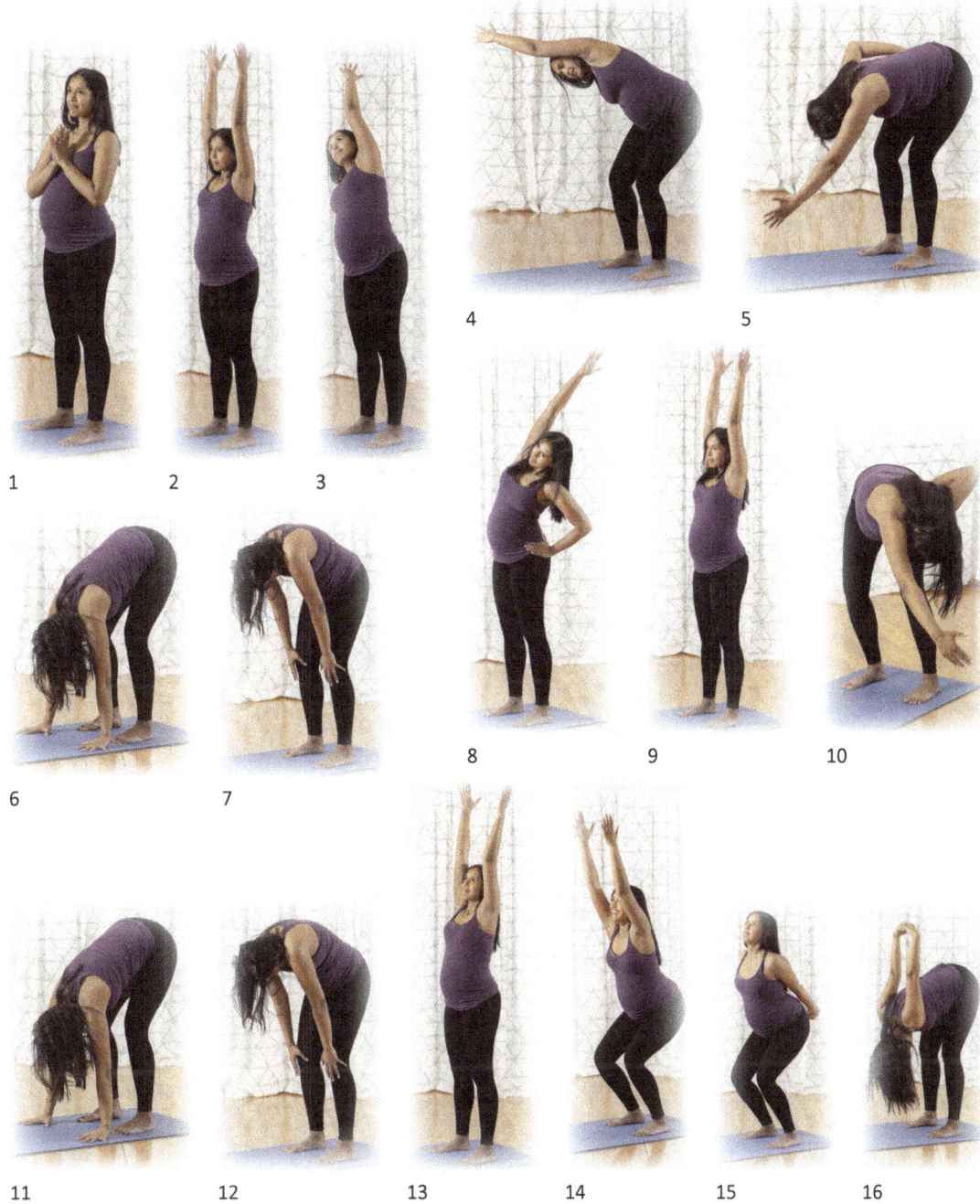

Earth Salutation continued

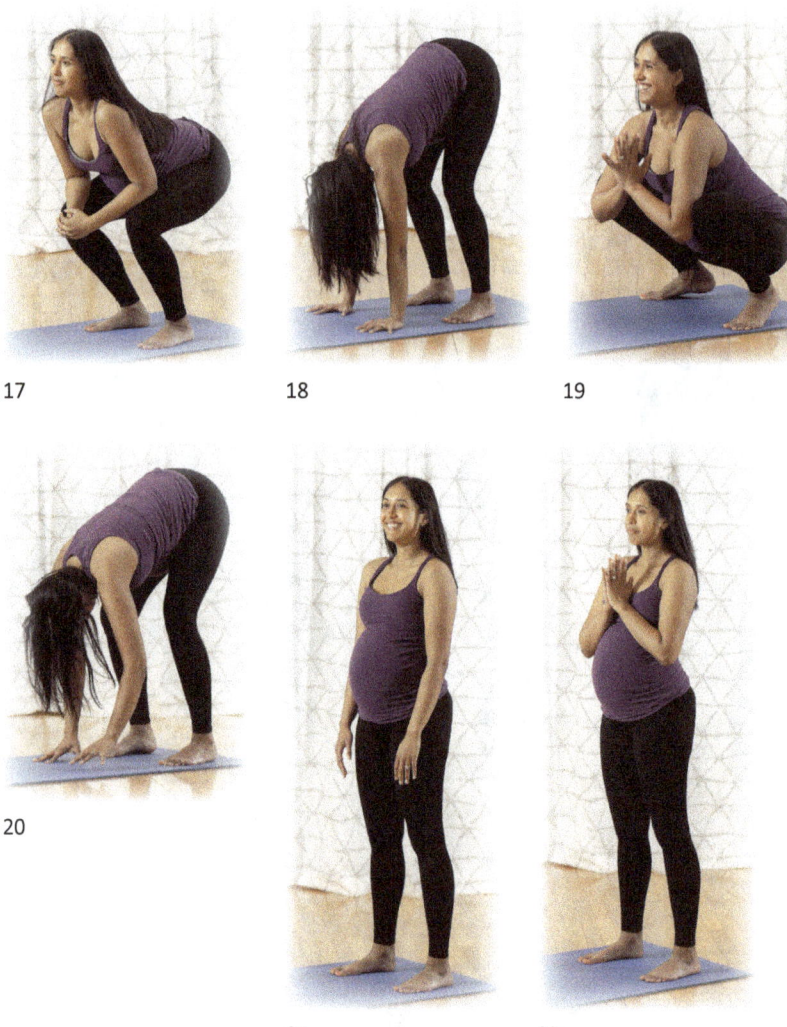

17

18

19

20

21

22

Low Lunge Vinyasa
(This series can be combined with earth salutations for a longer flow)

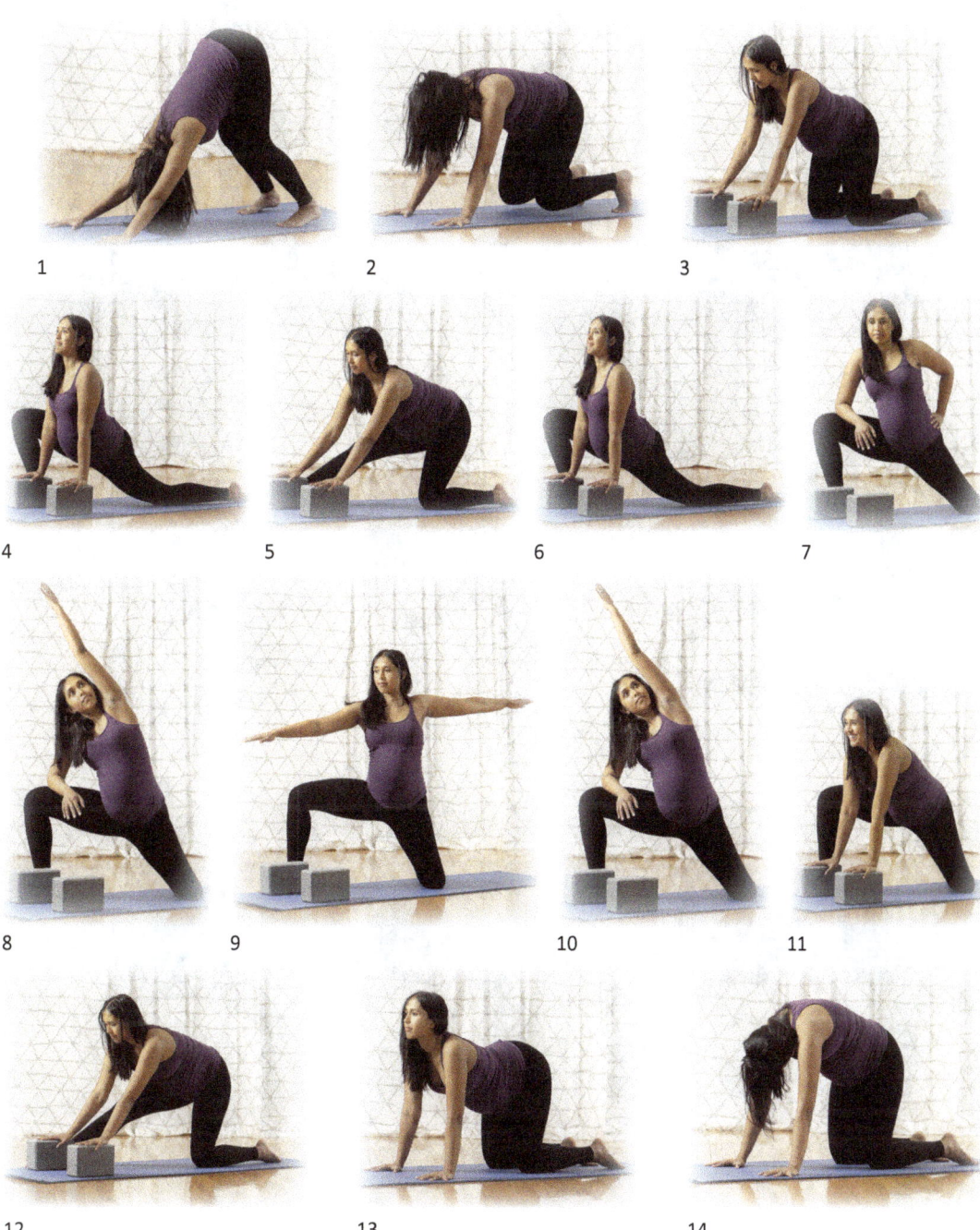

1

2

3

4

5

6

7

8

9

10

11

12

13

14

Standing lunges/Warrior sequence
(These can be combined in numerous ways — Be sure to practice both sides)

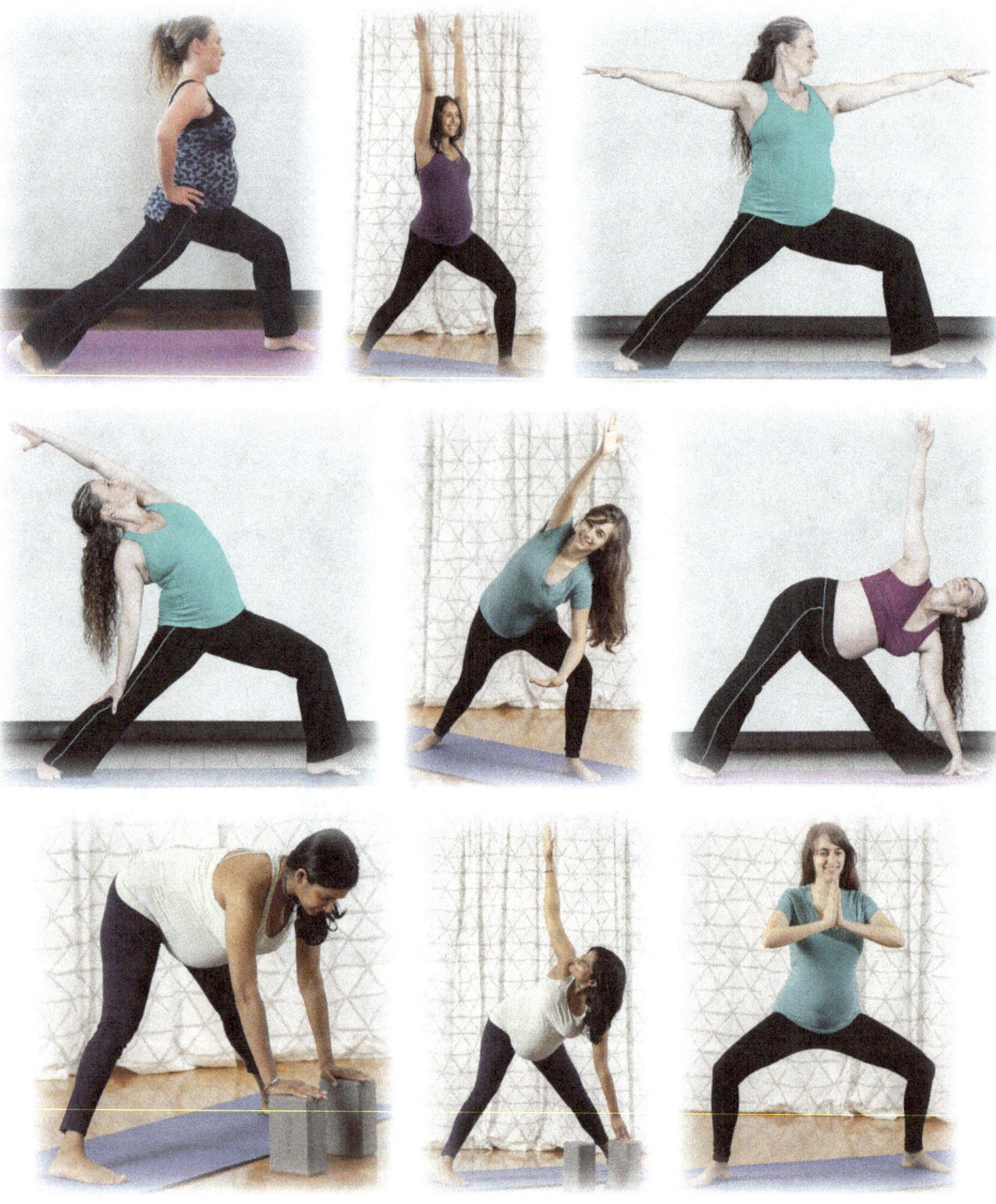

Spinal mobilization and twists—kneeling Ardha Chandrasana sequence
(Repeat on the second side)

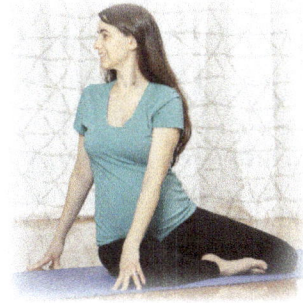
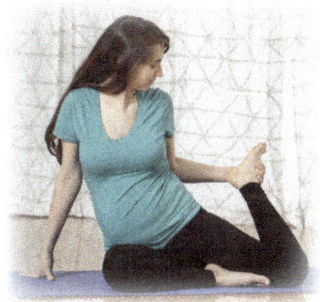
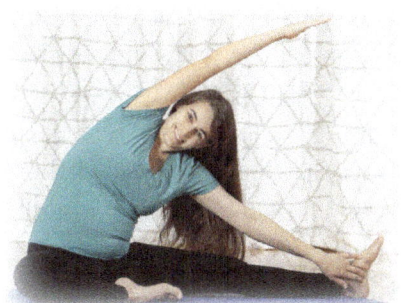

1

2

3

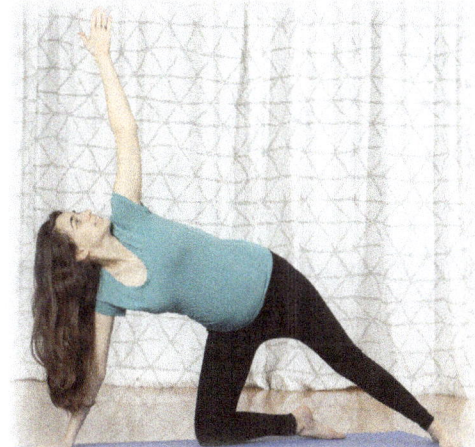
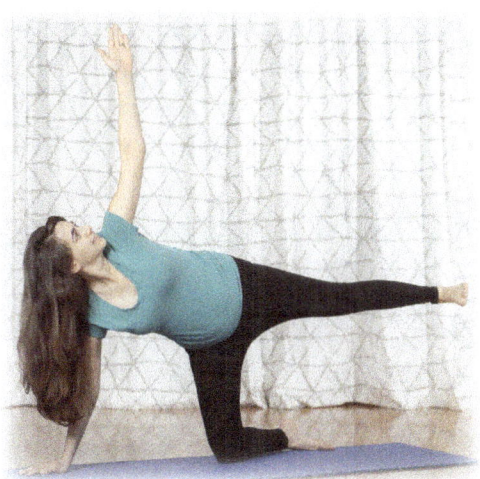

4

5

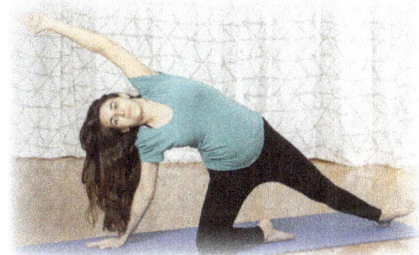
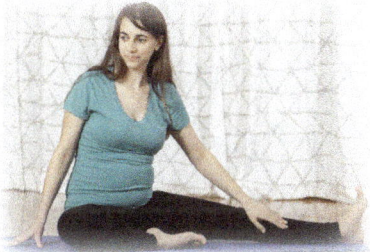
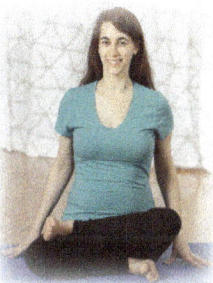

6

7

8

Aches and pains

I always approach aches and pains during pregnancy as signals that the body is out of balance somewhere, which causes too much or too little tension to be held in a specific area. Addressing the complaint may require stretching the area or developing more strength in the surrounding areas to help take the pressure off a specific spot.

With a system as complex as the pregnant body, we can't always know for sure what the exact cause is. But we can explore different shapes and movements to discover how the body tissues respond to being placed in different shapes. Ultimately, your own inner teacher is the best guide.

Suggested postures

Low back pain

- Side bends (Janu Sirsasana, Reverse Warrior, Seated side bend)

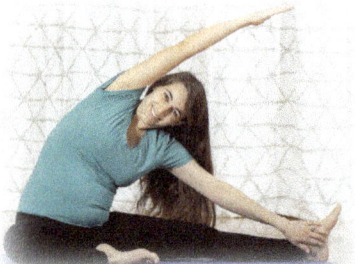 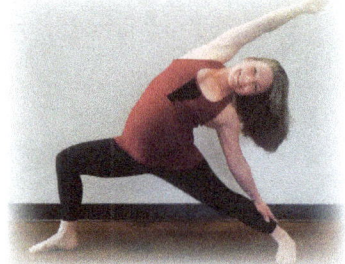 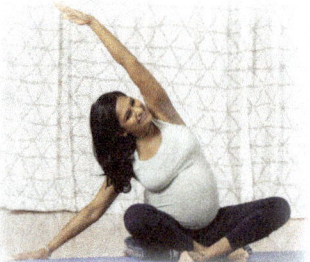

- Twists (Windmill, Janu Sirsasana B, Marichiasana)

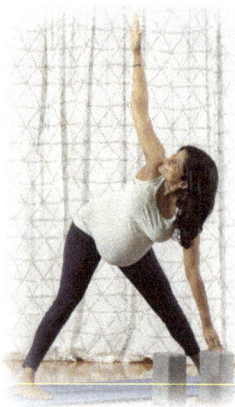 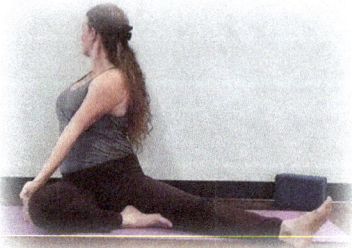 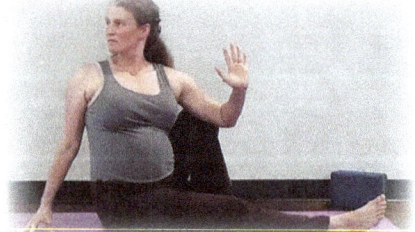

- Backbends (Bridge, Upper Back Bolster, psoas stretch, Cat/Cow)

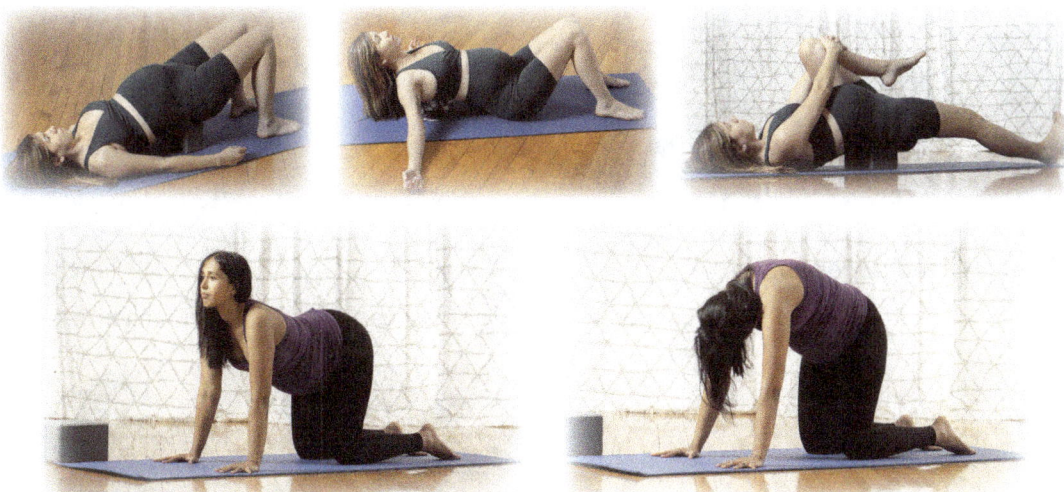

Hip/pelvic pain

- Hip openers (good for sciatica) (Baddha Konasana, Ankle to Knee, Goddess Squats, pelvic floor breathing)

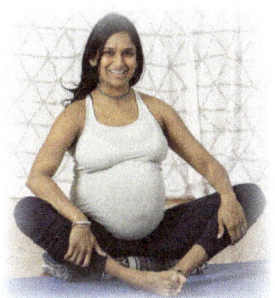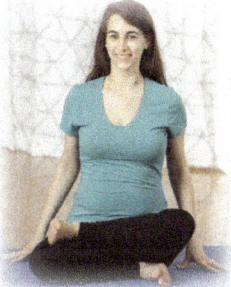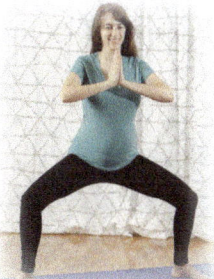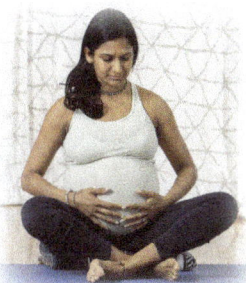

- Hip stabilizers (good for SI pain or PSD) (Goddess Squats for SI pain but not PSD, wall squat with block or strap, clamshells)

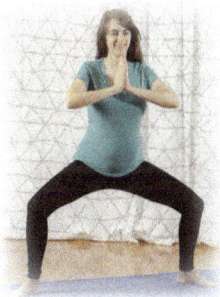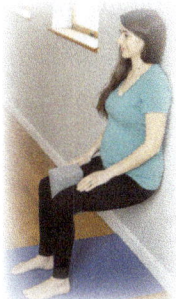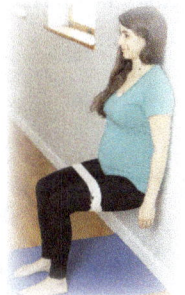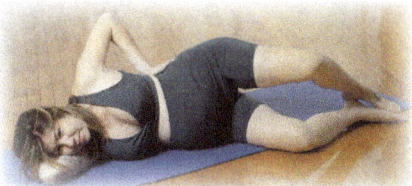

- Mobilizing hips (Cat/Cow, Skandasana, Anjaneyasana)

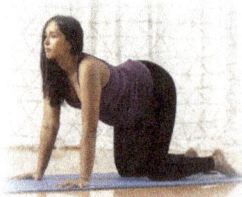 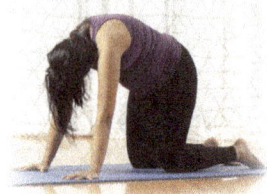 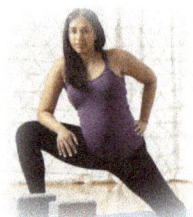 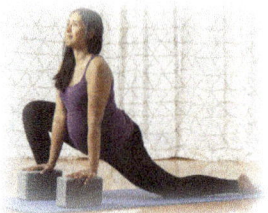

Shoulders and upper back

- Shoulder openers (chest opener with strap, Garudasana arms, Gomukhasana arms)

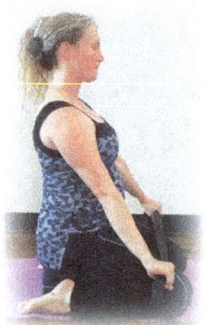 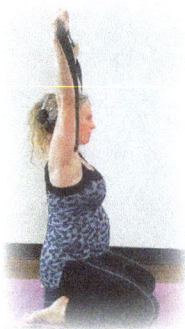 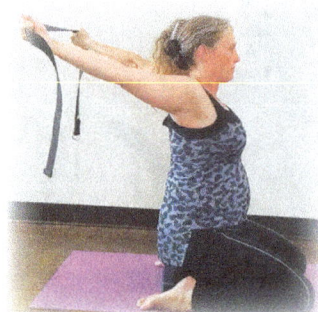 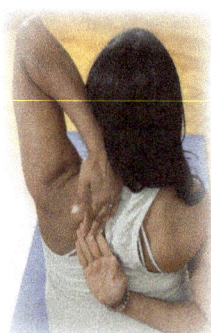

- Upper backbends (Upper Back Bolster)

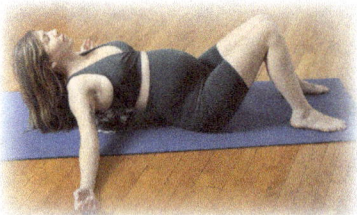 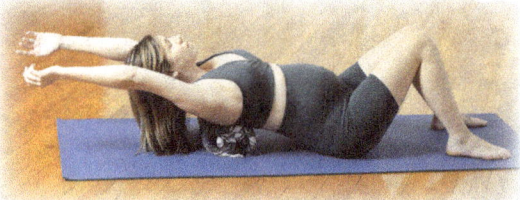

Lower body

- Leg stretches (calf stretches, Prasarita Padottanasana, Parsvottanasana, Supta Padangusthasana/Utthita Hasta Padangusthasana, Downward Dog)

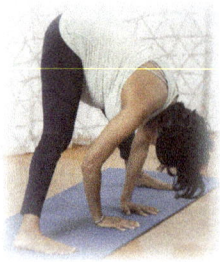 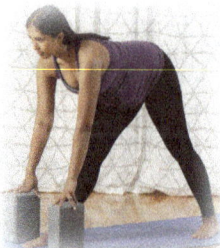 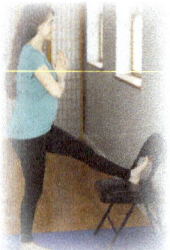 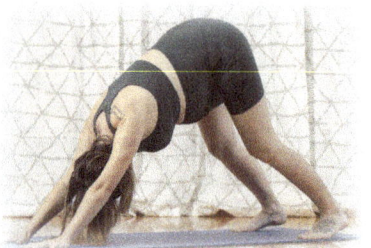

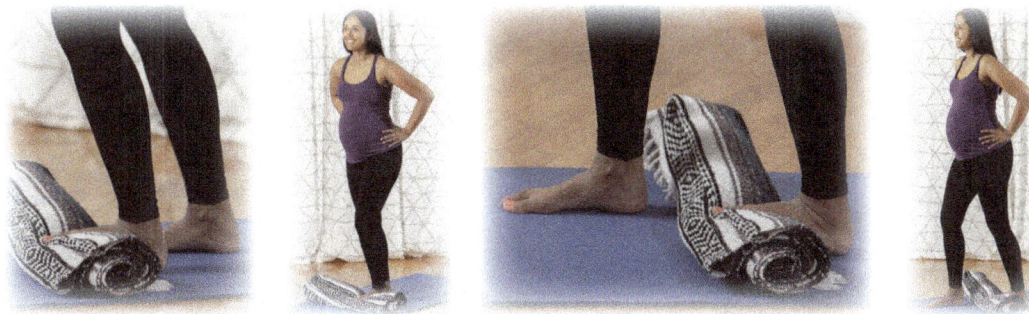

- Strengthening (Anjaneyasana, Warriors 1 and 2, Goddess Squat, Vrksasana)

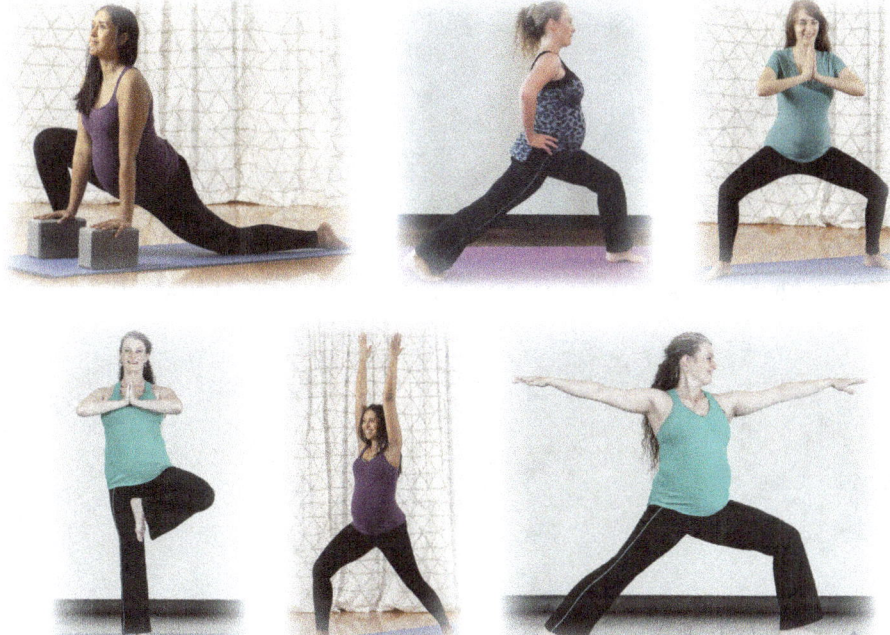

Rib pain/shortness of breath

- Side bends and bolster work

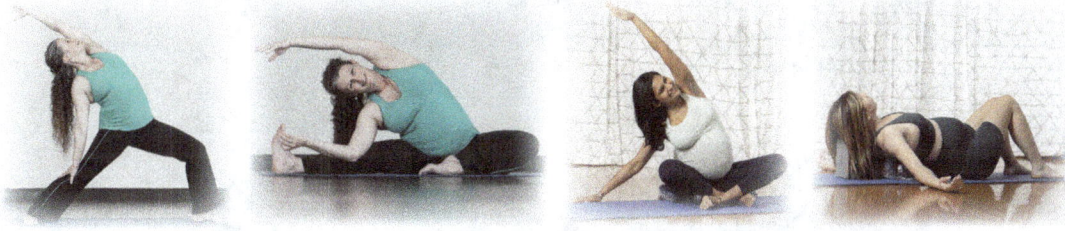

Heartburn

- Anti-heartburn poses (anti-heartburn pose, Urdhva Hastasana)

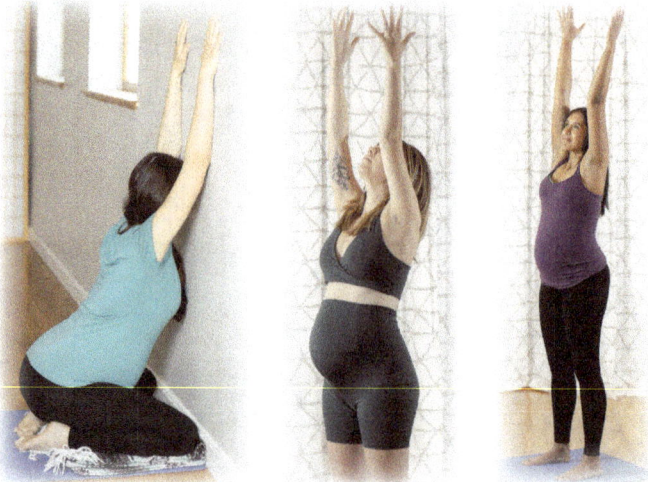

Sensitive wrists

- Wrist stretches and hand modifications (wrist circles and modifications)

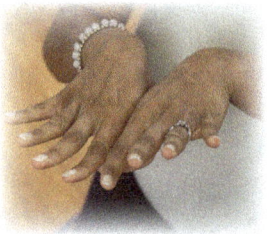 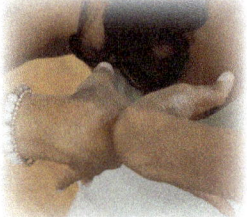 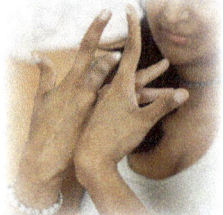 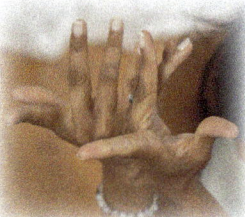

Fatigue

- Restorative postures

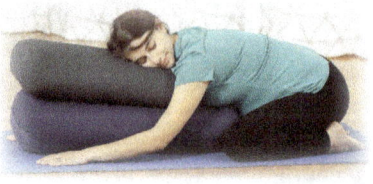 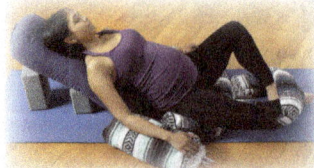 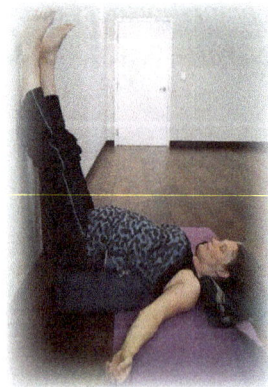

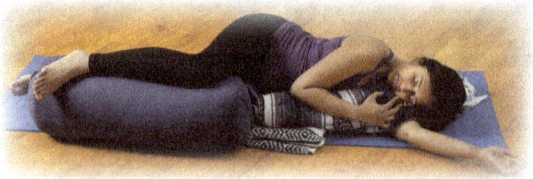

- Pranayama

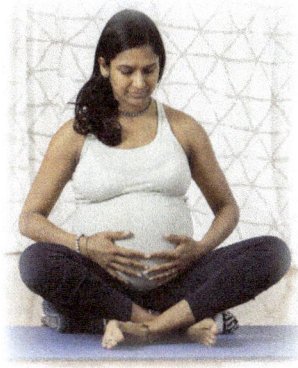 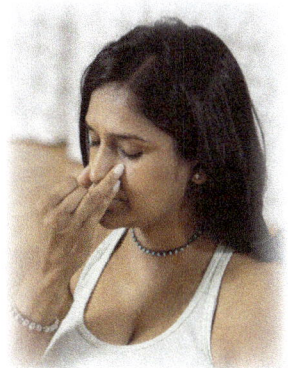 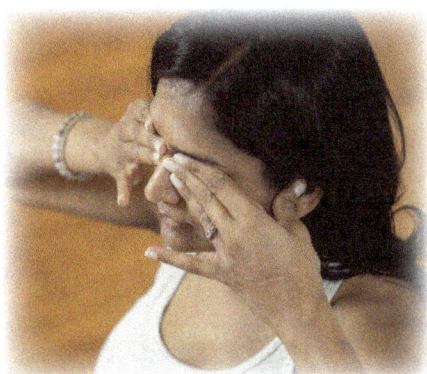

- Shavasana

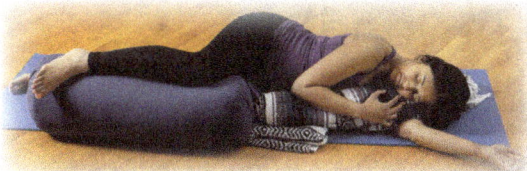 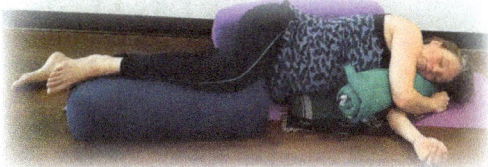

Ultimately there is no one practice that will ensure a specific type of birth experience. But by cultivating a sense of coming home to your body and embracing who you are in the moment, you can gain the stability, compassion, and awareness to ride the waves of pregnancy, birth, postpartum, and life in general with greater grace and ease. And ultimately isn't that what yoga is all about? "Yogas chitta vritti nirodha." Yoga is the quieting of the fluctuation of the mind.

Birth (and beyond)

"In birth preparation your first task is to empty your mind of expectations and judgments that narrow the possibilities for coping with pain, surprises, and the hard work of labor. Being "empty" will allow you to receive, moment-by-moment, the messages conveyed by your body, mind, and heart."

— Pam England, *Birthing From Within*

12 — Childbirth Education: The Missing Link and What You Need to Know

The way I see it, the most trustworthy knowledge about women's bodies combines the best of what medical science has offered over the past century or two with what women have always been able to learn about themselves.

—Ina May Gaskin

It's halfway through the second day of teacher training. A group of teacher trainees sits before me in a makeshift circle. Some rock side to side, feeling their sitz bones; others peel back tape lines stuck to yoga pants to indicate femur bone alignment. We have just finished exploring our own pelvic anatomy and postural patterns, discussing pelvic bony anatomy and the muscular network supporting the upper and lower body. Now we are about to diverge from the pure discussions of yoga asana and anatomy and venture into the world of childbirth education, medicine, and the physiology of labor.

Whether it's focusing on connecting with a baby or learning to cope with strong sensations, yoga during pregnancy inevitably confronts the reality of preparing both physically and mentally for the upcoming experience of labor and birth. A prenatal yoga class (or practice) by its nature involves more than modifying the shape of *asana* or omitting contraindicated postures.

When I first began training to teach pregnant women, I foolishly thought it would mainly be learning how to adjust postural shapes. What I quickly realized was that prenatal classes were often sprinkled with tidbits of childbirth education. Having an understanding of the birth process was integral to teaching well. These bite-sized childbirth morsels offer the opportunity to shift how we might think about the birth process, to delve more deeply into working with the sensations of labor, and to explore what it means to be fully respected during that process. In short, understanding the birth process turns a prenatal yoga class into an invitation to take the practice off the mat and into the labor room.

This chapter will not encompass everything that would be covered during a full childbirth education class. Discussions about epidurals, hospital triage, vaginal exams, and cesareans are beyond the scope of this book (and to some degree beyond the scope of a yoga class). But if you think conversations about the process of labor and birth are beyond the scope of a prenatal yoga class, think again. In exploring the changing sensations within our bodies, we inevitably begin to consider the upcoming process of birth and the choices we have available in that process. While many pregnant yoginis strive for a "natural birth" (that is to say, one without interventions or medication), there are others who choose differently for various reasons. Ultimately there is no one right way to give birth—except for the one that is right for you and your baby on the day they arrive in your arms.

I often find that during yoga classes, especially in check-in-discussions about the physical process and sensations of labor, coping strategies and the inherent physicality of the process become lively discussions. Understanding the science gives context for each new sensation—sensations which might be quite foreign and confusing if we didn't have the context of the physiological changes happening internally. I hope this chapter gives you some empowering information to better understand the physiology of labor and how yoga practice can impact your readiness for labor, birth, and that final transition into parenthood.

Pelvic organ anatomy

Hopefully the earlier chapters of this book have given you an understanding of the key bones and muscles, but if we're going to talk about pregnancy, we need to understand the organs involved, too. So, let's go back to the pelvis.

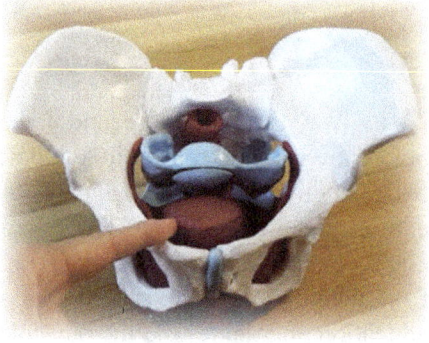

The pelvic organs are nestled tightly together within the bony pelvis. From front to back we find the bladder, then the uterus, and finally the rectum resting against the sacrum. The bladder, a hemispherical muscular hollow organ, is located just behind the pubic bone. Its function is to collect and store urine and to then empty it during urination. The urethral sphincter—fibers at the base of the bladder—are interwoven with the pelvic floor. That's why a common (though not fully accurate) instruction to stop a stream of urine is a method for activating the pelvic floor in Kegel exercises. The bladder sits slightly below the uterus, and as the baby's head descends into the pelvis, it begins to compress the bladder, which explains why there is an increased urge to pee towards the end of pregnancy.

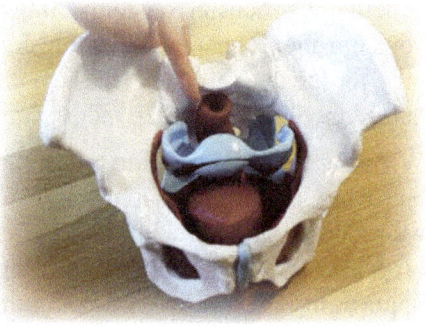

On the back side of the pelvic bowl we find the rectum, another hollow, muscular organ located at the end of the colon. Its job is to collect and store solid waste and to void it when the pelvic floor indicates. The rectum has two sets of sphincter fibers located at its end, one entwined within the pelvic floor and one deeper inside. Because it is behind the uterus and baby, the rectum is not usually as compressed by baby engaging in the pelvis, but it does become compressed as the baby moves out of the uterus during the pushing stage of labor. That's because the angle of the cervix points towards the back of the pelvis—hence the feeling of wanting to poop as the pushing stage of labor begins. The baby's head presses on the same nerve bundle that a full rectum presses on and in fact triggers the same expulsive reflex.

Last but by no means least we come to the queen of the pelvic organs: the uterus! A hollow organ nestled between the bladder and the rectum, the uterus is identified as triangular or pear-shaped. In good alignment, the uterus rests forward against the upper side of the bladder, with the rectum resting against the back. We also have the fallopian tubes extending from the upper third of the uterus and branching out towards the ovaries just beyond.

When no pregnancy is present, the uterus rests in the middle of the pelvic bowl, supported by a network of ligaments as well as the pelvic floor. Remember the pelvic dreamcatcher from Chapter 5? From the back of the cervix, the wide utero-sacral ligaments extend to the border of the sacrum. Running parallel with the utero-sacral ligaments, the broad ligament extends around the front of the abdomen like an internal support band. From the front and side, we have the pubocervical ligaments and the cardinal ligaments. The whole network supports and guides the alignment of the lower uterine segment.

Guiding from higher up, two ropey ligaments known as the round ligaments extend from the uterus over the pubic bone attaching into the front labia. These ligaments provide contact points to maintain the central placement of the upper uterus within the pelvic bowl and support its weight. As the baby grows, these ligaments help guide the uterus to remain centered within the body. Think of a hot air balloon held to the ground by tension lines to keep it upright as it inflates.

The uterus is made of three layers of muscle fibers. While I'm going to describe these fibers as separate "layers," they actually interweave with one another to create an integrated system within the uterus, similar to the interdigitation of the muscle layers of the pelvic floor. The outer uterine fibers run in vertical lines from the base to the top of the fundus (the domed top of the uterus). A middle layer runs diagonally in and around the uterus, encircling the blood vessels of the placenta with loops and "figure eights." Finally, the innermost layer consists of concentric circles that are wider at the top and get closer together towards the base. It is this inner circular layer which forms the cervix at the base of the uterus, literally creating a sphincter to hold the baby in during pregnancy. When we talk about the cervix changing during labor, we are describing the muscular opening at the base of the uterus.

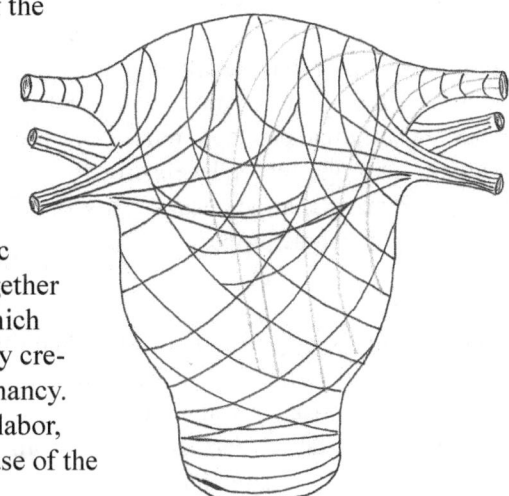

Physical changes during pregnancy for mom and baby

Before we get to talking about the changes during pregnancy, we should cover a bit about something many of us learned about in high school health class—though probably not in much detail—the menstrual cycle. I have often marveled that high school health classes often do not give girls enough information to fully understand their own cycles!

The menstrual cycle involves several hormones which prepare the body for pregnancy every month. Following the end of menstruation, estrogen levels begin to rise, increasing the blood-rich lining of the uterus. At the same time, follicle stimulating hormone (FSH) has been stimulating several follicles within the ovaries to "ripen" their eggs in preparation for ovulation. The egg that is released during any given menstrual cycle actually began ripening nearly 3 cycles earlier (so it really is one full year from the time the body begins stimulating the egg to the birth of the baby from that egg).

Around 14 days into this process (the exact number can vary based on the individual and a number of environmental considerations) a hormone called luteinizing hormone spikes, triggering the final release of the ripened egg from the ovarian follicle. The egg tumbles out and is swept into the fallopian tubes to begin its journey towards the uterus and, possibly, fertilization. An egg is only viable for 24 hours, so if it does not meet sperm within that window, it will die on its own.

Given the short window of viability, the female body usually assists any sperm which might be hoping to meet the egg. A few days prior to ovulation, the body changes the consistency of the mucus within the cervix, taking it from sticky and inhospitable to slippery, like egg whites. The slippery mucus also affects the pH of the environment, making it more likely that a sperm will survive. These changes allow sperm to live up to five days in the hospitable cervical fluid, as opposed to 1-2 days in the sticky version, making it more likely that a sperm will meet an egg while the egg is still viable.

Following ovulation, the follicle that produced the egg has an additional job. It begins releasing a hormone called progesterone, which will help the body maintain the uterine lining should the egg become fertilized and need to implant. The follicle, now called the corpus luteum, will continue to produce this hormone for 12-18 days. If there is no further signal from the body that conception has occurred, then the corpus luteum ceases progesterone production. As progesterone levels drop, the uterus begins to contract to release the inner uterine lining and menstruation occurs. Once the lining is shed, the body begins to increase estrogen levels and the whole process resets.

Conception

That is, unless the egg is fertilized! When this happens, sperm meets egg, usually in the upper third of the fallopian tube. The two merge to form one complete cell, which then begins to divide as it moves towards the uterus. Referred to first as a zygote and then a blastocyst, within 10 or so days of fertilization this ball of cells comes into contact with the uterine endometrium (lining) and burrows into the uterine wall. Some women experience slight bleeding at this point known as implantation bleeding.

At this moment, the mother's body sends out a hormonal signal to the corpus luteum to continue producing the life sustaining progesterone for the uterine lining. By 14 days (assuming a 28 day cycle, which again can vary), the blastocyst will be well-embedded. It then begins developing into the placenta at the point of attachment and into the fetus where it is not attached. The two, placenta and fetus, are eventually connected via the umbilical cord and surrounded by the amniotic membranes. By week three, blood vessels have formed to carry fetal blood to and from the placenta. The baby's blood never mixes with the mother's; rather, fluid exchange takes place across a permeable barrier. However, nearly everything carried by the fluid will cross the placenta (nutrients, hormones, water, waste, drugs, viruses, etc).

At the end of the first trimester, the placenta has developed enough to take over progesterone production from the corpus luteum. This is one of many reasons why some miscarriages occur at the end of the first trimester. If this handoff from follicle to organ does not go smoothly, the body can get confused and begin shedding the lining it was meant to maintain. The first trimester is also the period of the fastest cell division for the baby, as cells differentiate into placenta, baby, body systems, and brain. And the body is increasing levels of the hormone relaxin throughout the first trimester, to soften connective tissue for implantation and to maintain a relaxed uterus through these crucial months of initial development to avoid accidentally menstruating the growing fetus.

First trimester

For moms, the first trimester (0-12 weeks) involves a series of major internal changes but little outward visibility. Many women report feeling extremely fatigued during the first trimester due to the hormonal changes. The body's base temperature is slightly elevated due to the continued production of progesterone—though mom may not feel it. This is one reason that pregnant women are told to avoid saunas and hot tubs; the other is that elevated body temps during the first trimester can increase the risk of defects occurring during this time of rapid cell division. The increases in progesterone and relaxin can also lead to feeling slightly out of breath, as the hormones impact connective tissues and fascia around the diaphragm. Relaxin reaches its highest level around week 12 (Advanced yoginis, take note: you are at your most flexible at the end of your first trimester, and not in a way you want to take advantage of!).

The infamous "morning sickness" often does not emerge until 6-7 weeks, and it should be noted that despite the name, this can be a whole day affair. My own experience was quite mild, and most closely resembled the nausea I had previously experienced with hypoglycemia (low blood sugar). In my case I found that constantly eating was one way to keep it at bay (a slightly comical solution, as it meant I was sneaking cookies in the middle of teaching yoga classes). I know some students whose morning sickness was so severe that they were only able to keep down saltines and ginger ale for the first 12 weeks and some who required medication to cope. For others, it never materialized. It depends on the pregnancy.

The first trimester can also be a time of both excitement and anxiety. If baby was planned, there may be an increased protective drive. Or you might experience a quiet excitement, as though you are harboring a delightful secret (and you well may be!). For other mothers, these early weeks may be fraught with worry, especially if the pregnancy was preceded by other miscarriages or involved fertility treatments. I have seen students who found it challenging to connect to their growing babies during this time, out of fear that they would have to grieve them if the pregnancy didn't continue.

I have also seen even longtime yoginis cease all yoga activity during the first trimester; having now conceived, their instinct is to avoid all movement until they are certain the pregnancy is established. While understandable, this is not usually necessary, and some gentle movement and relaxation could actually be beneficial for maintaining a healthy state of body and mind as the body adjusts to the growing baby within. As one first trimester mom said in tears following a yoga class, "I didn't realize how much I was resisting feeling this baby, and how much tension that was creating in my body, until I let myself imagine she was actually here with me."

Second trimester

The first trimester is the formation period for your baby, the second trimester is when things develop. By the end of the first trimester the baby's internal organs have mostly formed but are not fully developed. Baby begins to swallow amniotic fluid and pee it back out, maintaining the amniotic fluid balance for the rest of the pregnancy. Around 16-22 weeks, mom may begin to be able to feel the baby moving inside. Called "quickening," this sensation can feel like fluttering or even gas bubbles. But with attention and time, these movements are more clearly recognized as belonging to baby. If the placenta is attached to the front side of the body (anterior placenta), these movements may be muffled and less noticeable, as the placenta provides a cushion between the abdominal wall and the baby's movement. I wasn't aware of my baby's movement until almost 22 weeks due to an anterior placenta.

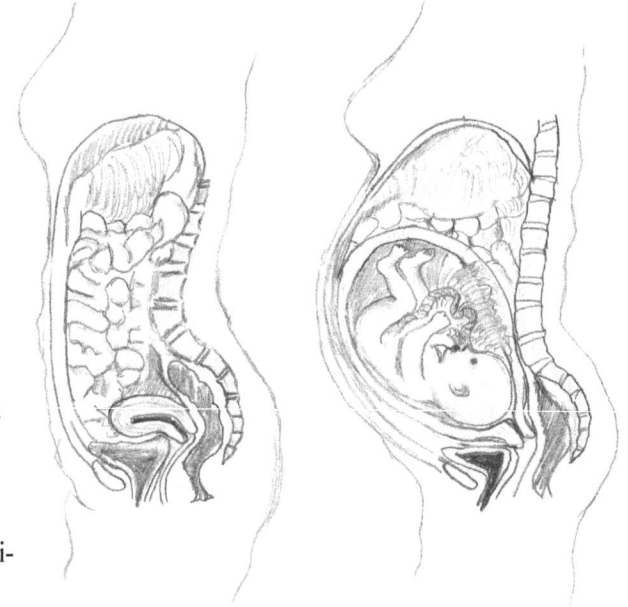

By 24 weeks the baby is fully formed, and modern medicine has developed to the point where, though not yet fully mature, they could potentially survive outside mom's body with assistance. The bones begin to harden, movements become stronger, and they are covered with fine hair (lanugo) as well as a white, creamy substance called vernix which protects their skin from the amniotic fluid.

The second and third trimesters are when the internal changes in mom's body begin to be outwardly visible. The organs within the pelvis are tightly packed together before pregnancy. If a baby is also going to develop and grow within this container, something will have to adjust by the end of the first trimester. Cue shifting abdominal organs! The base of the uterus remains contained by pelvic bones and fascia, so the only real space the body has is above the uterus in the abdominal cavity. By the second trimester, the uterus is too large to remain contained within the original pelvic bones, so the top (fundus) pushes upwards, shifting the intestines and other abdominal organs up into the diaphragm.

The result is a series of postural shifts that occur as the body adjusts within the field of gravity. The spinal curves deepen, and as we saw in Chapter 2, the angle of the lower back may seem more pronounced than in a non-pregnant body. This change does not necessarily need to be corrected, as it is the body's way of adjusting to its changing center of gravity. The breasts often increase in size and begin producing colostrum, the nutrient-rich food that will feed the baby until breast milk is produced. By the end of the second trimester (28 weeks), the stomach, intestines, and liver all crowd up against the respiratory diaphragm, which can lead to feeling short of breath and an inability to eat large meals, especially if mom was naturally short-waisted or carried tension in the intercostal muscles between the ribs. Side bends, anyone?

Second trimester is also when the blood volume in mom's body begins to increase. By the time we reach the "due date," her body will be carrying 150% of her original blood volume to accommodate for her needs as well as baby's. To compensate for this increased fluid, mom's body dilates the blood vessels and drops the overall resting blood pressure. This is so the fluid increasing within the closed system of the body doesn't cause a sudden increase of the resting blood pressure. As discussed in Chapter 10, this can lead to lightheadedness and dizziness if mom stands up quickly.

During second and third trimester, the uterus may also begin practice contractions. Referred to as "Braxton-Hicks," these contractions are usually mild and should not be cause for concern. Like a marathon runner doing short training runs, they are a way for the muscles to begin coordinating the movements they will perform during labor. The only reason to worry is if they become strong and regular or come very frequently (more than six in one hour). If you experience these symptoms, check with your care provider about how to proceed. Overall, the second trimester is often a fun time during pregnancy: the hormones of first trimester begin to level off, nausea and vomiting (hopefully) decrease, and energy levels often return.

Third trimester

The third trimester begins on week 28 of pregnancy and lasts until the baby's birth. This final period is when the baby primarily focuses on growth, maturing fully and developing the systems they will need to survive outside the womb. The lungs usually mature around 36 weeks, and the baby may begin doing practice breathing movements which can lead to temporary spasms in their newly activated diaphragm muscle: hiccups! Around weeks 24-28, the baby's head becomes heavier than its body, which usually initiates a turn into a head down position.

For mom, the third trimester primarily builds on the changes begun during the second trimester. But this time is also when the compound impact of the increased weight, the shift in the center of gravity, postural imbalances, and the prolonged hormonal shifts begin to take a toll. Small imbalances from earlier in the pregnancy now start to manifest—illustrating where adjustments are needed. In yoga classes, third trimester is often when students mention increased tension, discomfort, and other physical ailments. These aches and pains are not due to any major change within the body but are more likely the result of existing fascial and movement imbalances that had not previously been recognized. Practice-wise, modifications during the third trimester tend to become more personalized and dependent upon what each student is working with. One mom will need to release tight hip rotators for pelvic mobility; another will need to develop strength to create a stable pelvic bowl.

Summary of changes to mom and baby during pregnancy:

Changes for Mom	Changes for Baby
0-12 weeks	**0-12 weeks**
• Progesterone, estrogen, and relaxin increase • Relaxin at highest level by 12 weeks • Energy reserves may fade • Nausea may appear around 6-7 weeks • Body base temperature slightly elevated 0-12 weeks	• Cells rapidly dividing • Implantation • Development of body, limbs, eyes, organs, and other system differentiation • By 12 weeks baby begins swallowing and excreting amniotic fluid • By week 12, ultrasound can also show limbs, body, toes and possibly sex organs
12-28 weeks	**12-28 weeks**
• Increased weight on the front of the body can lead to postural shifts • Mom can feel the baby move (quickening) • The uterus may begin practice contractions called Braxton-Hicks. • Breasts begin producing colostrum • Blood volume begins increasing. (150% by the end of 40 weeks) • Blood vessels dilate, and static blood pressure drops • Energy may return as hormones level off. • Nausea usually disappears • Linea negra (darkened line) can appear along center of abdomen • Possible leg cramps—can be from baby drawing calcium for mom's bones	• Eyes move to the front of the head from the sides • Ears move into position • Baby can suck their thumb and grasp umbilical cord • Baby can hear sounds from outside world • Organs fully formed by the end • Body covered with lanugo at 19 weeks (downy hair) and vernix by 27 weeks (white sticky protective covering) • Sex organs can definitely be seen by ultrasound • Bones begin to calcify • Fingernails begin to form • The eyes open (they are nearly always dark blue at first)

28-40/42 weeks	28-40/42 weeks
• The uterus moves up into the abdominal cavity, pushing the abdominal organs up against the diaphragm. • Compression against diaphragm can lead to shortness of breath and heartburn • The ribs begin to expand sideways to give space for the baby and abdominal organs • Energy reserves begin to fade as the body must now support two full lives • Increased blood volume can lead to swelling in the legs and feet • Baby turns head down and settles lower into the pelvis • Hormones begin to prepare the body for birth.	• Baby's head becomes heaviest part, encouraging a head down position • Body begins adding fat stores • Practice breathing movements are present and sometimes hiccups • Responds to outside sounds and knows the sound of their parent's voices- especially mom • Liver begins to store iron • Lungs mature • Active movements now easily felt • Baby's position can be evaluated by palpation • Baby begins to find position from which to start birth

Preparing for labor

But of course, what we're preparing for during prenatal yoga isn't just the shifts that take place during pregnancy. We are preparing for that fundamental shift into parenthood, defined by the process of labor and birth.

As the pregnancy nears its end, the body takes several steps to prepare for labor. Following the turn to head down, the baby will often descend further into the pelvis, usually between 36 and 40 weeks. Due dates are set at 40 weeks of gestation, but a normal human gestation range is 265-300 days, or 38-42 weeks. So while the calendar date may be a nice reference, there is actually a birth month—not a single day—during which the baby might emerge. Only about 5% of babies are actually born on their estimated due dates. Watch for signs that the body is getting ready to clarify how close the actual birth day might be.

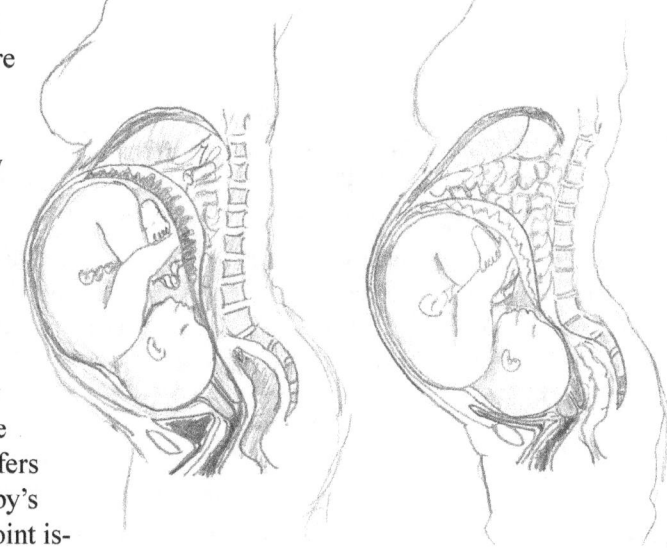

Signs the body
is getting ready for labor

Lightening/engagement

Engagement occurs when the baby descends into the lower bowl of the pelvis. Technically, engagement refers to the position where the top of baby's head becomes level with the midpoint ischial spines in the pelvis. Once engaged, it is less likely that a baby will rotate head up again. Instead, their movements will focus on getting aligned in the starting position for labor.

Most babies will settle into position by 36 weeks, then drop into the pelvis over the next month. For some women, this drop is a dramatic movement, resulting in increased downward pressure in the pelvis and much greater breath capacity as the organs move down away from the abdominal diaphragm. For others it is a more gradual process, only recognizable in hindsight. Not all babies descend before labor, especially second or third babies who may wait until contractions begin to settle into the lower pelvic bowl.

Increased Braxton-Hicks/warm-up contractions

As the baby begins to settle closer to the base of the uterus and the cervix, Braxton-Hicks contractions may intensify. These warm-ups can begin as early as the second trimester, but they are usually mild and unremarkable. As the baby gets closer to the cervix, however, these practice contractions may increase in frequency. While they may occur somewhat closer together, Braxton-Hicks contractions are not progressive—meaning they do not build in intensity or come in ever more frequent intervals. If that happens, they are no longer warm-ups, and labor may have started.

Cervical changes

As the body prepares for labor, the cervix may also begin to show some changes. Throughout the pregnancy, the cervix has been mainly high and in the back (posterior) of the pelvis. As the body begins to prepare for labor, the position and consistency of the cervix begins to change. It slides forward in the pelvis, making the distance from the opening of the cervix to the pelvic floor shorter. Hormones called prostaglandins begin to release, and the cervix begins to soften and eventually thin out from the pressure of baby's head above it.

If one were to feel the cervix at the start of the third trimester (or any time before that) it would have the consistency of the tip of your nose. With prostaglandins, it softens to be closer to the consistency of your earlobe, and if we were to feel it as the body goes into labor, it might resemble the inside of your cheek. This softening makes it easier for the cervix to thin and possibly open 1-2 cm before labor has even begun. Obviously we are not going to see this softening during our yoga classes (please, NO cervical checks during yoga!), but I have had many a student in late third trimester come to class right after learning from her care provider that her cervix has opened.

However, this does not necessarily mean the body is going to go into labor early. As a doula, I once had a client whose cervix was nearly 6 cm opened before labor even began—and stayed that way for two weeks! What we can infer from the opening is that the warm-up contractions might at least be well coordinated, so the body might be more efficient when labor does finally begin.

Colostrum

By the start of the third trimester, endocrine changes within mom's body have begun to produce colostrum in the breasts. This yellow, oily substance serves as the baby's first food and has been shown to be highly rich in both nutrients and antibodies, which helps babies get a jump start on their immune system. By the end of the third trimester, mom may be able to self-express small drops of colostrum by squeezing her nipples. (Save this in a freezer-safe container if doing so. Every drop contains vital nutrients, and babies don't need much to be satiated in the beginning. This should also be done carefully, as strong nipple stimulation could bring on contractions.)

Mucousy-brownish or bloody discharge

From the moment of conception, the cervix has been sealed closed by a thick mucus to prevent any bacteria from entering the uterine environment. As the prostaglandins begin to shift, the consistency of this mucus also changes, becoming more liquid. For some women, this mucus begins to drip or fall out in the days leading up to labor. It is sometimes tinged with blood due to the capillary beds at the edge of the cervix leaking as things soften. As a doula, this was always what I wanted my clients to call me about. If they were lucky enough to see it, they usually had between 2-7 days before they would need me to join them.

Signs of labor

Labor does not necessarily begin with a single moment. While Hollywood and television may give the impression that every labor begins with strong contractions and the water breaking, the truth is that most initial labor contractions are fairly mild and erratic. Only about 10% of labors actually begin with the amniotic membranes releasing before or during the early contractions. I have had five students seem to go into labor during my class. Two had their water break; two recognized they were having regular contractions; and one announced that she was in labor during the initial check-in. "It's my third, and I just couldn't be around the other two right now," she said. "I figured this was a safe place for me to breathe and relax." I believe we did a lot of squatting and other pelvic opening movements in the class, and she had the baby later that evening.

So, what are signs that labor has begun?

Hunger

Hunger is often a sign that will only be recognized in hindsight. Looking back after the labor, mom realizes she had an enormous appetite shortly before contractions became noticeable and more frequent. While it would be nice to think we could track labor's onset from your desire for a sandwich, the best outcome is in fact to miss the actual start of labor in order to remain relaxed and calm as the body begins to work internally. Nevertheless, consider this your reminder to eat and drink anything your body demands before and during the labor process.

Soft poops

We have lots of food going in, so we're going to have something come out eventually. As the uterus begins contracting more regularly, the rhythmic pulses massage against the rectum in the back of the pelvis, softening and eventually removing any matter which might lie in the baby's way. As a doula, I would often ask my clients who called in early labor how many times they had gone to the bathroom in the past few hours. Birth workers often say that they like to have things coming out of mom; doesn't matter what exactly.

Nesting urge

Like increased appetite, it can be difficult to pinpoint the urge to "nest" until after the baby has been born. Looking back, I had many clients recall an overwhelming urge to wash all the baby clothes the day before they went into labor, as if they knew they wouldn't be able to finish the task a few days later. It would be nice if we could use this drive to plan and initiate labor, but we're too complex for that. The upside is that if you feel like nesting, it usually involves some good simple movement, like bending and squatting, which helps keep the body supple and ready for labor.

Cramps/backache

Menstrual cramps are in fact uterine contractions, so the start of labor contractions can feel very similar. I have often observed yoga students saying a few days prior to going into labor that it felt as though they were about to get their period. Or, because the uterine ligaments attach to the back of the pelvis, they describe a tugging or pressure in their back. I remember one student commenting during a class check-in that she had been having a backache off and on throughout the day. When I asked her for more information, she explained that she was feeling some tightness and pressure roughly every 10 minutes for about a minute or more, and then it would disappear…I didn't say anything to alert her to the fact that she could be in labor (she was 39 weeks along) but spent most of the class doing movements to promote an optimal baby position and help her tune into her body. By the end of the class she reported that she realized the pressure was actually sweeping through her abdomen as well, and was it possible this was labor? (She had the baby early the next morning.)

An overview of the labor process

Although we have signals that labor is about to begin, why and when labor actually starts is still something of a mystery. There is some evidence that one of the hormones released by the baby may trigger a cascade of hormones in mom's body, culminating in the production of oxytocin (to create uterine contractions) and endorphins (the body's natural painkillers). Then there are prostaglandins, which soften and prepare the cervix to be ready to open. What we do know is that the labor process is generally divided into three stages:

Stage 1: Effacement and dilation 0-10 cm

In case you don't know the physiology, it's probably helpful to have a quick explanation of the labor process here. During the initial stage of labor, oxytocin causes the vertical muscle fibers in the uterus begin to draw upwards, gently pulling on an inner layer of circular muscle fibers. The pressure of these outer fibers pulling upward on the inner ones causes the inner fibers to release and open. At the same time, this movement gently nudges the baby's head downward into the opening cervix, flexing and rotating down through the pelvis, similar to the action of pulling a head through a turtleneck sweater, only upside down. The cervix gradually slides back into the wall of the uterus, first becoming thinner (called effacement) and then opening to a circle (called dilation), until that circle disappears behind the baby's head and the first stage of labor is complete. This is what care providers refer to as 10 cm dilated.[56]

Stage 2 : Descent, crowning, and birth

The second stage of labor technically begins when mom feels the urge to bear down with each contraction, although this stage is really a continuation of the action from the first stage. Once the cervix has opened around the full circumference of the baby's head and disappeared up into the wall of the uterus, then there is nothing to stop the baby from spiraling the rest of the way through the pelvis into the vagina and being born. The bones have plenty of space as long as mom can move and adjust as the baby spirals through. The outer uterine fibers continue to draw upwards in a wave-like pattern, but with no cervix to slow the process, the waves now move the baby down into the pelvis. This motion triggers the body's built-in expulsive reflex. That urge to poop? Same reflex!

Baby's head moves down through the open cervix while the muscles of the pelvic floor encircling the vagina pulse with the contracting uterus. Mom bears down in time with her body to help the birth process, and the baby spirals down through the pelvis. As the head moves lower, the urge to push becomes unstoppable. The head presses into the final layer of the pelvic floor, thinning and then releasing the perineum and vaginal outlet until the baby emerges into the world.

Stage 3: Bonding and the placenta

Finally, when the baby is in mom's arms, the middle, diagonal, looping uterine layer comes into play. These muscle fibers contract and tourniquet the blood vessels which feed the placenta. As these blood vessels seal off, the placenta detaches from the inner wall of the uterus. With a few more wave-like contractions and possibly some gentle pushing from mom, the placenta slides out of the body. During this time, the baby is orienting to the outside world, gradually crawling up mom's body and ultimately latching onto her breast.

First Stage of Labor

Specific signs that labor is beginning

The first stage of labor, the thinning and opening of the cervix, is primarily what we associate with the term "labor." This stage usually takes the longest time during the birth process. While we may not know the exact reason labor begins, as the process unfolds, several signs culminate to indicate that labor has, in fact, truly begun. These signals are:

---

[56] This is not to say that every woman opens to the round number of a 10 cm diameter circle, simply that the cervix can no longer be felt around the baby's head.

Progressive contractions

Contractions may start off mild and erratic, but as labor continues, the muscles begin to contract in a somewhat predictable pattern—and contractions increase in intensity and frequency. Contractions are always measured from the start of one to the start of the next, noting how long the contraction itself lasted and how strong the work felt during that time.

Early labor contractions can range from 5-20 minutes, and the length of the contraction itself can vary from 15 seconds to two minutes. As labor turns more active and settles into a pattern, the uterus often begins to contract approximately every 4-5 minutes for about one minute in duration. In other words, there is a one minute period of tension followed by 3-4 minutes of relaxation and feeling "normal" before another pressure wave begins. As labor continues, these intervals become shorter; just before pushing, there might only be 1-2 minutes between contractions, with each contraction lasting from 60-90 seconds. As with all things biological, there is some variation from person to person. I remember watching a video of a birthing woman whose contractions never got closer than seven minutes apart. Baby still came out just fine.

Bloody mucus

Again, we like things coming out of mom! The mucus that sealed the cervix closed through-out pregnancy continues to drop out as the cervix opens. The blood that may accompany the mucus is not a sign of injury but rather an indication that the blood vessels at the edge of the thinning cervix are stretching and leaking. The tissue is so soft during the labor process that just the pressure on the outer wall can lead to some blood being squeezed out. It is not painful or cause for concern. In fact, as a doula working with clients for home births (and thus not doing internal exams—that's the midwife's job), blood-tinged mucus was one of the best signs I would have to indicate that the cervix was changing.

Release of membranes/water breaking

While water breaking is rarely the starting signal for labor, it is common that as the cervix thins and opens and the baby moves downward, the combined pressure will overwhelm the amniotic tissues. The result is somewhere between a trickle and a gush of amniotic fluid. Many moms describe this sensation less like a faucet being turned on and more like a "pop" feeling inside, which comes with either a feeling of having peed their pants or a small rush of fluid. Often, this fluid is quickly stopped by the baby's head coming down more fully into the pelvis and pressing on the cervix. The release of membranes is one of the clearly identifiable signs that labor has started, or at least that the baby will likely be born in the next day or so. If labor does not start within that time frame, most women are advised to check in with a care provider.

Cervical changes

The two surefire signals that labor is in progress are a change in the effacement or dilation of the cervix and a change in the baby's station—the position of their head relative to the middle of the pelvic bowl. While mom is certainly able to check her own cervix (Hey, it's your body; you can do whatever you want! Though if your membranes have released, it's not recommended), most of us are not able to accurately self-assess what's happening internally, especially while coping with increasingly intense contractions. Usually a care provider will feel for these signals, either after mom has transferred to the hospital or after the midwives arrive at home for a home birth.

That said, there are ways to intuit whether the baby is descending through the pelvis based on the feeling during contractions. Sensations mostly in the lower abdomen and top of the pelvis? Baby is probably still high. Sensations more deeply internal—maybe slightly verging on pushing but not there yet? Baby might be down in the middle of the pelvis. Feeling that the body is instinctively and uncontrollably bearing down without your prompting? Baby is probably low.

Early labor

The first stage of labor is usually subdivided into three additional stages: early labor, active labor, and transition. Each stage has its own characteristics. Mom is generally considered to be in early labor when her cervix is dilated between 0-6 cm. Early labor usually takes the longest but is also often the mildest stage.

Contractions can range in frequency, length, and intensity, and it is often hard to predict when they are coming. Because they are fairly mild, most birth workers encourage moms to use this time to rest and find ways to distract themselves. If you spend too much energy when the surges aren't as strong, you're more likely to be exhausted when things get more intense. Ever tried meditating when you haven't slept well? It takes more effort and there's more resistance. Why create that situation for yourself during labor? The name of the game in early labor is distraction. Find something else to do until you can't do anything else; then call on your physical and mental stamina. Your body will absolutely let you know when it needs your attention.

Active labor

As the name suggests, active labor is when both mom and the contractions become more active. Active labor used to be designated by cervical dilation of 4-8 cm. Today, active labor is considered to start around 6 cm dilated, with the 4-6 cm range considered a "bridging" segment of early labor when the body is more fully establishing the labor process. Contractions often settle into a more predictable pattern, often lasting for about one minute and beginning every 4-5 minutes.

The cervix begins to open more rapidly, and coping mechanisms will probably involve more movement, positioning, vocalization, and deliberate breathing. This is when yoga positions might become helpful. Not because you need to do a Downward Dog (no one would voluntarily do that posture when birthing), but because shifting, swaying, and moving help change the internal dimensions of the bony pelvis and surrounding fascia, which helps create space for the baby to move down and open the cervix. This is also when opening the throat can be helpful for opening the pelvic floor. There is a neuromuscular connection between the vocal cords and soft palette and the vagina and pelvic floor. As renowned midwife Ina May Gaskin has often said, "loose mouth, loose bottom."[57]

Transition

The final phase of the first stage of labor is called transition. As the name indicates, this is when the body transitions from opening the cervix to actually moving the baby down and out of the uterus and into the pelvis. Transition is generally considered to occur when the cervix is opened between 8-10 cm.

Transition is usually the most intense phase of the first stage of labor. It is also usually the shortest, generally lasting 30-120 minutes. Hallmarks of transition can include shaking, nausea/vomiting (again, things coming out is good), strong and fast contractions, a lack of modesty, and a desire to escape or take drugs. If we were to pinpoint the stage of labor usually represented in film and TV, this would be it.

During transition contractions can sometimes stretch to 90 seconds long and come 2-3 minutes apart. That means mom may get only 30 seconds of rest before the next contraction begins. During this time, the ability to drop into deep relaxation and quickly focus becomes vital. Staying as fully in the present moment as possible can make a dramatic difference in your ability to cope. I've had several doula clients share that they felt like their body was beginning to push during transition, but they still had to release around that sensation rather than bear down with it.

While it is helpful to divide the first stage of labor into different segments, there isn't a big flashing light marking the shift from one to another. Labor is a progression, where some things are increasing while others are decreasing. In a progressing labor, we generally see the following.

Increasing	Decreasing
• Cramping (period-like) • Trips to the bathroom • Soft poops • Blood tinged mucus • Contractions increase in intensity, frequency, duration, and pressure • Need for relaxation • Inward focus • Vocalization **In Transition** • Agitation, chills/sweating, nausea, need to move	• Smiling • Sense of humor • Interest in talking or interacting • Talking through contractions • Comfort in a single position • Modesty • Being outwardly focused

---

[57] Gaskin, I. M., & Gaskin, I. M. (2003). Sphincter Law. In *Ina May's Guide to Childbirth* (pp. 167–182), Bantam Books.

As contractions gradually become more intense, moms will often be drawn deeper and deeper into themselves. I used to recognize this as a doula, especially when I was talking with clients by phone early in labor. If mom suddenly stopped talking during her contractions, and especially if I could hear her shift into a deeper and more controlled breathing pattern, I knew the sensation was becoming strong enough that it required significant focus—and that she would need me to join her shortly. Actually, the most typical progression would be that I would chat with mom by phone for an update, and we would agree to check in again in around three hours. Then one hour later I would get a call from her partner or support family member asking me to come and join because mom had stopped talking and was deeply in labor.

Second stage of labor

Once the cervix has fully slid open, the outer muscle fibers continue to draw upwards. But with nothing below the head, the baby now begins to slide through the opening of the cervix and into the curves of the birth path. This downward movement brings the head into contact with a bundle of nerves at the back of the pelvis which trigger the body's natural expulsive reflex.

For some moms, pushing is a relief because they can now be active in the process instead of having to simply breathe and release out of the way. That said, there is a misconception that pushing must be done in a highly active and forceful manner. While tactics like athletic position changes and holding the breath may speed up the baby's descent, they nearly always lead to more damage to the pelvic floor. In some cases, these tactics can compromise the available oxygen to mom and possibly baby.

At the end of the day, what moves the baby down through the cervix and through the pelvis is the same wave-like action of the uterine fibers that opened the cervix in the first place. Without the cervix below the head, it is the body, not an external action, which moves the baby down into the tissues of the lower pelvis. The baby takes a set of turns called the cardinal movements[58] to navigate the twists and turns of the birth path, thin and stretch the perineum, and emerge into the world. The idea that this process would require mom to violently strain into her bottom while holding her breath is somewhat laughable. The body got the baby this far; why would it not have a built-in process for getting them out? The reflex which brings the baby out is often referred to as the natural expulsive reflex, and we encounter it nearly every day when we go to move our bowels on the toilet. How hard do you have to strain in order to poop? Do any of us push so hard we burst blood vessels in our eyes? (BTW if you are, please stop! This is not the way the body was designed!)

If you're tempted to point out that poop is malleable while a baby's head is not, let me share that the baby's head is not in fact a single plate like an adult's head. Rather, it's a set of

---

[58] The cardinal movements are usually listed as: Engagement, Descent, Internal Rotation, Extension, External rotation, and expulsion, *www.medscape.com/answers/260036-172113/how-are-the-cardinal-movements-of-labor-characterized*

movable and moldable plates which are actually meant to slide over one another. Medical providers are well aware of the molding commonly found with newborn babies. The "caput" or "cone-head" shape usually subsides within the first 24 hrs after birth as the plates shift back into place. So again, there really isn't the need for forced straining to give birth.

Forget the dramatic pushing we often see in movies and TV shows. The body's true physiological response is far more internal—if mom is allowed to listen to her body's inner signals. I often marvel how, having allowed the body to open fully on its own, well-meaning medical professionals will suddenly become actively involved in directing pushing. Many of my doula clients describe the sensations of pushing as something their body initiated rather than something they started externally. "It was as though my body started to push," one mom said, "and I just had to go along for the ride."

If I were to describe how to follow the natural pushing reflex, it might sound like describing a bowel movement, in very soft, flowery language. For example:

Bring your body upright and draw a quick breath upwards into the chest, feeling the opening and expansion of the pelvic floor. Then, maintaining the pelvic relaxation, gradually begin to nudge that breath downwards, as though you could send it down the front side of your spine, around the curve of the sacrum, and then forward and out through the vagina (or anus if actually describing pooping). Don't hold your breath for more than a moment or two. Instead, use the downward pressure of the breath to release the muscles of the vagina and anus, allowing them to open like a beautifully expanding flower....

Another way to connect with this movement is to take a moment while sitting on the toilet. Imagine the pathway and angle the baby will take through your body, then follow the urge to move your bowels, breathing as your body naturally directs you to do. The actions are so similar that not only are people better in tune with things during the birth process, but many moms report they are also able to finish a trip to the bathroom much faster. Win-win for everyone!

Pushing positions

There are, however, some specific movements for pushing that are helpful to understand. In the natural birth community, it's generally understood that the classic position seen on TV (mom lying back, pulling her knees wide and tucking her tail) is not the most physiologically effective position for getting a baby to move through the pelvis. It isn't just the baby's head that molds during the birth process; the pelvic joints are able to adjust as well, stretching wider to make room for baby to move. Remember the hormone relaxin? All the way at the end of the pregnancy, it comes back into play! Depending on how you position the body and the legs, the pelvis can have more or less room at different levels. Want to make space at the top? Widen the legs and tuck the tail. (Hmm, isn't this what TV shows for opening the base...?) Need space at the bottom? Internally rotate the legs and arch the coccyx out.

Try this for yourself to better understand how different positions can change the internal dimensions of the pelvic structure.

Stand with the feet 2-3 feet apart and lean forward towards a table or the wall, hinging from the hips. Feel the impact on the space between the sitz bones. Now repeat this movement with the toes turned out and the heels drawn inwards. Do the sitz bones feel closer or further apart? Try it while actively tucking the tail and turning the feet out.

Now compare the external rotation movement to its opposite. Turn the toes in and the heels out, and arch the tail upwards while leaning forward. Assuming you are not burdened by excessively tight hamstrings, you will probably feel more space between the sitz bones with the internal rotation and anterior pelvic tilt than with external rotation and posterior tilting. Internal rotation of the thigh bone quite simply widens the distance between the ischial tuberosities (sitz bones).

Now take this knowledge and apply it to that mythical natural childbirth position, the squat. Sit into Malasana, bringing the knees wide, the heels in, and the tail under (note this is often how students with large bellies or tense lower backs and calves will slip into Malasana). Feel the space between the sitz bones. Now try bringing the feet parallel, even turning the thighs inwards while sticking the bum out. Yes, this will probably make the pose more challenging, but do you feel how it also widens the space around the tail and anus?

If you need a way to make the squat more accessible, there are three possible options:

- Allow the heels to lift and place a blanket under the heels for support.
- Place a block or other support (like a birthing stool) under mom's sitz bones.
- Add a partner or other solid support mom can hold on to, to offset the backwards weight shift needed to keep the sitz bones open.

As I often coyly ask students in classes, "Could you poop in this position?"

This action of making space in the back of the pelvis corresponds to the baby's path as they turn through the mid-pelvis and move into the pelvic outlet. If you want to move the baby out, you need to make space where they are.

The point? It is something of a testament to how well the birth process works that so many babies have been born using a position which closes the very bones they are moving through! The position often seen on TV (and which is still taught in many medical schools), with mom lying back and bringing the knees apart, in fact makes the pelvic outlet as small as possible. Additionally, lying back on the tailbone and sacrum locks these bones in position, so they cannot shift back to make more space for a baby moving through. While we don't need gymnastic positions like active squats or strained breathing, it could be helpful to move the pelvis to open the level where the baby sits. At the beginning of pushing, this might involve lying back (which opens the top of the pelvis, where baby may sit), but later on it might be helpful to shift to side lying or hands and knees, with the knees turned inward and the bum out to open the lower pelvic levels.

The baby does not typically slide straight through the pelvis in a single breath. The process of the second stage of labor is a rocking motion: simultaneously the baby's head molds a bit and moves down a bit; the pelvis spreads, and the pelvic floor releases. The rocking continues until all the dimensions of the head, pelvis, and pelvic tissues match up to one another, then the head slides through the pelvic outlet, thinning the perineum and opening the vaginal outlet. At this point, most medical professionals encourage mom to stop pushing (again, the body already knows what it's doing here), letting the outer skin have time to stretch and open as baby slides out.

Third stage of labor

The moment of birth comes with an enormous sigh of relief. The pressure of crowning gently builds until finally everything opens and molds the needed amount. Mom almost always lets out a giant exhale and might collapse back on the bed. Baby takes their first breath (and screams to be picked up). If there are no complications, baby is placed in direct skin to skin contact with mom. This contact begins the third stage of labor.

The third stage of labor is often focused on the birth of the placenta. I feel this stage is better characterized by the bonding and connection happening between the baby and their parents. Studies have shown that in their first hour of life, human babies go through distinct steps to orient themselves to their new surroundings; from what I have seen, so do the parents! Babies begin with a cry but often quickly quiet down when in contact with their parents. Gradually, they open their eyes, turn towards the sound of their parent's voices, and eventually even crawl up their mother's chest and latch onto her breast. All by themselves!

During this process, which might take 30-60 minutes, mom's body finally releases the placenta. It seems reasonable that the body wouldn't let go of the placenta until there was a physical indication that the baby no longer needed it. I have actually seen births where mom had to wait for skin to skin contact, and it was not until she could physically feel and hear the baby that the placenta released. With the physical birth process complete, the focus turns to meeting the baby in the moment they are in and getting to know who this new person actually is.

Navigating the sensations of labor

Everything I've just outlined describes the physiological and biological processes the body goes through during birth. This is what medical science is focused on, but these descriptions fail to answer an important question. What do contractions feel like? In my experience, this is the question most birthing parents would like to answer. And it is where yoga practice can have the largest impact.

Of course, the answer isn't easy to come by. Our perception of sensation varies from person to person. As a doula, I could look at a client and say she was moving well, making good sounds, and seemingly managing her labor, but there was no way I could know how she was experiencing the sensations from within her body.

Likewise, saying that someone's cervix is 7 cm open doesn't give any information about what their contractions might feel like during that time. Or what the rest between them might be like. We may say that contractions are getting stronger, but how does that translate to the felt sense within the body? The sensations of labor, and the ability to cope with them, are often a combination of several factors: the position of the baby, mom's mental state before and during labor, and the overall muscle and fascial balance within her body.

Fetal positioning

Not all starting labor positions are equal. A baby who begins labor with their nose facing towards their mother's back is more likely to descend into the pelvis smoothly than a baby who begins labor facing towards their mother's front. This is because facing back better promotes the chin flexing into the chest, which makes the baby's posterior cranium the presenting part of the head (the part moving through the pelvis.) Because of the structure of the fetal skull plates, this area is able to mold and shrink, offering a smaller circle than if the baby's chin were extended.

Said another way, when the head is lifted, the diameter of the head is larger than when the head is tucked. This means there is more pressure on the internal bones and tissue of the pelvis as the baby moves down through the cervix. Position a baby so their spine curves towards their mother's abdomen, and the chin tucks more easily, and the baby seems smaller as it is rotating through the birth path.

That path involves several twists and turns, called cardinal movements. The cardinal movements are engagement, descent, flexion, rotation, extension, restitution, and expulsion. These movements can begin before labor does, with the dropping or engagement of baby's head into the pelvic inlet. The head usually engages looking to the right or the left, as the top of the pelvic bowl is wider side than front to back. Once engaged, the baby descends further into the pelvis; ideally, this descent causes their head to flex into their chest. This flexion is easier if baby's spine is already curved; thus the preference for the spine being towards the front of mom's body, where the belly allows it to curve outward.

As they descend into the pelvis, baby comes into contact with the pelvic floor. Recall from Chapter 3 that the levator ani muscle opens front to back in the middle of the pelvis. This change in the orientation of available space—side to side now becomes front to back—leads to a rotation to align the baby's head front to back, ideally looking at mom's spine. In this position, the baby descends through the pelvic floor headfirst and begins to emerge out of the cervix.

If the head rotates to face the sacrum, there is less pressure on the internal pelvic bones, and the uterine muscles can work directly on opening the cervix. Mom feels strong muscular work but not necessarily pain. But if the head rotates to face forward, it is harder for the chin to remain tucked, and the wider circle of the head begins to press more firmly on the internal bony pelvic structures.

What does this feel like? Try pressing something hard against your shin bone. There is a sensation which might be described as grinding or pinching, which is very different from that of a muscle working. A mom coping with a baby in this position will have to navigate not only the strong crampy pressure of the uterine muscles but also the grinding sensation of bone on bone as the baby spins and descends.

Many of these labors are characterized by pain which does not dissipate between the contractions or which is localized in one specific area—often the front or back, depending on
where the bones are being compressed. Bone is living tissue, with nerves and blood flow just
like the skin, and it does not always like being squeezed. This is a time when movement or
position changes might be useful to open the internal dimensions of the pelvis and reduce the
pressure. If mom is able to work through the myriad sensations, then the body may be able to
open enough to allow baby to finish rotating to face mom's back.

As the head finishes descending, we come to the last three cardinal movements. Having
moved through the cervix, the back of the baby's head comes into gentle contact with the
inner edge of the pubic bone. This contact triggers a built in reflex which leads the baby to
extend their neck, gradually pulling their body under the pubic bone and over the perineum.
This action, in concert with the downward pressure from the uterine muscles, promotes
crowning and birth. Once the head emerges, there is a pause while the baby's shoulders rotate
to align with the pelvic floor. Once this final rotation, called restitution, is finished, the body
slides through (expulsion), and the baby is born.

Baby positions in the pelvis are usually referenced by
where the back of their head (the occiput)
sits relative to mom's body. OA, or occiput
anterior, means that the back of the head
is pointed towards the front side of mom's
body. OP, or occiput posterior refers to a
baby whose back of head is facing its mother's back. The head can further be directly
aligned with mom's spine or, more commonly, rotated slightly to the right or left
because of the shape of the pelvic inlet.
This means that the ideal position for
baby to begin labor is referred to as LOA:
left occiput anterior. In contrast, a less
optimal position, in which the baby would have
to rotate further and may run into some tight spots,
would be ROP: right occiput posterior.

Fetal Positions

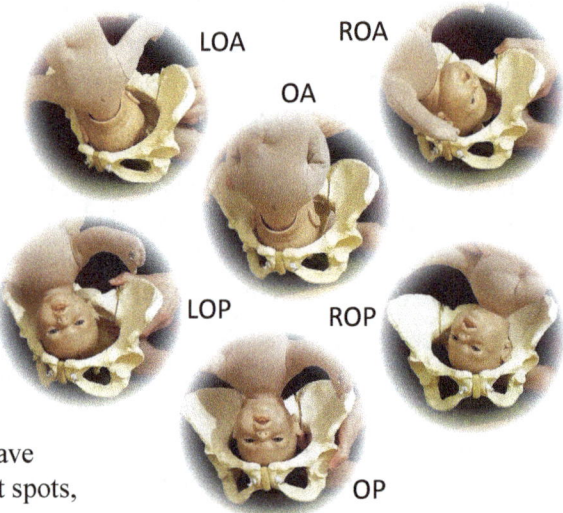

Many challenging labors involve a baby who has rotated "OP" or any orientation where the
back of the head is closer to mom's spine than her front. This is commonly called "back
labor" because the pain is often felt more keenly in the back. This name can be misleading,
however, since an OP baby can also press firmly on the inside of mom's pubic bone, which
would lead to consistent, unrelenting discomfort on the front of her body instead.

The OP position tends to create more pressure because the head is brought out of the tucked
position by the straightening of the baby's spine. It is much easier to curve the spine into flexion
when it is hanging into the curve of mom's belly (as it would be if baby was facing OA,) but in
an OP position the spine rests against mom's spine, which leads it to be more erect than flexed.

Try sitting up straight and bringing your chin to your chest. Now try the same movement with the upper back rounded in a slouch. The second version is far easier than the first. And a baby with a tucked chin is literally smaller inside the pelvis than the same baby with an extended head.

How can you tell which way a baby is facing? For centuries, midwives have used a series of hand movements which, when properly done, can show how a baby's body is oriented. And, because the baby's skull plates are not fused, the two soft spots on the head can be felt during an internal exam if the cervix is open enough.

However, you won't be employing either technique to assess your baby's position. Instead, moms can pay attention to where they feel the different movements in their bellies and what the characteristics of those movements might be. If you feel lots of kicks and wiggles on the front, it's probable (not guaranteed) that the baby's limbs are facing the front. Most babies do not hang out with their arms behind their backs. Something larger and more firm, however, could be the baby's backside. It's possible to track a baby's position by charting when and where you feel different sensations during the third trimester. You can then use that information to choose movement that encourages optimal positioning.

The body and mind during labor

Baby's position is one element that affects mom's ability to navigate labor sensations. Another important element is the nervous system, which can impact blood flow, muscle tension, and overall functioning of the body. As yogis, we quickly become aware that we are not a separate mind and body, but are rather a "mindbody." Just as the different energetic *koshas* of our being interplay with one another, the mind and body are constantly interacting as well. These interactions have a dramatic impact on the course of labor. Anxiety, fear, and negative expectations can lead to a self-fulfilling prophecy of pain and discomfort during labor in what's known as the Fear-Tension-Pain (FTP) cycle.

Labor is affected by the autonomic nervous system (ANS). This primal control system for the body is divided into the sympathetic and parasympathetic nervous systems. The parasympathetic nervous system is responsible for down-regulating the body's stress response and is meant to be functioning most of the time. We activate the parasympathetic nervous system by taking a restorative yoga class, soaking in a warm bath, or simply feeling safe and protected. Activation of this "relaxation response" speeds healing, lowers blood pressure, and promotes better overall body function.[59]

On the flip side, we have the sympathetic nervous system. The sympathetic system controls our "fight or flight" response. It's easier to identify when the sympathetic nervous system is triggered because it creates sudden, visceral bodily changes. Cortisol and adrenaline flood into the bloodstream, blood pressure rises, muscle tension increases, and blood is diverted

---

[59] Stahl, J. E., Dossett, M. L., LaJoie, A. S., Denninger, J. W., Mehta, D. H., Goldman, R., Fricchione, G. L., & Benson, H. (2015, March 13). *Relaxation response and resiliency training and its effect on Healthcare Resource Utilization.* PLOS ONE. https://journals.plos.org/plosone/article?id=10.1371%2Fjournal.pone.0140212

into the defense systems. The body readies itself to fight or flee—or freeze. "Freezing" is less commonly associated with the sympathetic nervous system, but this response is well known in trauma-informed and other therapeutic settings. The sensation is like hitting the accelerator and the brake on a car at the same time. Internal tension is running rampant, but it's impossible to move or speak. It is the "deer in the headlights" or the "play dead" option.

If the sympathetic nervous system activates during labor, it affects both the sensations of labor and mom's ability to cope with them. In a fight, flight, or freeze scenario, the uterus becomes oxygen-deprived because it is not part of the body's defense system. Muscle fibers that don't receive adequate oxygen eventually will not fire as strongly as they could. An increase in muscle tension causes the circular muscle fibers of the cervix to constrict while the outer muscle fibers simultaneously try to pull upwards to open. These two groups begin to oppose one another, firing together when they were designed to work synergistically.

What do you get when you combine oxygen-deprivation with two muscle groups fighting against one another? A baby's head that is strongly forced down by the outer uterine muscle fibers into a cervix that is resisting opening as hard as it possibly can. In other words, a perfect recipe for pain! The sensation is what a marathon runner (or even a 5K runner) might feel when they run out of glycogen and their legs begin to cramp and ache.

This type of pain would normally be the body's method for alerting you that something is wrong, so it's understandable that the emotional response to a sensation of cramping and tension would be more anxiety, which further activates the fight/flight/freeze response. Now add in the assumption many women have that labor is painful and has to be endured. Mom can easily end up in a situation where rather than examining or exploring the sensations she feels, she freezes, afraid that moving might make the pain and discomfort worse.

Generally, when we are afraid of something, we have an aversion to getting closer to it. This is true of animals, and it's true of human beings. This response has utility in a life-threatening situation. Suppose a bear walked into your birthing room (ignore the question of how the bear got up the elevator at the hospital). In this situation, your labor should completely stop so that you can either fight, flee, or, most likely, stand completely still until the bear goes away. Our minds don't easily distinguish between real bears and the perceived threats we might encounter. So we freeze and grit our teeth rather than moving. Ironically, movement could help indicate to our bodies that we are once again safe, and movement could also help reduce pain by shifting baby into a better birth position.

I've alluded to the Fear-Tension-Pain cycle already, but let's take a closer look:

- Fear leads to tension,
- Tension leads to excessive pain,
- Excessive pain (understandably) leads to more fear, which can then start a whole downward spiral.

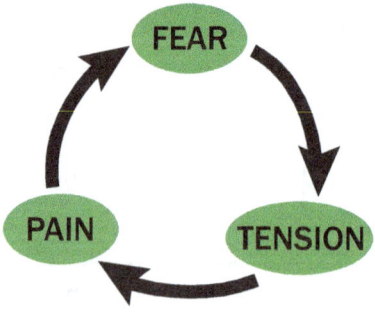

The result? A cervix that refuses to open, a mom who can't see how to work with her baby, and a labor that stalls out rather than continuing.

This, incidentally, is where the yoga practice comes into direct contact with the birth process. Yoga is the practice of stilling the fluctuations of the mind so that we can see clearly where we are. Through practice, we gain an ability to look past our initial fears and a willingness to explore sensation.

The way we talk about labor significantly impacts our expectations. Generally, labor and childbirth are described in vague terms. "The pain gets stronger." "Your body begins working harder." But none of these descriptions mention *where* the sensation might be. We can guess the abdomen—but no one seems to say that the sensation of a contraction is usually felt in the front of the abdomen, sweeping around and upwards through the belly—or that this sensation will change as the baby moves downward in the pelvis. It's all lumped into one bland category labeled "pain."

Imagine for a moment that as a new yoga student, the only thing you heard about Warrior 2 was that it was a strong pose for the legs. Now imagine doing Warrior 2 and having a strong sensation in your knee and your groin. If you took the time to examine your alignment, you might find that your knee was rolling inward, leading to pressure on the kneecap and interior groin, and that you could adjust to relieve the unintended pressure. But if you instead thought you were supposed to breathe and bear it, would you actually consider changing the shape? As a yoga teacher, I have helped many students discover that their knee and hip alignment wasn't optimal for their body and in so doing helped them realize there was a better way to practice the pose they were in that they had not considered previously. Some students have even come to love a pose they had previously loathed.

The same principle can be applied to labor. If we just accept that pain is inevitable, and don't consider that there are different types of sensations, then when confronted with unfamiliar and frightening sensations, we tense rather than release. The instinct is often to not explore the sensations further. This then leads to an increase in sensation from the fear itself, or a belief that we can't do anything about the sensation, as well as an increase due to a lack of movement. We fulfill the prophecy of a negative experience, then take it as confirmation that said experience was destined all along. In reality, we may have been getting in our own way.

I am not suggesting that we do not feel things during labor. Some of those sensations can be extremely uncomfortable, and you might even decide that medication to dull or decrease sensation is the right choice for you. This is a completely valid decision. But if we can't even look at our fears around the labor process and be open to the idea that our ability to be present and release has an impact on our experience, then we will most likely feel more discomfort.

Thoughts produce physical responses. Images, stories, comments, experiences, and beliefs produce thoughts. We each come into pregnancy with some idea of what we expect to encounter during the labor process. Faced with a seemingly inescapable situation, we become like a deer in the headlights and hope the "bear" will simply pass us by. And if you are "frozen" in your labor, there's an increased chance that more involved interventions might be needed. Prolonged delays in the labor process can lead to challenges for baby and possibly for mom. In some cases, an initial intervention can lead to the need for further interventions. While there is a time and place for riskier interventions such as assisted vaginal or cesarean births, most of us would prefer to avoid those options if possible.

Before your sympathetic nervous system gets too triggered reading this book, remember that there's another option. So far we have described what happens if we activate the fight, flight, or freeze response. What if we promote the parasympathetic side (rest and digest) instead? Rather than producing stress hormones such as cortisol and adrenaline, the body would produce hormones such as endorphins and oxytocin. Fabulous oxytocin! This hormone causes specific fibers of the uterine muscles to contract properly during labor. It has also been shown to be responsible for bonding and is produced in large amounts during orgasm. When the parasympathetic nervous system stays activated during labor, not only do large amounts of helpful hormones get released but the simultaneous tension and redirection of blood to defense systems doesn't occur. The uterine muscle fibers continue to receive enough oxygen and are able to function well and work in collaborative groups. The cervix can relax and open. Labor continues, and the baby comes into mom's arms!

How do we activate this side of the nervous system? By practicing activation regularly—such as with restorative yoga practices and meditation— and by reducing the anxiety-provoking images and ideas we have about the birth process. We can examine our own thoughts and stop speaking about the birth process as either a catastrophe ("And then the baby's heart rate dropped!" or "I thought I was dying!") or as a comedy ("I told my partner: you did this to me!!!"). None of these images and anecdotes will help mom be present and empowered in her own personal birth story. The HypnoBirthing® Institute sells a button that sums it up: "Only positive birth stories please. My baby is listening!"

Note: I am in NO WAY saying that if your baby is born via surgery that you are to blame. Let's stop thinking that we are somehow the problem in this equation. If you give birth via surgery, you will have done everything you possibly could, but you may not have known what you didn't know. And maybe you consciously choose this way to birth! This is part of working with labor. We control what we can control for, but then we must let go of the rest and work with the process of our personal labor journey as it unfolds.

My own son was born via surgery after a long labor at home. It wasn't until 10 months later that I learned about a myofascial release technique which could have resolved his position and allowed him to birth as I had wanted. I don't know if it would have truly changed things, and I know that I did everything I could at the time. But more importantly, during the labor process I had been able to work with the people around me. I was listened to, respected, and found ways to keep my nervous system as calm as possible, so that I could still enjoy and be present to welcome my baby into the world as he needed to come.

Body tissues: suppleness vs tension

Along with the baby's position and the state of your nervous system, the general tone and balance within the connective tissues of the birthing body can impact labor. Labor is a physical process, and although imagery and positive stories can do a great deal, we cannot think our way into a positive, workable birth experience. We need practices and postures that promote the health and tone of muscles, connective tissues, and organs. Through appropriate yoga *asana*, *pranayama*, and visualizations, we can help the body and mind prepare to enter the birth experience with as much confidence, balance, and readiness as possible.

Birth is the most profound letting go one can ever do. During the birth process, mom fully releases the tissues of her cervix and pelvic floor to allow the baby to emerge into the world. She also lets go mentally of her expectations to instead embrace the moment that is. No one is claiming that birth isn't a physical experience or that doing the "correct" *asanas*, *pranayama*, or visualizations will guarantee a certain birth outcome. But getting in touch with the body and mind, and acknowledging what medical science has discovered about how the body functions, is never a bad thing. It is hard to feel confident releasing if we have no framework to understand what is going on within our bodies.

There is also so much more to the birth experience than what I've included in this book. We have not touched subjects like induction, pharmacological pain management, or surgical birth. I recommend reading a book focused on childbirth for a deeper dive into these topics.[60]

At the same time, having an academic knowledge of birth is not the same as experiencing it. I once heard midwife Fiona Hallinan suggest during a Spinning Babies® conference that it is not the uterus contracting that births the baby but the release and "sigh" of the cervix between contractions. "What if we have been trained to think of this in the wrong way?" she asked. "What if labor contractions can't do their work without the release in between?" How we think about the birth process influences where we focus as we prepare. If we shift our focus to exploring sensation and unpacking misconceptions we may be holding, we can free ourselves to more fully work with the circumstances and sensations that arise as we birth.

---

[60] Recommended reading: *Ina May's Guide to Childbirth* by Ina May Gaskin, *Birthing From Within* by Pam England, *Mindfulness Based Childbirth* by Nancy Bardacke, *Orgasmic Birth* by Debra Pascale-Bonaro

13 — Om Births' Four Cornerstones to Working with Labor

There is a secret in our culture. It's not that birth is painful.
It's that women are strong!

—Laura Stavoe Harm

Birth is a major event. Whether it occurs naturally, with intervention, surgical, induced, or spontaneous, the process by which a baby emerges into this world involves many twists and turns, and a fair amount of physical and mental stamina. Even a planned cesarean section (C-section) is still major abdominal surgery. For all mothers, but especially for those intending to avoid medical interventions, the task of "facing" or "getting through" the pain and challenge of labor can be daunting.

It can be easy to make labor an experience about survival or "just making it through." But if we want to make this experience more positive, maybe even something we can embrace, look forward to, and (dare I suggest it) enjoy, we have to reframe the common conception of the labor process—it's not something to be endured but something that can instead be managed.

For several generations now, society has told women that we don't know how to birth. In some cases, we have come to believe it. There are very few views in Western culture that focus on working with the sensations leading up to and into birth. We make birth plans, think through support teams, take yoga classes, and educate ourselves about childbirth options, but none of these activities can guarantee a specific outcome or birth experience. Ultimately, birth is a huge unknown, and while we can prepare plans and contingencies (indeed, it can be good to do so), the best preparation we can give ourselves is to consider how to work with whatever comes up in the moment. Reframing how you think about labor can significantly shift how you view the outcome of your birth experience. As is sometimes said in *shamata* meditation practice, "Everything is workable. . . if you keep working with it".

The four cornerstones I'm about to describe are adapted from a plan I encountered while training for an Ironman Triathlon. Faced with a daunting and quite frankly terrifying physical distance, I was heartened to find what a trainer called "the four keys to racing the long-distance race." Rather than training regiments, these were principles to apply both during preparation and on the day of the event. When I became pregnant, I realized much of my birth preparation was following the same format, which led me to develop the Four Cornerstones to Working with Labor.

I am not suggesting that you, or any pregnant woman, should have run or have the inclination to run something like an Ironman Triathlon. I simply found these points to be invaluable when thinking about my own labor, and I firmly believe that they are applicable to any mom preparing to give birth, even if she is not the least bit athletic.

Cornerstone #1: It's about mental attitude. It's not about pain!

Ask someone the first thought they associate with childbirth, and they usually say pain. This idea has been reinforced for years. Story after story mentions the pain, sometimes focusing on it almost exclusively. Certainly there can be pain during the labor process, but here's the key to this cornerstone: Your experience isn't about the pain. It's about your mental attitude towards it.

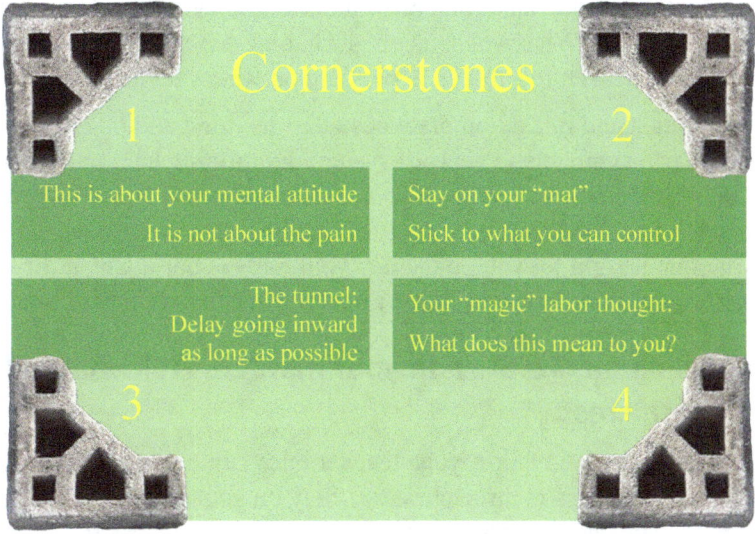

How we conceive of sensations dramatically changes how we experience them. Imagine going to the doctor for a shot. You could spend the hours leading up to the visit worrying about how big the needle will be, trying to remember the sensation of being pricked, even pinching yourself where the needle will go to anticipate feeling the stick. In fact, this was my strategy as a child facing vaccinations. But 99% of the time, the sensation of being stuck is not as bad as you expected. In fact, your fear of the sensation was worse than the actual experience.

Now apply this same thought process to the sensations of labor. For first-time moms, the added challenge is that you don't know exactly what labor will feel like, so you don't have a sensation to compare it to. Which seems more productive: spending months worrying about how to manage the supposedly excruciating sensations or dealing with the anxiety so you can simply experience what you are experiencing when the time comes?

You might be tempted to treat labor like a vaccine, and imagine that it's a great idea to "psych yourself out" so that your actual labor won't be as bad as you had expected. But working through and addressing your fear is less stressful for the duration of the pregnancy and helps make the sensations of labor more manageable.

Remember the impact of the nervous system in the Fear-Tension-Pain cycle? We want to remain in the parasympathetic nervous system as much as possible, so we avoid creating excessive tension which can impede the normal function of the uterine muscles. What triggers one side of the autonomic nervous system over the other is the thoughts and attitude towards the situation. How someone focuses on sensation has a dramatic impact on how the body then responds. This is why mental preparation is so key! I'm not going to be so extreme as to claim that labor doesn't hurt (though there are women who say it didn't). Mom will certainly feel something strong during the birth process, but how we frame our attitude towards this sensation can impact whether we activate fight or flight or rest and digest.

The process of birth is a huge physical endeavor, one which the body does not accomplish via brute force. No matter how strong the uterine muscles are, they must still work in tandem with one another, and the baby must still rotate through the pelvis. The process of working with these conditions requires mental focus. It is crucial to become familiar with your thoughts about the labor and birth process and everything that surrounds bringing a baby into the world. What we focus on is what increases. The same experience could be hell to one person or heaven to another, depending on where we allow, or even direct, our thoughts.

Meditation and relaxation practices offer the mind and body time to rest in the healing space of the parasympathetic nervous system. Examining habitual thoughts allows us to release doubts and fears that do not help us feel empowered and able to work with our situation. You have to find what works for you personally. There is not one right way to birth, except for the way that is right for you on the day your baby is born. But at the end of the day, getting to know your mind has a dramatic impact on the experience of birth.

Cornerstone #2: Stay on your mat. Control what you can control, and let go of the rest.

A good friend and fellow yoga teacher once summed up a great approach to mental attitude during yoga class in three phrases: "Stay on your mat! Don't get on someone else's mat! And don't let anyone else get on your mat."

1. **Stay on your mat:** Stick to what you can actually control, which is your own experience.
2. **Don't get on someone else's mat:** Don't try to copy someone else's practice. Don't try to copy someone else because they are thinner, faster, or more flexible. Don't try to copy someone else who seems better or more together in some way. That is *their* practice and their *dharma*. Never try to live someone else's story.
3. **Don't let anyone else get on your mat:** Don't let someone else tell you what your practice should look like, feel like, or be like. Even your teacher can't know how a posture feels within your body. Don't disregard your own internal intuition which says to stop, back up, or do something different. While you can choose to explore a challenge that a teacher may offer, don't place your trust in their judgments and feelings about your practice.

These principles can also be applied to the birth experience. In the process of working with labor, the second cornerstone is this idea of staying on your mat. There are things we can control during the process of labor, and there are things we cannot. Be mindful of what you can control and what you must let go. What is actually your own experience to have, and what are you grasping for or allowing in? Control what you can control, but let go of the rest.

So what are the things you can control? Well, for starters, your own reactions. That's decidedly challenging because it requires looking at your habitual patterns, then being willing to sit with uncomfortable situations long enough to start making different choices. A mindfulness practice is important here. This is meditation in action, where the practice of observing and seeing our thoughts more clearly gives way to a small gap, and the chance to choose a different action or to not react. As an often quoted Buddhist joke goes, "Don't just do something. Sit there!"

Your reactions are the most important part of what can be controlled during labor. When you are conscious of your own mind, you can decide not to be annoyed by that negative birth story you may be trying hard to avoid. You can see the thoughts that arise when you hear about other people's negative and possibly traumatic experiences. You can choose to entertain those thoughts or let them go and focus on being confident in the experience you are going to have. And you can clearly see if you are actually letting the thoughts go or if those stories are still affecting you. Just because we say we're fine doesn't mean we are.

However, we can do more than choose our responses to other people's comments and birth stories. If you are planning a natural, holistic birth experience, why hang around other moms who are telling stories that bring up anxious thoughts? You have choices: ask them not to share, or don't associate with them during your pregnancy. If you don't feel totally supported by the people around you, go find another group or establish clear boundaries around what you are willing to hear.

I'm not suggesting we avoid information or birth in ignorance. By all means, go and research the common practices where you are planning to give birth. Learn who you will be birthing with and what options are available to you. Solicit stories from people if you wish, but watch how their stories make you feel. You don't need every gory detail of someone's traumatic or sensational birth imprinted on your mind before your own experience. Your own birth may be completely different from theirs. And regardless, how does hearing their story help you in working with your own? It's not as though you can scare yourself into having a good birth experience. Remember the Fear-Tension-Pain cycle?

This curation also applies to books, blogs and any other information you encounter about the birth experience. Carefully consider your sources. Is the person writing or speaking with an ulterior motive in mind (like selling a book or having an exciting story)? Is their information based on evidence or anecdotes?

If you are taking a childbirth class (which I encourage!), be sure to evaluate carefully before selecting one. Not all classes are created equal, and it can be hard to tell which classes take a supportive stance on working with your labor and which simply encourage you to "be a good patient" and follow the instructions of your care providers.

Also be mindful about who you share your birth plans with. I have often heard moms in my prenatal classes confess that they had to stop telling their families about their plans for an unmedicated birth. They were constantly met with the response, "Oh, why would you want to go through all that!?" or some variation thereof. This is not a supportive response, and I applaud my students who felt empowered enough to create their own mental shields against those judgments. (My husband also confessed that when I was pregnant, he appreciated my position in the birth field. He didn't feel the need to defend our decisions to his non-birth-world colleagues. "She's been teaching this stuff for years," turned out to be a great push-back against incredulous colleagues. Then he'd stop telling them about our birth plans altogether.) All of this is to say: stay on your own mat! Notice when you can control things, and make the changes that create the most support for you and your preferences.

However, just as the perfectly conditioned marathon runner doesn't control the weather on the day of the race, there will be things during both pregnancy and labor you don't have control over:

- The *exact* position of your baby when your labor begins. You can influence it, but you can't control it fully.
- Exactly when your labor will begin and how it will start (inductions can take days and are not always successful)
- The judgments of other people with whom you share your birth preferences (doctors, family, friends, colleagues, and others)
- Comments that strangers may make about your body shape
- Whether your family is overly involved or not involved enough
- The length of your labor, possible special circumstances, or birth complications which could arise.
- Countless other circumstances specific to your individual life.

Given that you can't control those things, worrying about them is a waste of time and energy. You could be spending those resources getting to know your mind and feeling confident in yourself. Being willing to speak up about your needs during labor is absolutely key to being able to work with whatever comes up.

There is one area where you both do and don't have control during the birth process. You often cannot control the exact doctor or midwife who will attend to you during labor, unless you have chosen a solo practice OB or a homebirth midwife. That said, just as you choose which teacher's yoga class you go to, and which studio you practice in, you can exercise discernment around who you choose as your care provider, which childbirth classes you participate in, and which hospital or birth facility you wish to enter to give birth. Studies have shown that, if mom wishes to avoid a C-section, her first consideration might be the hospital where she plans to give birth.[61] As lead researcher and OB Neel Shah states, "the likelihood

[61] Shah, N. (2019, September 25). *The rise of C-sections – and what it means - US news & world report.* US News. https://www.usnews.com/news/healthiest-communities/articles/2019-09-25/the-rise-of-c-sections-and-what-it-means

of getting a cesarean is largely driven by the choice of hospital." Hiring additional support such as a doula could also be the difference between a birth experience that is traumatizing and one that feels workable.[62] Choose your birth team carefully, and be aware of which door you will walk through in order to give birth. Put your "mat" down in a place where it will be easiest and most supportive for you to "practice."

Cornerstone #3: Delay "the tunnel" as long as possible.

I know what your first thought was. "Tunnel? She must mean the birth canal." No, not that tunnel. I'm talking about the tunnel of focus that comes when we become fully absorbed in something. The place where we shut out everything else and are left only with our thoughts and feelings. The tunnel is the place where mom begins to fully engage with her labor.

People talk about the pain of labor, the intensity, the need to focus. But the truth is that the beginning segments of labor are often much easier than the movies and stories make them seem. During the early phases of labor, contractions are often irregular, mild, and sometimes only a few seconds long. The body is figuring out the whole process and finding out what rhythm works best based on the amount of oxytocin and movement available to the baby.

But there is a point when things usually become intense. Sometime during active labor or transition, most women instinctively close their eyes, turning inward and calling upon their own inner strength and resources. But here's the thing. The tunnel is usually pretty dark. It might also feel hot, cramped, or scary. But your baby is waiting at the other end, and every laboring mother, regardless of the interventions or supports she may have during labor, will have to pass through it. The tunnel can't be avoided. But you may have some measure of control over how long you spend in it. We all have our own tunnel "lengths," and while you can't know exactly how long the tunnel will be, you do have some impact on how long the tunnel feels. If you spend early labor breathing deeply, rocking and swaying, and visualizing the birth you want to have, you'll probably expend more energy than you need to during this time. The tunnel may begin sooner than it needs to, but the endpoint doesn't change. Result? You just made that tunnel longer than it needed to be. Oops! You will never know how long your time of intense focus during labor would have been, but if you waste energy at the start of labor, it makes the later stages harder and longer.

This is the part of working with your labor that is a little counterintuitive. You do all this work to get ready, to set your "mat" out in the right space, get the best team, clear negative thoughts, condition your body, and learn effective breathing. Then, when labor actually starts, you want to delay using all of it. That's because everything you do early in labor affects how things feel later on. The more fatigued you become, the more challenging it becomes to focus.

For early labor, the name of the game is DISTRACT! Find any way you can to occupy your

[62] Trueba, G., Contreras, C., Velazco, M. T., Lara, E. G., & Martínez, H. B. (2000). *Alternative strategy to decrease cesarean section: Support by doulas during labor.* The Journal of perinatal education. https://www.ncbi.nlm.nih.gov/pmc/articles/PMC1595013/

mind. Sleep, or at least nap. Eat and drink so that the body and mind have fuel. Watch movies (Happy ones! We want oxytocin!). Read books. Go for leisurely walks. Do yoga! Snuggle with a pet or your sweetie!

Whatever you do, don't get into wondering whether this is "it." Believe me, birth isn't something you can miss. Your baby won't suddenly fall out of your pelvis without you noticing. To return to the racing analogy I introduced at the beginning of this chapter, you don't want to "go out too fast." If you try to sprint through the beginning of your labor, you'll be exhausted by the time the real work kicks in.

Early labor is the perfect time to stay on your mat in a different way. I'm going to add an addendum to that Buddhist joke: Don't just do something, sit there—*and get interested*! Yes, you're distracting yourself, but as the sensation of the contractions begins to increase, see if you can combine mindfulness with yoga. Get curious about what the sensation actually feels like. Let go of any thoughts about why it might feel that way for a moment, and just feel. Is it a squeeze? Pressure? Tightening that sweeps around your midsection? Where does it start? And does it stay the same?

If you can become interested in the internal sensations you experience, some of which may be quite unfamiliar and confusing, you can stay more relaxed because you do not add additional tension to the feelings that are already present. If you do notice yourself tensing, attempt to let go of whatever conscious tension you are adding.

As labor starts to require greater focus, your attention will be drawn further and further inward. This happens organically, not through force. Eventually, all you'll be doing is breathing and focusing as you ride through the intensity of the contractions, then relax and rest in between. You've arrived at the opening to the tunnel. You don't choose when to go in; you just realize you're there.

Once you're there, be there. Allow your mind to drop into the deep meditative focus you might have been practicing. Let your body move or remain still, whatever feels instinctive to you. Watch thoughts come and go, over and over again. In its deepest state this phase can seem very close to sleep. Some women even snore between contractions (I've seen this happen even when contractions were just four minutes apart!). While the contraction is happening, do whatever your body needs; as it fades, allow the mind to drift back into deep mindfulness practice and rest.

Delay the start of the tunnel as long as possible, but once you sense yourself at the entrance, get as interested as you can and go in.

Cornerstone #4: The "magic" labor thought: What does this mean to you?

Once you're in the tunnel, what keeps you moving forward? You'll have to discover your own reasons. Every woman has her own reasons for wanting the birth she chooses. Don't wait until you enter the tunnel to think about what inspires or empowers you. The basic questions to answer are: What does this all mean to you? Why did you choose to give birth in this particular way? In the dark of the tunnel, what will keep you going? I have heard moms express these reasons for desiring a certain type of birth:

- Best outcome for baby
- Personal empowerment
- Previous trauma
- Inspirational birth story/video
- Shared experience with someone
- and so many more

So there you are in the tunnel, investigating each sensation, watching thoughts come and go… and maybe beginning to feel like this is more difficult than you expected—or that you simply cannot navigate it any longer. At that moment, maybe you remember that women have been birthing babies for thousands of years. It feels inspiring to place yourself in this lineage, so you meet the next contraction with the mantra "Women have done this since the dawn of time," or "My body was made to birth." Maybe that thought carries you for a while.

But after 30 minutes, you might get a bit tired of saying it. So then you have another thought, something focused more on your own persona: "I am strong," or whatever speaks to you. I had a student who admitted that part of her reason for wanting a natural birth was to prove her own mother wrong about how the birth process could unfold. Her magic labor thought at one point was literally "I'm not going to have my mother's birth!" (which we reframed as "I can have my own birth experience" to give it a more positive spin). It doesn't matter what you choose, as long as it's meaningful to you. You'll want to have several thoughts or reasons to fall back on; one single inspiration may not be enough.

And none of this means you are locked into one version of the birth experience. It may be that in the moment of working with your labor you decide that an intervention would be appropriate. This is completely fine! I have actually seen some birth experiences become fully empowered when the birthing person chose to have an epidural or a surgical birth. The choices were made from a calm, centered place with the best information they could have at the moment.

Many childbirth classes will use the acronym BRAIN to help in deciding around interventions. When considering if something is right, take a moment to ask what might be the **B**enefits? The **R**isks? The **A**lternatives? Then ask for privacy while you check in with your own **I**ntuition about whether this feels like the right step for you (or would you rather try something else?). Finally, ask what might be the **N**ext steps, and what if you did not do this thing **N**ow? Then having considered your options from a calm place, I always suggest informing your care team of your decision with a **S**mile, so you are expressing yourself in a cooperative rather than combative manner.

BRAIN(S) may lead you to deviate off of your original birth "plan," which is still part of working with your labor. Make the best choice you can, and then work with that. Second guessing or looking back is a recipe for depression and regret, neither of which serve us in labor, motherhood, or yoga.

14 — Preparing for Birth with Yoga

"...with yoga a pregnant woman can find the means to make the most of the months of pregnancy as well as the experience of birth and motherhood...Yoga allows her to pause and become quiet so the she is able to receive this gift and be empowered by it"

—Janet Balaskas, *Preparing for Birth with Yoga*

In some ways, this whole book is an exploration of preparing for birth with yoga. So why is there a chapter dedicated to this topic? With all the various components of anatomy, physiology, meditation, breathing, and movement, it would be easy to lose track of which practices are specifically beneficial in preparing for labor and birth.

I submit that preparing for birth with yoga actually has two aspects. One is the preparation with yoga throughout the pregnancy. The other is how to use yoga during the birth itself. In this chapter, we will examine the practices and meditations that promote balance in both body and mind to encourage a smoother, easier labor and birth. And then we'll look at what positions, movements, breathing practices and meditations could be helpful in navigating the twists and turns of labor and birth. Through such explorations, you can discover how to quite literally get out of your own way and make space for the baby to descend and be born.

Preparation: the body's "training" plan

The analogy of labor as a marathon is common in childbirth circles. Although I alluded to it in Chapter 13 on the Four Cornerstones of Working with Labor, I have some issues with this analogy. It can conjure up images of extreme physical exertion, intense pain, dehydration, and cramping—and potentially make the practice of birthing a child seem outside the realm of ordinary people. Not everyone feels or is capable of running a marathon. But the female body is designed for the birth process.

In other ways, the marathon analogy does work. When training for a marathon or any challenging physical endeavor, there is an amount of, well, training! You don't embark on a difficult athletic activity right after getting up off the couch. You do the physical work, prepare the mind, and—as any athlete will tell you—personalize the training plan, so you can be ready for the day when you step up to the starting line.

I'll reiterate that no yoga practice, no matter how well executed, can ensure a specific birth outcome. And no one movement is guaranteed to work for every labor and birth. There are too many variations in our bodies, in our movement diets, and in our babies for a one-size-fits-all program. But what is certain is that a longtime yoga and meditation practice encourages mental and physical flexibility, which is useful no matter what turn labor may take.

Let's briefly recap the body's changes and needs during pregnancy and labor. Hormonal shifts give the body's connective tissues greater pliability and flexibility. As the uterus grows it pushes the internal organs upwards and adds weight to the front of the body. The breasts also increase in size. The body's center of gravity moves forwards as much as 4 inches by the end the 40 weeks of gestation. As a result, the pelvis often tilts forward, and the curves of the spinal column become more pronounced to provide more shock absorption.

Areas that tend to become tense and require release:

- The hip flexors, such as the psoas, iliacus, and quadriceps
- The hip stabilizers, such as glutes, hamstrings, calves and lower back muscles
- The pelvic floor muscles, which come under stress from the increased weight
- The upper back, neck, and shoulder muscles, which come under stress from the growing breasts and belly

Areas that tend to become overstretched or weak, thus requiring additional strength and tone:

- The hip stabilizers, such as glutes, hamstrings, and lower back muscles
- The pelvic floor muscles
- The abdominal wall
- The upper back, neck, and shoulder muscles

Notice that several groups of muscles fall into both camps, needing to strengthen and also to stretch. One of the key components to using yoga for birth preparation is finding the middle ground of overall muscle and fascial tone. A body with great mobility in one area will frequently hold excessive tension elsewhere, an attempt to compensate for the lack of support in the more mobile places. Aches and pains during pregnancy can often be windows into where the body has shifted out of balance, and restoring that balance does not always mean stretching an area out further.

While it may seem paradoxical, the long-term solution for something like hip pain or sciatica could actually be strengthening the gluteal and piriformis muscles so they are better able to support the SI joint and posterior hip nerve bundles. Yes, the area needs to stretch—because you cannot work a muscle which is already in a contraction—but once released, the muscles also need to work. Excessive tension and mobility both lead to joint compression, and during pregnancy there is an even more profound impact on how the uterus and pelvic connective tissues sit together. Movement now can help ease labor later.

The basic movements included in Chapter 11 on home practice are a great starting point for addressing key areas and nudging them towards balance. I usually suggest that pregnant students think of these like macro nutrients, with the specific yoga foods being their choice. But just as we need a well-rounded food diet, so too does our daily movement need to encompass some of the following actions.

Basic yoga movements to prepare for labor

- Back muscle chain mobilization and toning (calf and hamstring stretches as well as spinal muscle release and strengthening)
- Hip mobilization (hip circles standing, sitting, from Table, or supine if in early pregnancy, Cat/Cow)
- Hip strengthening and stretching (Ankle to Knee, Baddha Konasana (active and passive), Wall Squat with blocks)
- Pelvic floor toning (strengthening active Malasana, stretching Prasarita Padotanasana, pelvic floor breathing)
- Psoas release (Bridge pose, Anjaneyasana, direct psoas release on block)
- Side bending and release (Parivrtta Janu Sirsasana, Windmill, Reverse Warrior)

This sequence is also included in Chapter 11 as a suggested place to begin when exploring practice on your own.

Preparation: the mind's "training" plan

Preparing the body for labor and birth is part of the picture, but it is not the whole. Consciously placing feet and hands in the practice of *asana* promotes the deeper side of using yoga for birth: preparing the mind. If you've picked up this book with a longtime yoga practice under your belt, you already know that yoga is a practice of the interplay between the body and the mind.

I often have students in childbirth education ask what positions they can use to prepare for the labor process. I like to point out that they need to prepare the mind and body equally. A yoga practice for labor and birth involves not only toning and balancing the body but also getting to know your own mental patterns and thoughts; honing and cultivating the mindfulness that allows you to stay present amid strong emotions and charged situations. As mindfulness teacher and pioneer Jon Kabat Zinn says, "Mindfulness is the awareness that comes from paying attention in a particular way: on purpose and non-judgmentally in the present moment."

With consistent practice, you can come to not only better know your own mind but to also build the mental stamina to address fears, habits, and preconceived ideas about the birth process. You gain the fortitude to ride the waves of labor contractions moment by moment.

A yoga student of mine once described how her mindfulness practice intersected with the birth experience. She said she became intensely aware of her internal monologue during and between the contractions. "Now it hurts," she would say to herself during the contraction. "Now it doesn't hurt," she would say in between. She credited her ability to stay fully in the moment with not needing further medication during her 12 hour induction and labor.

Mindfulness is getting to know your own patterns of thought and reactivity. In Tibetan meditation traditions there is the concept of *gom*, which means to become familiar with something. I often recommend students start practicing 5-10 minutes of mindfulness a day to become familiar with those pesky *chitta vritti*, or "whirling fluctuations" of the mind. Even one minute, done regularly, can affect how you interact with your thoughts. And there are quite a lot of thoughts when it comes to the process of birth and welcoming another human into your life. Being able to observe these thoughts without criticism or judgment makes an enormous difference in how you engage with the labor process itself. As HypnoBirthing® founder and creator Marie Mongan wrote, "Thoughts produce beliefs, which in turn create feelings, which then lead to actions and responses." Getting familiar with your thoughts can literally impact what you feel during labor and afterwards.

The elements of a basic meditation practice are simple:
(recording available at www.ombirths.com/ombirthsbook/mindfulness-meditation-instruction)

- Take your seat
- Place your attention
- If your mind wanders, acknowledge it wandered and come back

Come to a seated position that has a quality of wakefulness to it. The spine is upright and strong, but at the same time, the front of the body is soft. The chest is open, but the shoulders and belly are relaxed. Hands rest palms down on the legs.

If you are seated on the floor, have the legs crossed loosely in front of you. If it is challenging to sit on the floor and maintain an upright posture, then you might sit on some cushions or yoga blocks. You could also kneel, again making sure the posture is comfortable for your knees, ankles and hips. If you prefer, or if it is more appropriate, you can sit in a chair, in which case be sure that the feet are planted on the floor fully and that the back is again upright. These postures are equally effective, so don't think of the chair as a remedial option to the more classic cross legged seat. We often see this seated position simply because that is how Buddha's culture tended to sit at the time. There is nothing inherently more enlightening about lotus over Western style chair-sitting.

Establish your posture, feeling the solidity of the base, as though your body were buried up to the waist in sand at the beach. With the steady base, the upper body is able to feel lighter and more open. Soft and resting, just as it is. Palms rest easily against the thighs. Having established your upright posture, maintain an open eyed gaze. We aren't drifting off into la-la land with this practice; we are getting to know this situation here and now. But if there is a lot to look at, begin by reining the gaze in to a comfortable distance (traditionally 4-6 feet) so you can stay concerned with your immediate experience instead of the traffic going by outside.

The eyes are open, but with the soft, slightly downward gaze, the lids might close a bit. We are aiming for a soft focus, allowing the gaze to rest on whatever happens to be at that comfortable distance in front of us. No need to stare militantly or bore holes in the floor with your eyes. Just let the gaze relax and rest. This is step one, taking your seat.

Step two is placing your focus. The focus could be anything you choose: the feeling in the right foot, the sensation of the left earlobe. Or it could be the sound of a fan in the room—the actual sound, not thoughts about it.

For our purposes, we're going to use the traditional focus of the breath. This is the normal, everyday breath, not any special pranayama from a yoga practice. Use whatever breath you were breathing before I said anything about focusing on your breath. Be sure, however, that you are working with the sensation of the breath, not abstractly watching the breath come in and go out, but really getting up close to the feeling of it. This could be feeling the air moving in and out at the tip of your nose. Some people find it easier to feel the full cycle of the breath through the body. Whatever you choose, attempt to stay with the feeling of the breath just as it is. It comes in, goes out, and comes in again. It's been doing this for the whole day; we are simply becoming aware of it at this specific moment.

You will probably realize almost immediately that while you sit and feel the breath, thoughts come up. Some will be more pointed, able to be heard clearly, while others may be an indistinct hum in the background, like the noise at a cocktail party. Let me make one thing very clear about this technique: this is NORMAL and it is not a problem!!! Contrary to what many people may say regarding meditation, we are not trying to "clear the mind" in this practice. We are not even trying to stop the thoughts from coming up. Good news everyone! You don't have to stop thinking to be able to meditate!

So here's the third step in this practice. The thoughts will come, and if you don't give them too much focus, they will keep on moving, like traffic passing on a road. You may, however, notice that you have gotten caught up by a particular train of thought that has effectively transported you down the track (possibly a good distance). When you notice you have wandered, and that you are no longer feeling the sensation of your breath—at that moment of noticing, apply the third instruction, which is called "labeling." Here's how it works. When you realize you've become lost in thought, take a moment, metaphorically turn towards the thought and see what pulled you away (just briefly), and then mentally label it "thinking." Having labeled that train of thought, get off the train. Go back to the "station" where you are sitting, and bring your attention back to the next breath.

That's it. Take your seat. Place the attention on the breath, and when your mind wanders, gently label it as thinking and return your attention back to the next breath.

Inside of this foundational practice are all the tools you need to prepare for the birth experience. Returning to the present moment after clearly seeing where you have mentally wandered off is an amazing tool for changing your responses and coming to better know your own preferences and challenges. It is all too common to get lost in thought or spend time trying to solve a particular problem instead of trusting the answer to arise. Starting meditation practice can be like trying to see a forest but not realizing you are already sitting in one of the trees. You have preferences, history, and possibly trauma that might intersect with the birth experience. By coming back to the moment you are in, you may find the mental stamina to work with those feelings and release them if you can, or if not, to recognize them for what they are and respond accordingly.

Of course, this is no small feat! If it were easy, everyone would do it! With that in mind, here are a few expanded meditations that can be helpful when working with deeply held beliefs or ingrained storylines. These practices also cultivate compassion towards yourself, your baby, and possibly even the people who are challenging the birth experience you would like to have, if such challengers exist for you.

Dropping the storyline script (www.ombirths.com/ombirthsbook/meditation-dropping-the-storyline)

Take a comfortable seat, or lie down in a position which is supported and grounded. Bring your attention to the sensation of the body and the sensation of the breath softly moving in and out. Perhaps take note if there are sensations coming from the baby, but then gently return your attention to the immediate experience of breathing in and out. Just feel the breath.

As you are sitting or lying down and feeling the breath, there will probably come a moment when you realize you are no longer aware of the breathing. That your attention has wandered, and you are now off on a train of some thought which has possibly carried you quite far down the track. At this moment, realize that you are in fact once again present because you recognized that you weren't feeling the breath any longer.

You could simply shift your focus back to the sensation of breath right away, but in the moment of realizing you got caught up in a storyline, there is also a subtle feeling that might be accompanying the thought. Rather than hurriedly returning to the breath, take a moment and mentally turn to look at the storyline which grabbed your attention. Feel the attraction or aversion to it, and whatever emotions might be arising in the body—actually feel them if you can—even for just a second. Notice where they reside in your body. Notice any desire to continue solving the problem or replaying the "movie in your mind." Sometimes it's hard to stop processing a juicy storyline, but for this moment, see if you can. It's not forever, and you can come back to that particular thought later if you really need to.

But for this moment, having turned towards the thought and seen just a glimpse of it, acknowledge that it is again just a thought. Having labeled it, there are three micro-movements we can apply. We can drop the storyline. Just put it down and effectively "get off the train of thought." Then shift the focus back to the sensations of the breath and the body. There may be a lingering feeling from the emotions of that thought. See if you can let this fade as well, and simply begin again, feeling the inhale and the exhale.

The instruction here is very similar to the basic meditation practice I outlined first. The key difference is that in this meditation, you take a split-second pause to note what it was that grabbed your attention, and then feel what it feels like to let go of that storyline and return to the direct moment you are in. Recognizing the feeling gives you a chance to see where there might be some strong emotions tied into your thoughts. Emotions are thoughts which have not yet been given language or energy which has not yet been put into words and form. Feeling that inner response gives insight into places you might be ignoring and helps generate compassion for yourself and those you interact with as you prepare to welcome our baby into your life.

Metta meditation

Along with dropping your internal storylines, conditioning the mind also involves cultivating gentleness towards yourself and the world around you. In doing so, we begin recognizing our interconnectedness with one another, which helps generate a greater sense of compassion. When we can see our connections with others we are less likely to put up boundaries, which makes for a much more cooperative environment as we navigate the uncertainties of labor and birth.

If we can cultivate compassion towards ourselves and then towards our larger circle of interaction, we open the possibility for more connection and less reactivity, which helps maintain a positive environment throughout not only the birth experience but also throughout the pregnancy and into postpartum. We begin to see people as wanting to collaborate rather than conspiring against us. Just as your perspective can trigger the stress side of the nervous system or stimulate the relaxation side, developing a sense of compassion helps you let go of internal storylines—and might allow you to release during the intensity of birth itself. It's hard to feel safe and secure if you have decided that your nurse is working against you. But if you can see her as a person, one who might be tired from a long shift or fearful of what a supervisor might say (and unable to drop her own internal storyline), you might soften towards this person. It doesn't mean you allow someone to abuse or restrict you, but you might assert yourself differently, perhaps in a way that results in more cooperation and support.

Cultivating compassion starts with yourself. As many yoga teachers have said, "If you want to cultivate peace in the world, begin with your own home." From there, gradually widen your circle to include the people you care for, and then those you might be struggling with, those you don't really know, and finally, all beings everywhere. This practice is often taught using mantras, which I have included here. But I have found that a more powerful way to practice is to imagine the mantra coming true and observing how I respond to that image.

The 4 mantras are:

- May you be happy
- May you be healthy
- May you be safe
- May you live in ease

Further instruction *(www.ombirths.com/ombirthsbook/meditation-metta-compassion-practice)*

Begin sitting or lying in a comfortable position, one which has a quiet internal dignity but does not require much effort to hold. If sitting, let the spine be strong but the front body soft and relaxed. The hands can rest down in the lap. Gently close the eyes if it feels safe to do so, and bring your awareness to the inner experience of this moment. Feel the sensations of your breathing, simply moving in and out. There is no need to change this rhythm. It was working just fine before you started noticing it. Sit for a few moments, just feeling yourself where you are, as you are.

Now sitting or lying quietly, in your mind's eye picture yourself as you would like to be. And as you imagine this, quietly say to yourself internally "May I be happy." As you say this, what image can you bring up? What would it look like to be happy right now? What would it feel like? You don't have to actually feel happy as you imagine it, but see if you can be open to the possibility that you could be happy, and notice what that would mean for you. Maybe you see a scene, or perhaps you just get a felt sense in your body. And of course, notice if it is challenging to bring up this wish for yourself. This, too, is good information and good practice for compassion.

Now from happiness, internally say for yourself, "May I be healthy." Notice what images this brings up. Maybe you see yourself being physically active or growing in your pregnancy smoothly and strongly. Maybe this image has a mental health component to it, and maybe it is just an internal feeling, a sense of physical health throughout your being. Let yourself experience what it would mean to be healthy for you.

And now from that feeling of health and wellbeing, internally wish for yourself, "May I be safe." And notice what images or feelings this brings up. Is it a picture of being protected during your birth? An image of having advocates around you or being in a place where you know everyone has your best interests at heart? Maybe it is a picture of being able to lock out bad forces or an internal sense of safety and security. Whatever arises, including a sense of anxiety: just notice. Can you feel compassion for this person (yourself) who is living in this state?

And from feeling and imagining safety and security, internally say to yourself, "May I live at ease." And again, what does this bring up for you? What would it look like if you were living at ease right now? Would this be a picture of relaxing in the sunshine? Or laughing with friends and family? Maybe it is just a feeling like taking a deep breath and being able to sigh it out. And what does it feel like to imagine this for yourself? What would it mean if you could step into this picture?

Sit for a moment, feeling what it feels like to wish these things for yourself. Then take a deep breath and sigh it out, releasing the images and returning to the direct experience of sitting and breathing as you are right now. Having sent loving kindness towards yourself, shift your attention to a being who you love dearly. This might be your baby, or a family member, or a beloved pet. This is someone for whom you usually have no trouble feeling kind towards, who always seems to open your heart a little bit. (If you can't think of anyone, think of the cutest baby animal you've ever seen.)

And holding this being in your heart and mind, imagine saying to them, "May you be happy," and watch what arises if you imagine them being truly happy. "May you be healthy." What does true health look or feel like for this being? "May you be safe." What would safety look like for this being right now, even if you don't really know where they are at this moment? "May you live at ease." What does ease look like for them? And as you send these thoughts in their direction, what feelings arise in your own body? How does it feel to hope for happiness and ease for a beloved being? Sit for a moment with this feeling. Then take a deep breath and sigh, and bring your awareness back to the direct feeling of being right now.

Now if you feel so inclined and want to strengthen your compassion muscle, call to mind a being with whom you might be having some challenge. This need not go all the way to someone you are genuinely angry with or who has hurt you. It could just be someone with whom you are currently having some static, or someone who you do not usually wish good things for. If all else fails, imagining someone from the other side of the political aisle will usually create the necessary mental muscle work.

Holding this challenging person in your mind (and heart if you can), can you say for them, "May you be happy?" And what does it look like for them to truly be happy? What does it feel like for you to wish happiness towards this person? "May you be healthy." How does that look and feel? "May you be safe." Again, what does this look like? What would it feel like for them? What does it feel like for you? "May you live at ease." What might you envision here? How does it feel to wish this for this being? What are you noticing in yourself? Feel this for a moment, and then take a deep breath (I usually need a deep one here), and with a good sigh, release that image and come back to the immediate experience of the moment.

Finally, can you extend these loving generous thoughts out beyond the circle of only those we know? In whatever way you can, imagine all the different people, animals, and beings living on this planet. Those you like, don't like, feel neutral towards, and those you don't even know. Be sure to include yourself in this group, as you are also a human being on this planet. Send the wish out as far as you can imagine: "May all beings be happy." What would that feel like? What if all beings lived in happiness? "May all beings be healthy." What if there was no more sickness or injury? What would that look like? "May all beings be safe." What would that mean? What would disappear if that were the case? "May all beings live at ease." And how does it feel to wish for that for all beings? Sit for a moment, just feeling. There is no right or wrong way to feel when imagining this. Just notice where you are.

And then taking a final deep breath in, and giving a long sigh out, return your attention to where you are at this very moment and what it feels like to simply be in your body right now. Notice if there are thoughts or judgments lingering from any of these visualizations. As we would in straight mindfulness practice, take note of what they are, but then recognize they are simply thoughts—just as this whole meditation was. Let the thoughts go, shift focus back to the sensations of breathing, and once again feel the direct sensation of air moving in and out. Sit for as long as you like, feeling whatever it felt like to wish happiness for all the different people and beings your life has touched or will never touch. Then simply drop the practice and resume your day.

For some, this practice can feel a bit beyond their ability to actually create. How could we possibly create happiness for all beings just by thinking of it? But in turning our thoughts towards a larger picture, we may find that our internal dialogue shifts slightly. I have seen couples who practiced this meditation in classes report that after they did it they felt more gentle towards one another. Some even found themselves able to discuss deeper issues they had around birth or parenting which they had been fearful to bring up; they had assumed they would be met with resistance rather than cooperation. I remember one student who returned from a conversation about her birth plan with her doctor, saying, "I suddenly saw this person as just another human being who was trying to do his best and was scared I was going to ask for something unreasonable. It changed everything, and I was able to have a much deeper conversation where we both came to an understanding of what I needed to feel supported during my birth and what constraints my doctor was working with under the hospital setting."

I always wonder what might happen if we imagined all our relationships from a place of love and compassion. Almost as an additional birth verse to the John Lennon song: "Imagine there's no conflict. I wonder if we can. No birth fear or trauma. Just love and holding hands." Call me a dreamer, but I'm not the only one.

Yoga Nidra

Yoga Nidra, or yogic sleep, is a process of using progressive relaxation to bring the nervous system into a state of deep release and stillness. I have found several meditation practices in other traditions that follow the same pattern. Mindfulness-based stress reduction (MBSR) courses utilize the progressive body scan, and hypnosis scripts for birth use a progressive relaxation segment to bring the body into deep rest before embarking on further visualization. Consistent practice of both physical and mental relaxation can help establish a mental pathway which is then more easily accessed during labor and birth. In short, practicing daily relaxation helps keep the nervous system in a more relaxed state, which then reduces the activation of the Fear-Tension-Pain cycle in moments of stress.

Yoga Nidra is a state of consciousness between waking and sleeping, like the "going-to-sleep" stage. The body is completely relaxed, and you become systematically and increasingly aware of your inner experience by listening to a specific set of instructions. Yoga Nidra differs from meditation in that the mind is left to float in awareness rather than returning to a single point of focus (such as the breath). The goal is to remain in a state of light *pratyahara*, with four of the senses withdrawn and only the hearing still connected to the instructions. Yoga Nidra is among the deepest possible states of relaxation while still maintaining full consciousness

During Yoga Nidra, mom finds a comfortable position, usually using bolsters and props to fully support the body. From there, either the teacher or a recording takes her through a body scan, moving in a particular pattern. While this progression is ideally done fairly slowly, it does not have to be. Deep relaxation can be achieved by moving relatively quickly through the body if necessary. Once in deep relaxation, scripts sometimes move through a range of alternating sensations: hot/cold, light/heavy, and so on, bringing the awareness to internal rather than external experiences. For pregnancy, the visualizations could also include images of health and wellbeing for mom and baby or riding waves of sensation, as during labor.

Like the mindfulness body scan and the hypnotic induction process, Yoga Nidra seeks to bring the student into a state of alpha wave brain activity, where the mind is aware of the surroundings but focused solely on the sensations of the body. We pass through this alpha wave state whenever we fall asleep or wake up. Hypnotic states also include theta wave brain activity (the kind we experience during REM sleep), which is just short of the delta wave, or deep sleep state.

The main difference between hypnosis and Yoga Nidra is that after the progressive body relaxation, a hypnotic session would then incorporate imagery designed to suggest something to the subject's mind. Yoga Nidra, on the other hand, simply rotates through sensations and awareness, allowing the mind to remain relaxed and open. Basically, Yoga Nidra can be thought of as hypnosis without any overt suggestion planted in the subconscious. However, because the mind is wide open and aware of things said, even if all other appearances may be otherwise, one should be very conscious of the environment and secondary sounds which might distract or shift the focus during Yoga Nidra.

(recording available at www.ombirths.com/ombirthsbook/yoga-nidra)

Find a position which is comfortable for you now, where you are fully supported and it takes no effort to be here. Ask yourself if you could be 5% or 10% more comfortable in this position. What would that feel like? Feel your breath flowing easily throughout your body: a normal, relaxed breath without any specific control or pattern. Just your natural rhythm.

Now as I name individual parts of your body, imagine each of those parts releasing and becoming filled with a healing, rejuvenating light, as though guided from your breathing.

(said calmly but at a regular pace)

Bring your attention to the thumb of your right hand, your right index finger, middle finger, ring finger, pinky, the palm of your hand, the back of your hand, your right wrist, right forearm, elbow, upper arm, your right shoulder—relaxed and filled with the healing golden light of your breath. Moving down the right side of your torso, your right hip, right thigh, knee, calf, shin, right ankle, top of the foot, sole of the foot. The whole right side of your body, relaxed, and filled with the healing, golden light of your breath.

Now moving to the thumb of your left hand, left index finger, middle finger, ring finger, the palm of your hand, the back of your hand, your left wrist, left forearm, elbow, upper arm, left shoulder relaxed and filled with the golden light of your breath. Moving down the left side of your torso, left hip, left thigh, knee, calf, shin, ankle. The top of your foot, and the sole of your foot. The whole left side of your body, relaxed and filled with golden healing light.

Coming to the middle of your body, to your abdomen, your chest, your heart, your neck, your throat, the dome of your skull, your face, your jaw, relaxed and filled with the light of your breath.

Now imagine that golden light of your breath flowing down from the crown of your head, entering through the crown chakra. Gradually filling your body with calm, peaceful energy. Feel it fill your face, your shoulders, your arms and your heart. Now imagine a grounding, earthward energy entering through the roots of your feet and wherever you are in contact with the earth. See this energy flowing up your legs and hips, coming to meet this golden light in your center around your belly and your baby. Joining heaven and earth within your body. And your heart takes this mixture of heaven and earth and sends it out throughout your body to wherever it is needed, wherever your internal wisdom guides it to be. See your radiant, luminous energy body pulsing with the light of heaven and earth mixed together. Maybe feel baby's energy within that flow.

And now bring your attention back to the room, and the feeling of your whole body, and know that your body is healthy, complete, and whole just as it is. When you are ready, open your eyes.

Breathing: The intersection of mind and body

The breath is the physical expression of our nervous system, and as such, being able to use the breath is a powerful tool in calming the potential fear response during labor. There is a reason that Lamaze, the Bradley Method®, HypnoBirthing®, and general natural childbirth classes all have a breath component. Harnessing the breath helps stimulate the parasympathetic nervous system and can literally move the abdominal and pelvic floor muscles out of the way of the contracting uterus, creating more space for baby to be born. And the breath is always happening in the present moment, so using specific breathing techniques can be an invaluable practice for preparation and during the birth process.

By controlling the movement and pace of the breath, the yogis say we literally control the life force within our bodies. Whether or not you believe that, there are specific breathing practices which can be useful to practice ahead of and during labor as a way of calming the nervous system working directly with the movement of the uterus during contractions. I recommend using one of these *pranayamas* at least daily for 1-2 minutes.

Calming Breath

This breath was covered on pg 178 as one of the basic breathing practices for yoga during pregnancy. This breathing pattern is useful anytime during pregnancy to calm down reactivity in the nervous system, and also helpful to re-establish a calm state between the surging muscle contractions of labor.

Bring attention to the natural rhythm of inhale and exhale through the body. Begin to internally count the length of the inhale and exhale. It doesn't matter what the numbers are at the moment. Simply get a sense for your current internal rhythm. Once you have whatever the numbers are, gradually coax the exhale to become 2 counts longer than the inhale. There are no set numbers for this exercise; though inhaling for 4 and exhaling for 6 seems to be popular when moms are relaxed. Continue to breathe this way for several minutes feeling the body and mind relax. When you let go of the breathing and return to normal, notice the impact overall.

Full Body Breathing (contraction variation)

This *pranayama* is a combination of the Full Body Breath described on pg 178 and the more audible Ujjayi breath covered on pg 179. The 360 degree expansion of the Full Body Breath helps move the front and side abdominal muscles off the uterus as it contracts during labor. During this muscle contraction, the uterus changes shape and shifts forward against the abdominal wall. Breathing to expand the front sides, back, and base of the abdomen makes more space for the uterine muscles to do their work and can sometimes reduce the intensity when the uterus surges back and forth as it contracts and releases.

Clear any leftover breath in the lungs by taking a short inhale and exhaling through the mouth with a sigh.

From this new empty space, close the mouth and feel the breath move down into the center of the body, expanding the front, sides, and back of the abdomen on the inhale. Additionally, feel the muscles of the pelvic floor release downwards as though expanding like a balloon. There may be a subtle whispering sound as the breath moves in, but the back of the throat and soft palette should remain open. The breath is quiet, as though you were whispering a secret to a dear friend.

Once the center body feels full, allow the breath to seamlessly flow upwards into the ribs and chest and then, finally, up under the collar bones. The feeling is almost as though filling the torso three times with breath, taking as long as possible to do so. With the body completely filled, allow the breath to escape in a slow but steady exhale, as though releasing from the top of the head through the vagina and down to the toes.

Soft lips/"horsey" breath

Another helpful breath variation focuses on releasing the muscles around the jaw and throat. Remember many midwives refer to the neuromuscular connection between the muscles of the jaw and the muscles of the pelvis and vagina with the phrase "loose mouth, loose bottom." This variation on Full Body Breath combines a full abdominal expansion with a flutter of the lips and jaw muscles on the exhalation to promote further relaxation.

Begin as with the Full Body Breath, inhaling slowly and feeling for the expansion first of the abdominal center, then the side ribs, and finally the top of the chest and collarbones. On the exhale, allow the breath to escape through both the nose and the mouth. The lips should not be pursed but rather barely parted, as though holding a piece of tissue paper between them. As the breath escapes the lips may flutter, creating a soft sound like a horse exhaling. The cheeks will flare out and may also flutter as the lips vibrate. The softness of the lips should extend back to the back of the throat, and the teeth are gently parted (not clenched). Once the exhale is finished, let the lips close slightly and repeat the full body inhalation.

The aim here isn't to create a sound but rather to make the facial muscles as loose and relaxed as possible. Releasing up top helps to release in the base of the pelvis, which assists the cervix in sliding back as the outer fibers of the uterus draw upwards around the descending baby's head.

"Pushing" breath

You'll recall from Chapter 12 on childbirth education that there is an internal expulsive reflex which moves the baby out. This means we do not need to be holding our breath or straining to push our babies out. Instead, find a way to use the breath rather than hold it.

Tune into the sensations in your body. As the uterus begins to contract, take a deep but fast breath into the upper chest—like you are getting ready to do something. Feel the opening and expansion of the pelvic floor. Then, as the pressure builds and maintaining the pelvic relaxation, gradually begin to nudge that breath downwards, as though you could send it down the front side of your spine, around the curve of the sacrum, and then forward and out through the vagina. Use your breath to assist the natural reflex of your body. When you need to breathe again, repeat the quick, deep inhale and nudge baby further. Relax as the contraction releases.

Yoga in the birth room

It's one thing to practice yoga *asana*, *pranayama*, and meditation ahead of labor; it's quite another to actually use them when labor arrives. No matter how much you have practiced, the moment when you recognize labor has begun always has some emotion attached to it. When doula clients called me during early labor, I could often hear the mixture of excitement and trepidation in their voices. "Is this really it?" "Have I prepared enough?" "What do I do next?" It would be nice if labor came with a roadmap, but the truth is that as labor begins we don't know exactly how things will proceed. We have only the moment by moment sensations to guide us in how to move, breathe, and lean into the experience. This is where the mental and physical yoga practice come together.

The start of labor is a dance between focused curiosity, deliberate relaxation, and distraction. As labor progresses, the sensations shift and change, building in intensity. At this point I usually guide my doula clients to start getting curious about the sensations themselves: to yoke the mindful awareness they have cultivated through their prenatal yoga practice with the movement of their breath and body to see where the path begins to unfold for them personally.

Yoga during labor is always a combination of mental and physical practices. The mental focus and attention you craft during pregnancy can help you more readily drop the storylines in your head and come back to the direct experience—pleasant, unpleasant, or neutral. If labor proceeds smoothly, then nothing further needs to be done beyond moving as it feels right to do so. Plenty of women spontaneously move their bodies during labor in the way that feels best and that ultimately supports them during birth. Doing so requires a safe environment, where mom feels supported and disinhibited, where the body can truly be the guide.

But it isn't always obvious which way the body needs to open. Sometimes it can be helpful to think about where the baby is in the body and how that area of the body might release to get out of the way. If there are challenges in the labor—excessive pain, slowing contractions, a cervix that does not dilate, or a baby that does not seem to emerge, movements from the yoga practice may help create the space needed within the body far more effectively than gritting your teeth and trying to breathe. While there are sensations in labor which are uncomfortable, I tell my childbirth education classes that if they feel something that is genuinely painful (grinding, breaking, tearing; not just tightening), they should not ignore it or assume it is "just part of labor." Pain is the body's way of telling us something is wrong, and that holds true even in the intensity of labor.

I've heard childbirth instructors say that during the first stage of labor, and in the pushing phase as well, there isn't much one can do to help the contractions work better. That no yoga posture or breath will increase the strength of the uterine muscles working, and all mom can do is to get out of the way and let things work. This advice is often taken metaphorically, as guidance to remove mental blocks like fear or leaning into the sensations of labor.

But through the yoga practice, this advice becomes far more literal. By changing the position of your body, you change the internal shape of your pelvis. You can literally get out of the way by physically moving the bones into different positions, creating space for the baby's head to move down into the cervix and for the cervix to open smoothly beneath that pressure. While making space to move out of the way may not always be comfortable, I have often found that by creating the space for labor to continue, the contractions also become more manageable.

Laurel (not her name) was a yoga student and doula client of mine whose labor had progressed slowly and steadily but seemed to be hitting a snag about 8 hours in. She initially managed the contractions by rocking on her hands and knees on her bed, but she soon found that she more enjoyed walking back and forth outside on the steep hill in front of their home. She described some of the contractions as a "wave of pressure that started in the front and swept around to the back." She was clearly able to breathe through these contractions, and she rewarded herself with a piece of dark chocolate between each one (I went through so many bars of chocolate at this birth!).

But she described other contractions as a searing pain that began in her back and then focused into her sacrum and SI joints. For these contractions, it took support from both myself and her partner to cope. They were far more uncomfortable and often met with a big hug (as well as more chocolate) at the end. As labor gradually intensified, I suggested that she circle her pelvis, focusing in particular on tucking the tail when the contractions were more intense. This didn't seem to help immediately, but over time, the sensations shifted until they were mostly happening in the front of her body. What we discovered later was that her daughter was trying to engage into the top of her pelvis and was rotating front to back, looking for the widest space.

When baby was facing forward (not the optimal position) her head was grinding into her mother's spine and was more extended, presenting a larger circle to the top of the pelvis. When baby rotated to face her mother's back (more optimal), her chin tucked into her chest and her head was more easily able to nuzzle into the upper pelvic brim. This meant less pressure on her mother's spinal bones and thus the sensation became just that of the uterus moving her down into the cervix. This downward sensation was far more manageable, even though the process of her moving into position was not. Once there, labor was able to continue much more smoothly.

Remember that babies are guided into a set of cardinal movements as they move through the three levels of the pelvis. They engage in the inlet, rotate around the level of the mid-pelvis and then emerge in the outlet. The levels are measured by what is called pelvic station, or where the top of the baby's head is relative to the posterior ischial spines in the back of the pelvis. Level with the ischial spines is referred to as being at "0 station." Being a centimeter above the spines is referred to as being "-1 station." And being a centimeter below is referred to as "+1 station." The stations continue into -2, -3 and +2 +3 accordingly. You will almost never hear someone say that a baby is +4 because that would be crowning, and +5 is outside the body.

Also remember that the top of the pelvis (usually referred to as the pelvic brim) is wider side to side than it is front to back. If a baby is trying to engage into the top of the pelvis but the brim is restricted (maybe by an overly tight psoas muscle pulling the sacrum forward), creating space means finding a way to move the top of the sacrum away from the pubic bone and deepen the upper circle. Or it could mean finding ways to release the psoas, which can itself create tension at the pelvic inlet. On the other hand, the outlet of the pelvis is wider front to back and bounded by the sitz bones, so making space there involves finding ways to move the tail, pubis, and sitz bones apart. Remember the exploration from Chapter 1 about how much the sitting bones move?

Sit or stand upright, and put your attention on your sitting bones and the diamond of the pelvic floor. Feel how much space there seems to be in a neutral position. Now actively scoop the pelvis under while rotating the knees apart. Do the sitz bones feel closer or farther apart? When I practice this in yoga classes I find most students report the sitz bones feel closer together.

Now try the opposite action. Turn the knees to knock against one another and arch the back to stick the tail shamelessly backwards. Do the sitz bones feel closer or wider? Again, when I practice this in yoga class most students report the bones seem to spread more fully in this position, where they seemed to close with the previous action. As one student commented, "I feel like I'm trying to poop in the woods."

The sitz bones are the base of the innominate bone (the bone composed of the ilium, ischium and pubis). Bringing the sitz bones and tailbones together moves the upper segment of the pelvis wider. Likewise, spreading the sitz bones and tail will subtly close the top level of the pelvis but open the base.

Tuck for the top

Helpful actions for opening the pelvic brim include active Cat pose where the tail scoops strongly forward as well as ways to release the psoas muscle, which crosses over the top of the pelvis and forms a sort of guidewire for the baby entering the pelvic inlet. In addition to the exercises found in Chapter 8, try single leg swings, which help soften an overly tense psoas line and calm the nervous system.

The pelvic tuck of Cat pose can also be done in a standing position. Even better, try a standing Cat pose with the legs turned out! It should be noted that this position should only be taken during contractions, since you need the power of the uterine muscles to guide the baby downward into the pelvis. And it may take several contractions for baby and pelvis to fully align.

Standing Cat/Cow movements or hip circles which incorporate a pronounced pelvic tuck can assist in gently guiding the baby and pelvic bowl into alignment. Hip circles can gently spiral the pelvic brim around the descending head, helping it to find the widest space to drop into. This is an interplay and a dance between the birthing person, her mind, and her baby. As a midwife I know once said, "There is only room for one head in the pelvis, and that should be the baby's head."

Walcher's variation

A position which can also help open the pelvic brim is called Walcher's position.[63] The Spinning Babies® program goes one step further by rotating the legs outwards to create what they call "Froggy Walcher's" position.

Walcher's position acts much the same way as the psoas release described above, but in this case both legs are extended. The sacrum rests against the edge of a bed or table, with the upper body lying back and the legs hanging forwards with the knees outwardly rotated. The result is that the ilium bones of the pelvis are dragged forwards from the weight of the legs but the sacrum remains fixed. As the top of the sacrum moves away from the pubic bone, it creates more room in the top section of the pelvis for baby to move through the bones and connective tissues.

Walcher's is a fairly dramatic position and is rarely comfortable for moms during contractions. But again, if the discomfort has been due to the baby's head grinding into the pelvic brim, then the sensations may change and become more manageable after using this position.

Sideways for the spin

Once inside the brim, the baby's head descends and then comes into contact with the muscles of the pelvic floor. Recall that these muscles open front to back, where the top of the pelvis was open side to side. It is not uncommon for some labors to seem to pause in the opening while the baby begins to make a 90 degree rotation to align with the mid-pelvis opening. Or it may be that the cervix opens but the baby doesn't seem to emerge. Baby's station in these cases ranges from -1 and +1.

Abby (not her name) was a second-time mom who opened very quickly for her birth at home. Five hours into labor her cervix was fully opened, and she began pushing. (It should be noted that watching her I wondered if she really felt the natural expulsive reflex, since the pushing didn't seem to come from inside but rather from an idea that she should be doing something).

After 3 more hours and with no sign of baby, we began trying other positions. Squatting, hands and knees, tucking, tilting—nothing seemed to change. After a quick consult, in which we discovered that baby was at the 0 station mark, I suggested we try something new: a side opening position where her leg dropped off the bed, which was similar to the action produced by lunging to the side with her leg on the chair. One release right, and one on the left,

---

[63] *Medical Dictionary.* S.v. "Walcher position." https://medical-dictionary.thefreedictionary.com/Walcher+position

and she stood up, exclaiming "I can feel her head!" The next contraction clearly involved an expulsive reflexive push. Her body took over as she bent forward onto my lap, pushing from deep within her body. Fifteen minutes later, her daughter was crowning and born while Abby was on her hands and knees.

When baby is moving through the mid-pelvis, it often involves accessing the pelvic floor on some level. Opening these deep muscles can require breathing along with release and opening. But something like a gentle side lunge, where one side of the pelvis is open and spreading and the other side is dropped, can widen the ischial spines, creating more space for the baby's head to rotate, extend, and emerge through the pelvic floor.

During this time, yoga movements might resemble the alignment for Warrior 2 or Skandasana described above. This alignment can be achieved from hands and knees by bringing one leg out to the side at about a 45 degree angle and rocking back and forth. Another approach is to stand one foot onto a chair, facing open from the knee and possibly leaning on a partner. Gently rocking back and forth widens the pelvis in the diagonal direction and slackens one side of the pelvic floor, moving the bones and muscles out of the way for the baby to descend. The other name childbirth educators use for this position is the "Captain Morgan" stance, recalling the position of the pirate on the spiced rum bottle—and probably invoking a bit of humor. I know a midwife who almost birthed her second baby in the shower because she had lifted one leg up to shave her leg and the baby had simply slid right through. Move out of the way, and the body already knows what to do.

The leg-up pelvic position can also be achieved when lying down with the strategic use of some props. From side-lying, place a stack of pillows—or an elongated yoga ball known as a peanut ball—beneath the top leg, parallel and supported as you would for Side-lying Shavasana. From this position, roll the body and leg forwards so the belly shifts into the bed and the knee slides to the side. The position geometrically resembles the standing "Captain Morgan" stance turned on its side. This position could be appropriate for someone who has an epidural during labor when weight-bearing postures are no longer an option.

Butt out for the base

And then the baby comes down into the lower pelvis, bounded by the sitz bones, pubis, and tail. To expand and open the outlet, we come back to the actions that seem to widen the sitz bones and tail from prior explorations. There are often claims made in yoga circles that squatting can open the pelvis by as much as 2-3 cm, but that's only true if the femur bones are internally rotated during the squat.

The yogic pose for opening the lower level of the pelvis (station +1 and more) is either:

- a high squat where the lower back can arch and the pelvis can sit backwards
- a hands and knees position where the thighs can spin inwards with the pelvis in Cow pose
- If lying on the side, closing the knees together with the bum pushed back into an anterior pelvic tilt

Think about the position often shown for pushing on TV and the movies (and which I have often seen women coached into in many labor rooms). Mom is typically reclining with the legs spread wide and knees pulled back, being instructed to tuck her tail and curl around her baby in a C curve. These actions open the top of the pelvis, not the base! And they definitely do not create the sensation of "pooping in the woods." As one doula client quipped when a nurse told her to push like she was having a bowel movement, "Yeah, that's not something I would do in this position!"

And here's the best part of using yoga to change the shape of your pelvis: it works even if you have opted for medication or an epidural! The actions of tucking, side lunging, and internally and externally rotating can be achieved with props as much as with muscle action. Need to open the top? Play with outwardly rotating the thighs and supporting the legs with several pillows or the peanut ball. Need to open the base? Prop mom on her side with the knees together and the feet apart, and pull her hips back.

Yoga, birth, and medication

It is easy to assume that using yoga during labor and birth only applies to an unmedicated birth, but that's simply not the case. Using yoga in the labor room can mean recruiting *asana* to make space, but it also means leaning into the experience you have and choosing what is right for *you* in that moment. The real practice is sitting with whatever comes up. Can you be with your internal storylines and see them for what they are? Can you feel compassion for yourself, your baby, and the people around you? Can you find ways to be relaxed, even when the circumstances do not conform to what you were expecting or hoping for? Ultimately the answer is probably not, at least not fully. But can you then sit with this inability as well?

For some, the hardest work they have to do during labor is letting go of the birth they thought they were going to have so they can be open to the magic of the birth they are in. Being mindful in labor doesn't mean a perfectly smooth outcome. It means being able to calm the nervous system when you need to and making choices from a calm, centered, and awake place.

In preparing for birth with yoga, you are also yoking the practice of yoga with the medical options you have available and choosing which options best suit your personal situation. This may mean that your "yogic birth" involves an epidural—or helps you embrace a birth you did not plan or hope for. Birthing with yoga has room for all the possibilities that birth presents, but in each of them, we birth embodied in the moment as things unfold. Birth is NOW at its fullest expression, the deepest meditation practice one can do. When you add the physicality of the process, you have the ultimate "yoke" of mind and body, of medical and natural, of physical and spiritual, of beginnings and endings, coming together in a dance of transformation and wakefulness.

15 — As the Dust Settles: Postpartum

"If you were wise enough to know that this life would consist mostly of letting go of things you wanted, then why not get good at the letting go, rather than the trying to have? These exotic revelations bubbled up involuntarily and I began to understand that the sleeplessness and vigilance and constant feedings were a form of brainwashing, a process by which my old self was being molded, slowly but with a steady force, into a new shape: a mother. It hurt. I tried to be conscious while it happened, like watching my own surgery. I hoped to retain a tiny corner of the old me, just enough to warn other women with. But I knew this was unlikely; when the process was complete I wouldn't have anything left to complain with, it wouldn't hurt anymore, I wouldn't remember."

—Miranda July[64]

We spend a great deal of time preparing for the day the baby is born. Parents read books, take prenatal yoga and birthing classes, and carefully select care providers, birth facilities and attendants. Friends and family eagerly wait for the call saying that mom is in labor or baby has been born. Baby arrives, and everyone celebrates, and moms and partners go home and live happily ever after…

And then the REAL yoga begins.

It is hard to express the shift involved in the first few weeks and months following a birth. Suddenly, there is a new being that is completely dependent on its parents! The immediate postpartum period is a time of intense uncertainty, shifting, and all-out change for mom, partner, and baby. Feelings can range from total bliss to absolute despair—and everything in between.

The shifts are so dramatic that the first three to four months after birth are often referred to as the "fourth trimester." During this time, babies undergo dramatic growth, both physically and mentally. Mom's body and mind begin the long journey into postpartum recovery and rediscovery. A full exploration of the twists and turns of parenthood is beyond the scope of this book, but we can look at how the yoga practice might intersect with this time of profound transformation and explore what *asanas* are appropriate for a postpartum mother returning to the yoga mat.

Most yoginis return to their yoga practice around six weeks postpartum. Six weeks is when the medical community has determined that the body is ready to ease back into movement

---

[64] July, M. (2015). *The first bad man: A novel.* Canongate.

and exercise. In truth, this timeline is somewhat arbitrary. While the body does need time to heal following birth, the idea that you should only be lying or sitting around, not doing any movement for six weeks after giving birth, is misguided.

Around six weeks after delivery, the site where the placenta separated has healed and the uterus has returned to pre-pregnancy size. Birth providers generally step back from the role of primary care, expecting most postpartum issues to self-correct or be handled by other professionals. But if you have spent the past six weeks doing nothing, it is not reasonable to jump back into running, high-impact exercise, or even general population yoga. If birth were treated like any other major physical endeavor (or any other surgery, if you had a cesarean), you would emerge with a prescription for physical therapy beginning as early as 1-2 weeks postpartum. Or you might be sent home with a set of gentle exercises to help you regain and maintain mobility and strength in preparation for returning to fuller movement at the six week mark.

Many people are able to do gentle movements during the "six week wait", and likewise, many people are not ready for full exercise right at the six week mark. As a yoga teacher who works with pelvic floor issues, I often pull avid runners and athletes back from high-impact exercises that are not appropriate for most bodies six weeks out. And almost in the same breath, I encourage students only three weeks postpartum to become conscious of their posture and the movements they do throughout the day as they care for their babies.

How and when to return to movement and exercise is, as always, a personal journey. The timing depends on the circumstances around the birth, the movement patterns and level of practice pre-birth, and what type of practice you are attempting to restart. Restorative slow flow yoga? You might be ok. Mysore Ashtanga practice, CrossFit®, or running? Give it more like 3-6 months, with some preliminary work in the interim.

While it is advisable to give your care provider a call (and please do give them a call!), if you plan to return to the yoga mat before your six week follow-up, it is reasonable to consider gentle recovery exercises and mindfulness practices to cut through some of the post-birth fog that many moms encounter. Once we understand how the body heals after birth, we are able to make better judgments about how fast to progress and what is actually appropriate. This may require a slower return to prized activities than you expected (runners, I'm looking at you). But as the saying goes: slow is smooth, and smooth is fast. When we move slowly, things are smoother, and when things go smoothly, we ultimately move faster.

Immediate postpartum (in the dust cloud)

Immediately post-birth—no matter how fit you were or how easily labor progressed—there is a great deal going on, and the body needs some time for physical recovery. Right after the baby is born, the muscles of the uterus contract once again, this time squeezing around the blood vessels of the placenta and releasing it from the inner uterine wall. The placenta will usually fully release and be pushed out of the body 30-60 minutes after the baby (no bones in the placenta, so this part is far easier). The uterine muscles will continue to release and contract for the next 4-6 weeks, gradually shrinking the uterus back down to its pre-pregnancy size. During pregnancy the uterus grows to 15 times its previous size, and it takes time to shrink this organ to fit neatly back in the pelvis.

The shrinking of the uterus creates some post-birth bleeding, similar to a menstrual period. Each time the uterine muscles relax to recontract, any blood vessels which have not yet sealed off will leak a bit. This blood will then drip out in what is called a "lochia." Heavy for the first week or so, the lochia should decrease in volume over 4-6 weeks. It also turns from bright red to brown as the body sheds older cells rather than fresh blood. To allow the blood vessels to seal and the uterus to heal at the site of placental attachment requires rest. Return to activity too quickly, and you risk internal blood vessels and, in extreme cases, triggering severe conditions such as postpartum hemorrhage.

If you are returning from a vaginal birth, your bleeding should have completely ceased—not even a trickle—before you begin twisting or tugging on your muscles and fascia. Those who join my class earlier are encouraged to stick to very gentle exercises and be especially easy with any core work. If the uterus isn't fully healed and back to pre-pregnancy size, you don't want to squish or tug on it in any way. If you begin to increase your activity and lochia either increases or becomes bright red again, back off. The body is asking for more time to rest. If the bleeding does not decrease, or if you are soaking through multiple pads, call a care provider immediately.

For those who give birth via cesarean, the timeline for returning to exercise is a little different. At the time of this writing the US cesarean rate is 31.8%,[65] which means 1 in 3 babies is born via surgery. Following this type of birth, the uterus is not only healing at the placenta attachment site but also recovering from an incision—as are the muscles and fascia of the abdominal wall. Most yoginis who give birth via cesarean are advised to wait 6-8 weeks before returning to the yoga mat, compared with 4-6 weeks for a vaginal birth.

I encourage students returning from a cesarean birth to get clearance from their OB before attempting a full yoga class (meaning level 1). There are just too many things that need to reconnect to be able to fully self-assess prior to the six-week mark. Again, this doesn't mean cesarean moms should not be moving up until that point. Some movement could actually be helpful! But the full activity of a general population yoga class doesn't take into account the specific changes involved in recovering from major abdominal surgery.

The golden month: "lying in" practices

Many non-Western traditions have a post-birth practice of deliberately resting and taking time to rejuvenate. Ayurveda—yoga's holistic health cousin—talks about preserving the "golden month" following the birth for the mother and baby. During this time the mother is nourished with warming foods and teas to rebalance her energy and restore her internal *dosha* balance as she takes care of the baby.

---

[65] Osterman, M. J. K., Hamilton, B. E., Martin, J. A., Driscoll, A. K., & Valenzuela, C. P. (2022, February 7). *National Vital Statistics reports - Centers for Disease Control and ...* National Vital Statistics Reports. https://www.cdc.gov/nchs/data/nvsr/nvsr70/nvsr70-02-508.pdf

Other cultures incorporate specific rituals such as "closing the bones" ceremonies or traditions of belly binding, where long strips of fabric are wound around the mother's abdomen to assist her body in regaining tone and containing the internal organs. These practices should not be conflated with the Western obsession with regaining a flat stomach or narrow waistline (cue eye roll). The focus is much more on containment, and for some women, the feeling is like having a constant hug around an area of their body which can feel quite disconnected post birth.

In contrast, Western culture often overlooks this time of rest for new parents. While it may seem nice to have a parade of visitors meeting your little one, it can leave you feeling exhausted—especially if you have to take on the role of host. Not to mention that babies are born with full personalities, and parents need the time and space to find out who the person they brought home actually is.

I often point out in my childbirth classes that the individual tasks of caring for a baby may not be all that trying in and of themselves. Sure, changing a diaper is a new experience, but it only takes a few minutes once you get the hang of it. The same goes for washing breast pump parts or changing yet another outfit covered in spit-up. But together, these tasks add up. And babies don't have an off switch; they typically eat every 2-3 hours, including through the night. On minimal sleep, the barrage of little tasks keeps coming. And we haven't even touched on the time mom will spend nursing if she decides to breastfeed! So when exactly are parents of a new baby supposed to wash dishes in preparation for a family visit?

To get the idea of how casual the immediate postpartum period might be, I offer a challenge to my childbirth education classes: after the baby comes home, see how many days you can go without wearing pants. After a few laughs, I find this begins to get the point across—of how inward this time is, how little activity should be expected. Incidentally, this is also a great test for deciding whether a friend or relative should come visit. If someone requests to come visit the baby, the answer might be "Sure! Oh, but I won't be wearing any pants." If the visitor balks, they aren't the right person to come by at this time. Maybe ask them to visit after you've had some time to adjust to your new baby.

(I should mention that I employed this 'no pants' time with the birth of my own son. While it was very helpful, my father might have been slightly uncomfortable with me being only half clothed: he spent quite a bit of time admiring the flowers people had dropped off. But he did his best and was still good emotional support. Times change, but I acknowledge that some grandparents may find it challenging to work around certain states of undress.)

Many couples opt to not have any visitors at all for several weeks. Others might employ a postpartum doula to support the family as they find their rhythm and settle in together. Remember, you're not the only one learning during this time; babies go through incredible changes during the first four weeks of their lives (and afterwards).

There could also be significant emotional processing you need to do after giving birth. While your birth experience may have been everything you wanted, it also may not have been. According to one study,[66] 34% of women report the birth process is either physically or mentally traumatic. Even the easiest birth requires time and healing.

Plus, there is a new dynamic between mom and partner. Who are they now as parents? The saying goes, "it takes a village to raise a child." But in our increasingly individualistic culture, moms are often left alone to cope with the dramatic shifts of their bodies and minds, along with the changing needs of their children.

The fourth trimester is a time of spiritual and mental groundlessness, referred to in some spiritual practices as a *bardo*. Everyone's sense of self is in a state of flux and rediscovery, and parents can completely lose both their competence and their compassion. Conversely, they may find aspects of themselves they didn't know existed. And this transformation doesn't stop when baby reaches the four-month mark. Birth changes us profoundly. At the same time, there is something that endures and remains amid the changes in body shape, movement ability, energy level, and identity. Where better to lean into yoga practice than at a time when your very sense of self seems to be shifting as well?

Leaning into yoga practice may simply mean reflecting on the incredible changes you have gone through or incorporating mindfulness into the everyday activities of childcare. I often joke (sort of) in Baby and Me yoga classes that any posture can become a yoga practice, but the most important posture we need to learn is the ancient pose of "holding baby *asana*" or that intense awareness practice of "changing diaper *maitri*." And don't forget the *vinyasa* of bouncing coupled with walking meditation and shushing *pranayama*! I mention these in jest, but the point is worthwhile—as new parents, our yoga has stepped off the mat. We must find ways to relax and practice without requiring the world to be perfect before doing so.

As the dust begins to settle and slightly more predictable patterns begin to emerge, movement and more formal *asana* practice may become possible. The first step might be taking a few minutes in one restorative posture at a time (often involving baby in the pose). But gradually, you may be drawn back to your mat, ready to explore this new body you have come into.

Working with awareness of how the body has shifted and focusing on balancing specific areas can help you find a sense of grounding, both physically and mentally. This is not about working out immediately after birth in an attempt to "get your body back." It's about developing functional strength and coordination as the body recovers from the immense physical task of growing and birthing a baby. No other physical endeavor of this magnitude comes without therapy protocols for recovering and returning to full function. Postpartum women have been shortchanged, but we can strive to do better.

Practices 0-6 weeks postpartum

As I mentioned earlier, please check with your care provider by phone before beginning any movement you feel concerned about. They know your pregnancy and birth story better than any book.

---

[66] Soet, J. E., Brack , G. A., & DiIorio, C. (2003, March). *Prevalence and predictors of women's experience of psychological trauma during childbirth.* Birth (Berkeley, Calif.). https://pubmed.ncbi.nlm.nih.gov/12581038/

The first six weeks after giving birth is a time of focused rest but not of total stillness. As you adjust to the requirements of caring for an infant, you can also begin recovering and caring for your healing body. I said it before, and I'll say it again: after a major surgery or even a major athletic event, there would be 1-2 weeks of dedicated rest, followed by exercises intended to help the body return to normal functioning. The same is true of birth.

With that in mind, you want to reconnect to your physiology in ways that will lead to lasting and maybe lifelong functionality, support, and strength. Many of the same exercises that you practiced during pregnancy to prepare the body for birth will serve you well here, with some variations.

Note: Many of these exercises (and many general exercise programs for the core) involve lying on the floor on your back. One of the biggest mistakes I see newly postpartum mothers make is rolling straight down along the spine, or worse, kicking the legs to sit straight up from the floor (or in bed). This action loads the front abdominal wall (rectus abdominis) without providing deeper support from beneath—a recipe for exacerbating or even creating abdominal separation (diastasis recti).

Please: STOP ROLLING STRAIGHT UP AND DOWN! To come to the floor, lay all the way down on your side, then roll to your back. Take the same pathway in reverse to get up. No more kicking up to sit up in bed! I know how tempting it is to do this at 3 am when you hear the baby cry. But the more you can remember to roll to the side first, the more you give your deep core a chance to engage, and the less chance you have of needing Depends later in life. It wasn't just a pregnancy thing; this is a lifelong practice.

Pelvic floor breathing

This exercise can be done lying in bed with your baby in the first few days post-birth. I use it in classes to help students reconnect with the pelvic floor and abdominal "soda can."

Come down onto your back by laying down on your side and then rolling to your back. Lying on your back (baby can sit or lie against your chest if they are with you), bend the knees and come into constructive rest. Allow the inner thighs to release towards the floor, bringing the spine into a neutral curve, and drop the floating ribs into the floor. It is also helpful to place a folded blanket, pillow, or yoga block beneath the head to support the chest and reduce flaring of the lower ribs.

With the pelvis and spine in neutral, begin to deepen the breathing, noticing if the breath can move into the lower abdomen and pelvic floor. It is important to realize that this is not a forced deep breath, nor are we manipulating the pelvic floor in this instance. The alignment of the body brings the invitation for the breath to move deeper and touch the pelvic floor. If this movement feels elusive, put a pillow under the knees to support the legs, and place a weight (like a heavy blanket, or a bag or rice) across the top of the thighs. The added pressure can help to further release the groins and bring the breath deeper into the pelvis.

Once the pelvic floor/lower abdomen begins to move, simply allow the body to breathe for several minutes. The internal movement of the diaphragms will begin to awaken the deeper core muscles, bringing them online for later work. If you don't release the muscles, you can't strengthen them.

Engaged TA breathing

Once you have a sense of the breath moving into the lower abdomen and pelvic floor, you can begin activating the deep core stabilizing muscles we will need as we move into progressive core work. Engaged TA breathing is useful when undertaking exercises which involve lifting either the legs or head. If the TA engagement collapses and can't be regained, it signals that the body is stressed beyond what the muscles can support. The exercise has either been done long enough or is too challenging at the moment; in either case, the next step is backing off or moving into an easier variation.

Lie on your back in constructive rest with a neutral spine. Inhale, feeling the lower abdomen and pelvic floor expand. On the exhale, rather than allowing things to passively re-engage, actively draw the perineum up into the pelvis. Feel the muscles between the hip points (ASIS bones) draw together and the navel pull up and in as though lifting towards the heart. It is as though the pelvic floor was again a jellyfish and it is swimming up the spine, drawing the surrounding walls up along with it.

On the inhale, see if about 50% of this deep abdominal engagement can be maintained (the breath still moves deeply, but the lower abdomen doesn't expand as fully). On the exhale, engage the pelvic floor and deep core further. The key here is that the breath continues to be full, not shallow—and definitely not held. We are NOT trying to suck the navel back to the spine and hold it. This is counterproductive, and reinforces the myth of a flat stomach being automatically strong—which it isn't always! Practice engaging the internal corset of support around the abdomen for several breaths, then inhale, allowing everything to release and open.

Note: If you have determined your pelvic floor is in a hypertonic state, it will be critical to do good pelvic floor breathing and maybe even one of the release stretches from Chapter 3 before attempting to engage the deep core muscles. A muscle in a chronically contracted state cannot provide further strength until it first releases. After releasing the muscles, many people find that they are actually far weaker than they would have expected.

Psoas release: constructive rest

Deep beneath the surface abdominal support you'll find the spinal guidewire of the psoas muscle. Possibly one of the most powerful and misunderstood muscles in the body, the psoas can become intensely compressed and stiff post-birth, largely due to the postural shifts during pregnancy and the positions often taken when caring for a new baby. This stiffness can lead to pelvic

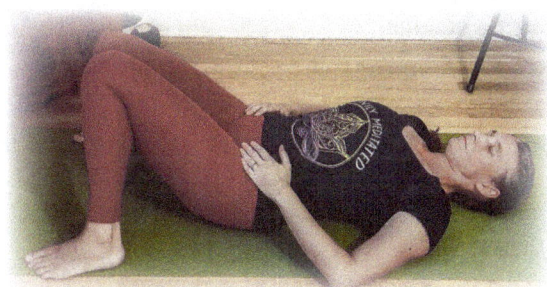

floor dysfunction, lower back tension, and a mismatch between abdominal diaphragmatic breathing and pelvic diaphragm movement. Psoas release is key to coordinating the back and deeper core muscles as well as relieving lower back tension and pain postpartum.

This release is more of an undoing than an active stretch. The psoas is intrinsically tied to our sense of safety and security, so forcing it to open usually results in resistance rather than lengthening. Having become contracted, the psoas needs a moment of rest in a slackened state to unwind internally. The trick with any release work is not to try too hard to let go. Release work is something we must allow. It cannot be forced or mentally willed into existence.

Begin by rolling to the side and coming onto your back. Bend the knees, and place the feet hip distance apart on the mat. Turning the toes slightly inward, allow the knees to rest against one another, creating a slight inward rotation in the thigh bones. A variation could be to place a yoga block (narrow width) between the upper thighs, allowing the femur bones to rest into the sides of the block. The pelvis should rest in neutral, with the lower back light but not lifted off the floor and the pubic bone dropped. If needed, place a pillow or yoga block under the head to relieve any neck tension or flaring of the lower ribcage.

Once the knees and hips are in position, place the fingers softly against the front hip points (the ASIS bones) with only the weight of the fingers resting (not pressing down). I once heard it described as having the weight of a nickel on the hip crease. With this subtle weight drawing attention to the groin area, inhale into the belly, and on the exhale focus on softening the space where the thigh and pelvis meet one another. It is as though dropping the upper most inner thigh section. There will be no movement of the pelvis, but you may feel a heaviness in the pelvis as the muscles let go. Rest here for 5-10 minutes if possible, allowing the architecture of the pose and the body's natural tendency to find internal balance to do the work for you.

Psoas stretch on a block or floor

I recommend waiting on this exercise until 3-4 weeks postpartum, especially if you have a cesarean birth, because the extended leg pulls across the lower abdominal fascia. Alternatively, you can practice this exercise earlier by removing the block and placing the hips flat on the floor.

Having softened the psoas and hip flexors in constructive rest, we can move into a more targeted stretch for the psoas muscle itself. This release involves using gravity to gently lengthen the front hip flexors and was also employed in the section on basic daily movement during pregnancy.

Note: If you experienced dysfunction or pain in the pubic bone during pregnancy and are less than three months postpartum or still breastfeeding, this pose should be done with caution and very gently. The asymmetry involved in stretching one side at a time can further strain a joint which remains loose for a while after birth. Check with a pelvic floor physical therapist before jumping into hanging asymmetrical stretches like this one.

Beginning in constructive rest, lift the hips and place a yoga block or rolled blanket beneath the sacrum (the yoga block should be on the lowest height). On an exhale, bring one knee in towards the chest, holding with both hands. On an exhale, extend the opposite leg out along the mat, reaching as far as possible. The knee may or may not straighten depending on the hip flexibility. Draw the lifted knee actively in towards the chest to increase the stretch, while at the same time imagine a weight pressing the extended thigh down towards the ground.

To focus even further into the psoas, internally rotate the extended leg so the groin deepens towards the floor. Breathe and hold the stretch for as long as feels comfortable—usually about a minute. To change sides, gently bring the extended leg into the chest and feel the difference between the two hips. Give the body a chance to absorb the change before stretching the second leg out and down towards the floor.

Pelvic rocking

Pelvic rocking is a great exercise for restoring spinal mobility and fluidity and for recruiting the subtle proprioceptive muscles that stabilize the deep core. This exercise, and the pelvic clock which follows, begin to engage the front abdominal muscles, the psoas and other spinal stabilizers, the deep glutes, and the pelvic floor.

For pelvic rocking, begin on your back in constructive rest with the knees bent and the spine in neutral. Inhale to release, then exhale and engage the supporting core muscles as described in the engaged TA breathing exercise.

With the deep core engaged, inhale and gently tip the pelvis forward so the top of the sacrum lifts slightly and the tailbone moves towards the floor. Maintain 50% engagement of the TA muscles throughout this movement. From the tilt, on the exhale, tuck the pelvis backwards, pressing the lower back into the mat and drawing the abdomen in and up towards the heart further engaging the TA.

The pelvic floor can be recruited as well, but because of the tuck of the tail the alignment does not lend itself to good overall engagement. The action engages the surface abdominals while the TA muscles support them from beneath. Be sure the upper spine remains fairly steady (no bottom ribs popping up and down) and the neck and shoulders remain quiet. On the inhale, maintain the core engagement and tilt the pelvis forward once again.

Repeat this movement 10 times, then take a break and allow the lower abdomen to release with the breath.

Pelvic rocking with a block

To help connect the lower muscle chain a bit further, place a block between the knees while in constructive rest. On the pelvic tilt, simply hold the block lightly, but on the exhale, tuck and squeeze the block actively with the inner thighs, feeling the action move up the core body. This action helps engage the adductor muscles that are fascially connected to the second layer of the pelvic floor. Continue with these motions, easing the pressure on the tilt, then re-engaging it on the tuck.

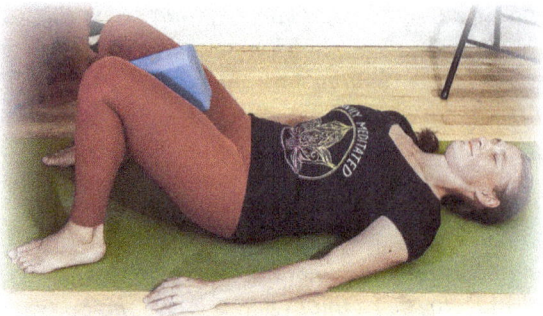

I recommend reserving this variation for when you are 4-6 weeks postpartum. Until then, use the gentler variation without the block. This action develops awareness of pelvic placement and begins recruiting the surface abdominal muscles, but it is not a progression into crunches or other head lifting exercises.

Pelvic clock

After getting used to the pelvic tilt, you can further develop proprioception (awareness of the body's placement in space) and pelvic stability by making more circular movements. I first encountered this exercise in a Feldenkrais Method® class in college and have since found it exceptionally helpful for creating deep core awareness, particularly for those with sacral instability or SI joint pain.

Begin lying on the back in constructive rest, lightly holding a block between the knees. The aim here is not to squeeze the block but to simply hold it for reference so the movement does not drift up into the knees.

From constructive rest, imagine an analog clock on the abdomen, with 12 o'clock at the navel, 6 o'clock at the pubic bone, 3 o'clock at one hip point and 9 o'clock at the other. Exhale and engage the TA and pelvic floor muscles as described above. Inhale and begin as you would for pelvic tilt, rocking towards the pubic bone, then exhale, tucking the tail to press the navel towards the floor.

From the tuck, and with the breath in a neutral rhythm, begin to circle around the "clock," moving from 12 to 3, to 6, and so on. Imagine rolling a marble around the circumference of the clock until you get back to the 12 position. This action will require one hip to press slightly into the floor while the other lifts up as you pass by the 3 and 9 o'clock positions. Continue circling clockwise several times, moving slowly and purposefully rather than moving as fast as possible.

After maybe five rotations, reverse the direction and roll the "marble" counter clockwise. The whole time, keep the knees as stationary as possible, and maintain the deep TA engagement, making sure the breath remains deep as well. At the end of the last circle, bring the pelvis to neutral and let the abdomen and pelvic floor release with the breath. Notice the effect of the exercise. Repeat if you like.

I have noticed, both in myself and in my students, that there are places on the circle which move very smoothly and other places where things feel almost stuck or uncoordinated. The circles may also feel different in one direction than the other. The movement may feel smooth moving from 6 to 9, but moving from 9 to 6 feels jerky and uncoordinated. This is good information, as it can illuminate where a joint might be out of alignment or where the stabilizing muscles of the glutes, obliques, and pelvic floor are not well integrated and thus not able to provide adequate support.

These foundational exercises can help bring awareness and integration into the deep core, the muscles closest to the internal organs which connect to the spine and support the torso. Good engagement at this level ensures that subsequent exercises target and develop the functional strength we need for lifelong health.

Prone breathing/Crocodile breathing

A way to access the pelvic floor, support the stretched-out front abdominal muscles, and begin gently opening the chest and shoulders is to rest on the stomach with the hands folded under the head, allowing the breath to move down into the abdomen and pelvis. The lift of the arms brings a subtle backbend into the thoracic spine—helpful for combatting "new parent posture." The soft pressure on the abdomen from the floor helps to contain the front abdominal wall and move the breath into the pelvic floor, promoting better function.

Begin this practice on a bed or other soft surface. If you are recovering from a cesarean birth, you should also wait 2-3 weeks after giving birth to undertake this exercise. The healing incision tissue can be sensitive and tender, and you want to give the tissue time to rethread.

Coming to your side, roll gently to face down on the bed or yoga mat. Allow the legs to softly rest on the floor, and see how it feels to be resting on the abdomen. It may have been sever- 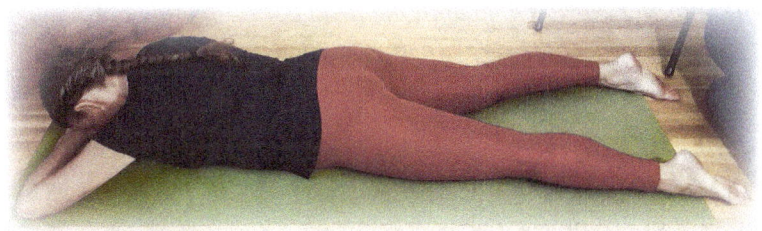 *al months since you were able to lie in this position. Bring the arms up and fold the hands under your forehead to rest the head in a neutral position. For those who feel tenderness in the breasts (which is common in the first few weeks), place a pillow under your shoulders to support the breasts away from the bed.*

Rest forward and feel the abdomen softly pressing into the bed or floor on the inhale, then receding on the exhale. Notice if you can also feel movement in between the sitz bones in the pelvic floor. This may be subtle for some, and we are not yet working with any pelvic floor engagement or toning. Simply let the breath and the positioning do the work.

When ready to come out, either bring the hands under the shoulders and press back into a wide knee Child's Pose or roll to your side and use your hands to press up to sit.

Slouchy Sphinx

This variation of Sphinx pose allows for further release into the upper spine—and is a nice modification for those with extremely tender breasts.

From Crocodile pose, walk the elbows back so they rest just ahead of the shoulders, with the upper arms perpendicular to the ground so they prop the shoulders and chest up off the floor.

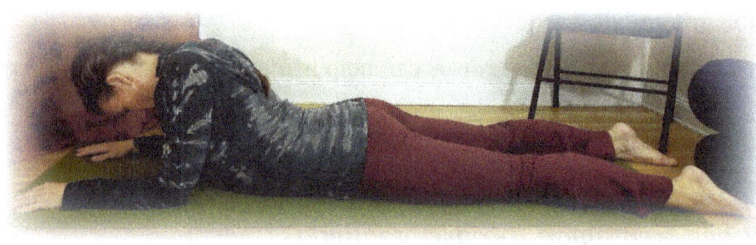

From this position, allow the shoulders to slump upwards towards the ears, sinking the upper back spine into a valley between the shoulder blades. Let the head and neck truly hang from the collar bones, sinking into the force of gravity. The feeling is of the thoracic spine hanging from the shoulders like the tension lines of a large suspension bridge.

With each inhale the ribcage can expand, and then with each exhale the spine can sink further. Because the roots of the neck muscles rest in between the shoulder blades, the hanging head and neck help to further release this area of chronic tension.

When ready to come out, instead of simply lifting the head from the chin, focus on beginning the lift from deep within the mid-back, as if your neck started at your bra line. Slowly draw the spine forward and up until the head floats up and back, as though you were being lifted from the backs of the ears. Then walk the elbows forward, returning to Crocodile, and either push back to Child's Pose or roll to the side.

Upper back bolster

This is perhaps one of my favorite exercises postpartum, and one which I teach in nearly every postnatal yoga class. This pose combines the passive spinal release of Slouchy Sphinx with a restorative pose and chance for stillness. And with slight modifications, it can be done while holding a baby.

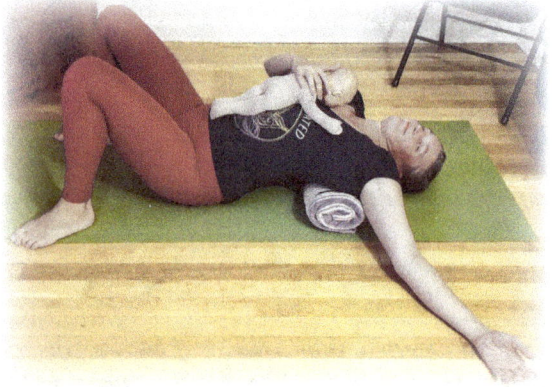

Begin by taking a yoga blanket or large beach towel and rolling it up into a moderate-sized bolster. The exact height will depend on your own body's tension and what feels workable for you as you begin to practice. For some moms, using a barely folded blanket is sufficient. Others have gone so far as replacing the rolled towel with a foam roller. The key is that you are able to breathe easily while resting. If the sensation is disturbing your breathing, lower the bolster.

Place your blanket roll about a foot behind you. Slide to your side, lowering your armpit onto the bolster (you could also hang out here for additional shoulder release), and then softly roll onto your back so the bolster sits roughly under the base of the shoulder blades. I often find having a yoga block or pillow under my head helps me ease into the stretch, and after a minute or two I am able to remove it to let my neck hang back.

If you are holding a baby, they can lie on your chest or sit up against bent knees on your lap. If you are not holding a baby, however, allow the arms to spread out from the shoulders in a "T" position. Feel the weight of the arms gently pull the shoulders down—as though someone were lightly pressing down on the heads of your arm bones. Check in with the breath, and feel how the body is responding to this passive backbend. If the lower back begins to hurt, bend the knees to release the psoas muscle. If this does not alleviate the discomfort, press the feet into the floor to float the pelvis and gently tuck the tail to release the contracting muscles. Having released them, see if you can float the pelvis back down to the floor. For many students, this lift-tuck-lower action is a periodic vinyasa as they rest, while the lower back figures out that it doesn't have to be holding quite so much. For others it is necessary to place a folded blanket beneath the pelvis to pad the sacrum against the floor.

This exercise is often surprising for new parents, who aren't aware of how stiff their upper spines have become until they are asked to bend. I remember lying back over a bolster several weeks after birthing my son and suddenly exclaiming, "Oh my God!" as I saw the difference only three weeks had made. Be patient. The body will remember its natural flexibility again.

To come out, avoid sitting straight up (yes, even if the baby is crying) because of the excessive strain that can place on a healing abdominal wall. Instead, bend the knees and roll to one side (hold baby to you if they are on your body). From the side, use your hands to press the floor away to come up to sit.

Use these exercises to rediscover how the body is functioning post birth and to relieve the tension patterns which develop from the daily demands of taking care of a newborn. From these foundational practices, you can gradually work back into more demanding asana, provided you can maintain stability and coordination.

Neck and shoulder rolls

Modern culture is plagued with activities that round the shoulders and pull the head forward, and very few of us take the time to pause and truly stretch the neck and shoulder muscles. This is even more true for new parents who have slumped into the "new parent" posture, with the muscles of the upper back and neck constantly pulled into a long and taut position. I confess I myself was guilty of not paying enough attention to my own upper back and neck during the hours of writing this book. It just doesn't come into our awareness when we're focused on other things (like a baby).

See if this sounds familiar: the shoulders and neck curl forward around the infant in your arms; the upper back slouches; the spine flexes; and, in some cases, the hips tuck under. It is almost as though adults are trying to create the same primary curve present in the baby's spine. And this posture is often held for multiple minutes, if not hours, at a time. If you were regularly working out pre-baby, I doubt you would ever go to the gym and hold a 10 lb weight in the crook of your arm for 30 minutes or more at a stretch—or while bouncing up and down.

Fortunately, neck and shoulder rolls are exercises that can be done almost anywhere, even with a newborn baby in your arms. You can even do them right now while you're reading!

Sit up (or stand), lift your gaze to focus across the room, and let the shoulders drop. Now with gentle movement, bring the right ear towards the right shoulder until you feel a stretch on the left neck muscles (we are not going for a chiropractic adjustment here, just a gentle stretch). Maintaining an upright spine, softly roll the chin towards the chest, feeling how the stretch moves around the base of the neck. From the chin on the chest, roll the left ear towards the left shoulder and observe the tension. Keep the chest lifted the whole time.

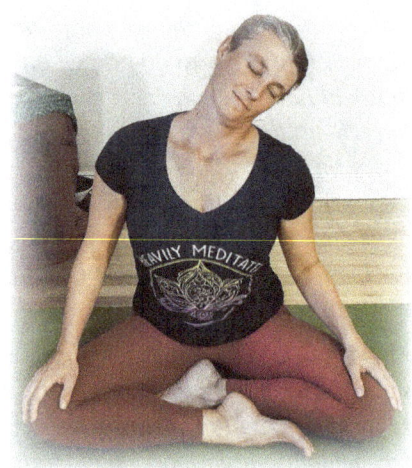

You can repeat this half circle or take the head towards the back and around to the right again into a full neck roll. If you are doing this holding a baby, give them a big smile as your head comes around their direction. *Babies often enjoy facial expressions, learning how to interact from the adults around them. Be sure to reverse the circling at some point.*

If you have the time, pick the shoulders up and circle them around to the back, squeezing the shoulder blades together. Then shift them down and forward before lifting them up and back again. We want to find the full circle, but emphasize the chest opening action, since we spend much of the day rounded forward. If you are holding a baby, you might need to roll one shoulder at a time—which is equally effective.

If your arms are free, an additional (and delicious) addition to the shoulder circle is to incorporate the arms into the movement. Begin by circling the elbows back, pausing in the back quadrant with the fingers up like goal-post arms to feel the opening across the front chest. Then continue the circling, gradually involving the whole arm.

I highly recommend this action following any long period of holding baby, whether that be a feeding session or just bouncing them to sleep.

Calf stretches

The calf stretch doesn't lose its value after the baby is born. Just as the back leg line can become tense during pregnancy, the same is true, and more so, postpartum. With the sheer amount of time spent in seated positions, it is not uncommon for people who have spent six weeks postpartum not moving their bodies to come back to the mat and discover their entire calf/hamstring/glute movement line is locked down.

Work calf stretching into everyday activities rather than trying to find time to do it as an individual practice. Place a rolled towel somewhere convenient around the house, and stand with the toes on the roll and the heel on the floor for about 30 seconds several times during the day. Little self-care movements can make an enormous difference in the immediate postpartum period.

Walking

While we are on the subject of stretching the calves, walking is a beautiful way to return to movement. We are not talking about power walking or even low-level cardio here. You simply need to get the body moving. Start by walking around the house (cesarean moms, be cautious of stairs for the first few weeks), then transition to taking short walks outside for a bit of fresh air. Research has shown that being in nature, getting natural light, and finding time for gentle movement can have a positive effect on postpartum emotions and overall mood.[67] If you are able to get a good friend to walk with you (someone who understands that you'll need a very slow pace), you'll get the added benefit of social interaction and community!

Returning to yoga practice

The most common question I get from prenatal yoga students is "When can I start practicing yoga again?" Whether you want to reconnect with a community, alleviate aches and pains, or manage repetitive stress injuries you've acquired during the early weeks with your newborn, the postpartum period is a great time to reincorporate yoga! The key is to move appropriately so the body can re-establish its own functional movement patterns.

It is important to think of returning to the mat as a holistic process, not a test of how much your body can do. Not every yoga student will need to wait six weeks to return to more involved exercises, but some may. As you move into coordinated movements aimed at strength building and classic asana, you want to respect the other demands on your body: milk production, sleep recovery, and learning newborn cues and cries, to name just a few. I recommend waiting 4-6 weeks post-birth (6-8 post-cesarean) before popping into a postnatal yoga class. Your postpartum lochia should be complete, and you should be free of other postpartum complications before you begin strengthening and fully re-balancing the system.

But this doesn't mean that you should think of postpartum yoga as just a generic level one class, possibly done with a baby. The postpartum body needs attention in specific areas which need to be in balance before you resume regular practice. If you take the time to fully connect your movements, your center, and yourself, then when you do return to your pre-pregnancy yoga class you can do so not only with confidence but maybe even stronger than before you became pregnant!

---

[67] Coventry, P. A., Brown, J. V. E., Pervin, J., Brabyn, S., Pateman, R., Breedvelt, J., Gilbody, S., Stancliffe, R., McEachan, R., & White, P. C. L. (2021, October 1). *Nature-based outdoor activities for mental and Physical Health: Systematic Review and meta-analysis.* SSM - Population Health. https://www.sciencedirect.com/science/article/pii/S2352827321002093?via%3Dihub

Areas of focus for postnatal yoga

Full core body

When I say core, I am not only talking about the muscles on the front of the abdominal wall. The core in this case refers to the deep support of the transverse abdominals, back muscles, pelvic floor, psoas muscle, and abdominal diaphragm; the network of muscles which actually attach to the spine and support the internal organs and structure.

Upper back

Along with the back muscles along the core, the upper back also needs attention. These muscles are often both long and tight from the "new parent slouch." Long, tight muscles are also weak, so the area between the shoulder blades and back of the shoulders needs to be released and strengthened.

Neck and shoulders

The neck muscles originate in the upper back, so they too are affected by the new parent slouch. I get requests for neck and shoulder releases in nearly every postnatal yoga class I teach.

Hips

The base of the core body is supported by the glutes and hip stabilizers. These muscles can become progressively tight and under-recruited from long hours of sitting or standing and swaying with a baby. Balancing the strength and tone of the glutes and other hip muscles can help yoginis return to more challenging *asana* and other forms of movement.

The postures and exercises you practice postpartum will depend on how far out you are from birth, the type of birth you had, and your ability to connect the different parts of the body to one another. Working back into certain levels of core exercises in particular may require waiting until you have developed deeper support.

Core body

The core body allows for coordination between the various muscle groups that bring support for more complicated yoga *asana* and other movement. During pregnancy, these muscles had to make dramatic shifts. Now, without the weight of the uterus and baby, they need to redefine their role. This means coordinating movement from the pelvic floor up while considering where the body might have developed tension or become weak. To function optimally, the core must support the front, side, back, top, and base of the body and be able to shift, twist, and jump without losing support for the organs contained therein.

While core exercises are important for good body function, avoid jumping back into vigorous exercise too quickly. There is a hyperfocus in the fitness world on returning to pre-pregnancy weight and restoring that "flat stomach" (which, did you really have that before pregnancy anyway?). This is a time of rediscovery and exploration of your new postpartum body. It was not just the baby's body that was created through the pregnancy. Your body was also remade in a new image.

While I fully understand the desire to get back to the body you had before (I still long for my pre-pregnancy abdomen!), it might be more compassionate and a little more realistic to find ways to acknowledge, if not love, the body you have now. And to those who achieved their "pre-pregnancy shape," that's wonderful! I hope that in doing so, you also found deep strength and compassion for who you are now.

Dealing with diastasis recti

Before diving back into core exercises, it is worth discovering for yourself how well the front abdominal wall stayed intact during pregnancy. For some bodies, the stretch and increased load during pregnancy on the linea alba of the rectus abdominis is more than the fascia can sustain, resulting in a separation known as diastasis recti. A study in 2016[68] found that as many as 60% of women in the US may emerge from pregnancy with a separation of their front abdominal line. Diastasis recti can occur anywhere along the linea alba, from pubic bone to the xiphoid process at the junction with the ribcage. For some it is fairly minor, and for others it is a wide split covering the entire front line. If you are working with diastasis recti it is crucial to support the surface abdominals and pay attention to places where the deep core is either not supporting (belly hangs) or is bracing outward rather than in and upwards as it is intended to (tenting during abdominal exercises).

To find out if there is a separation, lie on your back in constructive rest and place four fingers across the abdomen at the belly button with the fingers pointed at the pubic bone. Relaxing the abdominal wall, press down into the body towards the floor gently but firmly. (Yes, this will feel weird!) Keeping the pressure and the finger pressing down into the abdomen, exhale and lift 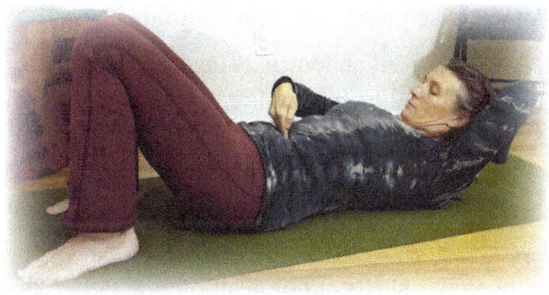 the head and shoulders as high as possible. This is for diagnostic purposes only, and not what you want to be doing when practicing!

With the head lifted, feel with the fingers around the belly button. Is there a firm muscle on the side? Then, palpating towards the center, is there a place where things seem to drop or a ridge where the muscle seems to end? This would be one side of a separation. Feeling across to the other side, see if you can find the other ridge. Diastasis recti severity is measured by how many fingers would fit between those two ridges. 1? 2? 3? More? If I am working with a student who is less than eight weeks postpartum I don't worry too much about a widening of

[68] Sperstad JB, Tennfjord MK, Hilde G, Ellström-Engh M, Bø K. Diastasis recti abdominis during pregnancy and 12 months after childbirth: prevalence, risk factors and report of lumbopelvic pain. *Br J Sports Med.* 2016;50(17):1092-1096. doi:10.1136/bjsports-2016-096065

two fingers or less, since with good abdominal toning and body mechanics, that may come back together. Someone with more than two fingers width however, I usually refer out for pelvic floor PT to augment their yoga practice. For some a two finger separation will come back together on its own, but I find that most students need to do some proactive modifications and mindful movement to ensure they regain the deeper control to bring this layer back together.

If dealing with an abdominal separation, you'll want to splint the surface abdominals to avoid making the split wider while regaining deeper control. Splinting can be done with a scarf, belt, or yoga strap wrapped around from the back and crossed over the abdomen at the widest point of the separation. Holding the scarf in each hand, on an exhale, pull the scarf tight around the abdomen. At the same time activate the TA muscles. The action of the scarf is to assist the muscles in bringing the surface together (as a spotter would in weight lifting at a gym). The scarf helps ensure that if the deep core becomes overloaded the force of the exercise doesn't shift into the separated abdominal layer. That said, the splint is a tool—not a crutch. So when using a splint, practice actively drawing away from the band rather than allowing the core to bulge into it.

Core exercises (beginning at 4-6 weeks postpartum)

The following exercises are intended to be introduced after practicing the immediate postpartum movements and after clearance from a care provider. At 4-6 weeks postpartum, you can begin adding on to exercises such as the pelvic clock and pelvic tilt (see pgs 305-306). The trick is to add the right amount of intensity; the deep core must stay stable and engaged.

An exercise may be too challenging if:

- The front abdominals push away from the center abdominal line (a phenomenon referred to as "tenting," where the abs lift upwards like the dome of a camping tent
- The pelvis shifts on the floor, rocking either right or left, (a signal that the obliques and transverse abdominals have not fully engaged), or
- The lower back begins to arch away from the floor (a sign that the psoas muscles are doing too much stabilizing)

If the pelvis shifts out of position, the pelvic floor is not able to offer adequate support, since the pelvic floor is strongest when the spine is neutral.

I recommend beginning with a few rounds of engaged TA breathing, pelvic rocking, and pelvic clock to awaken your inner awareness of the current pelvic position. Then progress into the following exercises. Note that none of these exercises involves lifting the head. Head lifts use the surface muscles of the rectus abdominis, which is the muscle group most likely to be overstretched during pregnancy. We'll get to these muscles, but only after we've awakened the deep core support.

Pelvic floor core exercises

Many of the exercises in the immediate postnatal time frame are focused on the pelvic floor. That's because without the floor, we can't build the walls or start embellishing the ceiling.

We need a strong foundation, and that strength comes from unwinding chronic tension and then building awareness from the ground up. The work you do during pregnancy isn't just for birth preparation; these exercises promote good lifelong habits, which translate into better movement coordination, less pain, and greater ease in returning to the yoga mat postpartum.

Pelvic floor breathing (review)

Lying on your back, bend the knees and come into constructive rest. Allow the inner thighs to release towards the floor, bringing the spine into a neutral curve, and drop the floating ribs into the floor. It is also helpful to place a folded blanket, pillow, or yoga block beneath the head to support the chest and reduce flaring of the lower ribs.

With the pelvis and spine in neutral, begin to deepen the breathing, noticing if the breath can move into the lower abdomen and pelvic floor. It is important to realize that this is not a forced deep breath, nor are you manipulating the pelvic floor in this instance. The alignment of the body brings the invitation for the breath to move deeper and touch the pelvic floor.

If this movement feels elusive, put a pillow under the knees to support the legs and place a weight (like a heavy blanket or a bag or rice) across the top of the thighs. The added pressure can help to further release the groins and bring the breath deeper into the pelvis. Allow the body to breathe for several minutes, then continue on.

Pelvic floor contraction

A longer version of this exercise can be found on pg 55.

Beginning with the pelvis in neutral, bring your attention to the space bounded by the sitz bones, pubis, and tailbone. As with the relaxed pelvic breathing, on an inhale, allow these muscles to relax and expand downward—possibly feeling the sitz bones widen slightly. On the exhale, actively draw all four points of the diamond towards the middle while lifting in the center at the perineum. The motion involves a contraction of the vaginal, anal, and urethral sphincters, as though you were picking up a pearl with the walls of the vagina. On the inhale, allow the muscles to release the pearl back downwards, feeling the pelvic floor spread once again.

Depending on the manner of your baby's birth, your movements post labor, and the relative tone of your pelvic floor before giving birth, you may find that postpartum you are more tense, more loose, or more uncoordinated than before. (To self assess your pelvic floor tone, visit the external pelvic floor massage instructions on pg 53-54.)

Hypertonic postnatal exercises

For those who find themselves on the tighter side, here are two simple exercises to prepare the pelvic floor for postpartum core work. Approach these movements gently and put your attention on bringing the breath deeper into the body rather than on finding deep stretch. This is generally accomplished by finding the alignment between the abdominal and pelvic diaphragm domes.

Overly tense pelvic floor muscles are quite common postpartum, especially for those who gave birth by cesarean. It's critical to get these muscles to release before trying to make them contract or bear weight. Remember, a muscle that is constantly tense can't contract further. Additional exercises for stretching overly tight pelvic floor muscles can be found on pgs 62-69 in chapter 3.

Prasarita Padottanasana with internal thigh rotation

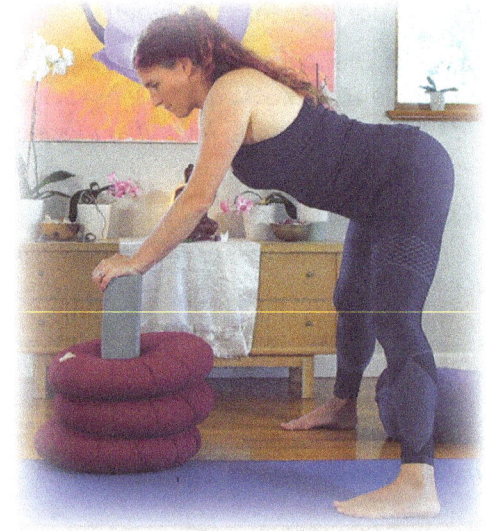

Step the feet wide, perhaps 3-4 feet apart, turning the toes slightly in and the heels out. Bending the knees and hinging from the hips, place the hands on a tall support. The goal here is not increasing range of motion (i.e., being able to touch the floor) but maintaining a neutral spine and moving solely from the hips. This will require elevating the hands on either tall height blocks or possibly a chair.

With the back long, lift the sitz bones without dropping the front ribcage to find a neutral spine. Focus on the feeling between the sitz bones, and allow the tissue there to soften and expand on the inhale. On the exhale, let that remain open. If you can't feel the breath in the perineum, check the alignment of rib cage to pelvis and try bending the knees a bit more while lifting the tail slightly. The feeling might be like a cool widening between the sitz bones rather than a pulling sensation.

Half Happy Baby

Since you are no longer pregnant, we can resume postures which are fully supine, which brings back Happy Baby, a pose that can help breathe space into the pelvic floor while stretching the glutes and hips. A caution to those with stitches post birth: please do not attempt this *asana* until all tissues have fully healed and the stitches have dissolved or been removed.

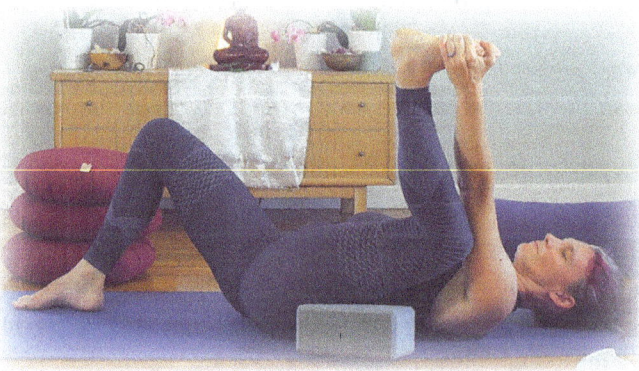

Coming to lie on your back with the knees in constructive rest, place a yoga block on the right side of your hip next to your waist. Bring the right knee in towards the chest, holding the back of the thigh with the hands. With the knee in, shift the knee towards the armpit and shoulder so the thigh presses the block (raise the height

to be workable for you), swinging the heel of the foot towards the ceiling. The leg is working to come to a 90 degree angle if possible.

If it works for your body, reach up along the inside of the lifted leg to grab either the inside of the ankle or the outside edge of the foot. It is also fine to continue holding the back of the knee, as the focus is not on the foot but on the hip. With the leg in position, rotate the pelvis to bring the right sitting bone and tailbone towards the floor. The action of bringing the leg in while tipping the pelvis forward lengthens the front to back fibers of the pelvic floor, while the slight lateral position of the thigh can access the sideways fibers of the perineum. The block under the lifted thigh helps anchor the pelvis down rather than allowing it to rock backwards and tuck under.

Breathe in this position for a few minutes, feeling the breath come low in the body. Then release the knee and hug both legs into the chest before switching to the second side.

Hypotonic postnatal pelvic floor exercises

To further engage the pelvic floor muscles in addition to the engaged "jellyfish" breathing of Mula Bhanda (pg 61) we can also revisit the inner and outer thigh toning exercises from the pelvic floor chapter. You can modify these exercises by sitting on the edge of a chair with good hip alignment (weight on the front of the sitting bones).

Adductor engagement

Sit on a firm chair or yoga ball with the knees at or below the level of the pelvis and the feet planted firmly on the floor. Place the weight on the front of the sitting bones so the pelvic bowl comes into neutral and stretch the spine gently upwards. With the pelvis balanced, place a yoga block between the inner thighs.

In your own time but following the tempo of your breathing, lightly pulse the knees against the yoga block, activating the adductor muscles of the inner thighs. The goal is to pulse for about 60 seconds to begin, then give the legs a break. Keep the toes relaxed on the floor. Relax and inhale, allowing the pelvic floor to drop, then exhale and engage upwards as though lifting something with the walls of the vagina, or like a jellyfish swimming upwards. What sort of response do you get?

Abductor engagement

Sit once again on the chair with the weight forward on the sitting bones. Take a yoga strap (or a scarf or belt if you lack an actual strap), and buckle it into a circle around the mid-thighs so it provides some resistance to the outside of the leg. It's important not to place the belt too high or too close to the knees.

Gently stretching the spine upright and relaxing the toes, begin to pulse the thighs outwards into the strap in time to your breathing. Focus on moving the upper thigh bones apart, as though trying to fit a yoga block back between the legs, rather than simply pushing the knees apart against the strap. It may also feel as though the sitz bones are trying to spread apart.

Pulse out with about 50% of the effort you think you could for 60 seconds, then relax and repeat. Try inhaling and letting the pelvic floor drop, then exhale and actively lift up and in, like a jellyfish swimming up through the water. What do you feel here?

Progressive postnatal core exercises

With the pelvic floor online and responsive, you can finally move on to the abdomen! We're still working on the deep center here, but the surface muscles can now join the party. Most of these exercises begin in constructive rest with knees bent and spine in a neutral position. Back floating ribs are in contact with the floor and should stay that way throughout the exercises. It may help to bolster up the head and shoulders with a folded blanket or pillow to reduce flaring of the front ribcage. Once positioned, activate engaged TA breathing before beginning the exercise.

Single knee lifts

In this exercise the lower leg stays on the floor, offering additional support if the deep core is not yet ready to bear the full weight of the single leg. If even this feels too challenging, stick with the pelvic rocking and pelvic clock exercises .

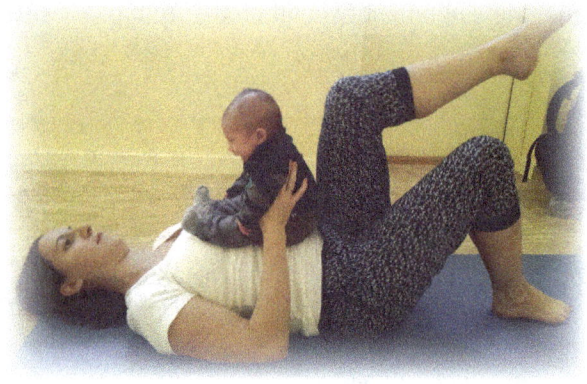

Lie in constructive rest with knees bent, spine in a neutral position, and the head supported. Baby can sit or lie on your belly if needed.

Begin engaged TA breathing to coordinate the deep core muscles.

On an exhale, draw in the pelvic floor and raise one leg to 90 degrees over your hip, keeping the knee bent. Maintain a level pelvis and avoid shifting from left to right. The goal is that the pelvis does not move at all. Keep the side waist drawn in around the middle and the navel moving in and up towards the heart. Watch for any abdominal "tenting," and return the foot to the floor if this can't be avoided. Inhale to return the foot to the floor, and repeat on the second side.

The action becomes a stepping motion, lifting and lowering each leg individually. The pace is meant to be slow, following the breath, which is better for building muscle stamina.

Heel slide variation

From the single knee lift, you can add a leg movement to recruit deeper pelvic and core stabilization. Unlike the previous exercises, this variation sticks to one side for several repetitions before switching to the other leg. This movement is adapted from a Pilates exercise, but it should be noted that the breath is not held or pulsed in any way.

Beginning with a single leg lift, exhale to engage the pelvic floor and raise one leg to a 90 degree bend off the floor. On an inhale, maintaining the core stability, bring the lifted heel to the floor and slide the foot out to extend the leg while pressing the heel into the ground as you slide. The feeling is as though pushing something heavy with the foot. Reach fully through the heel, elongating the leg at the top of the inhale.

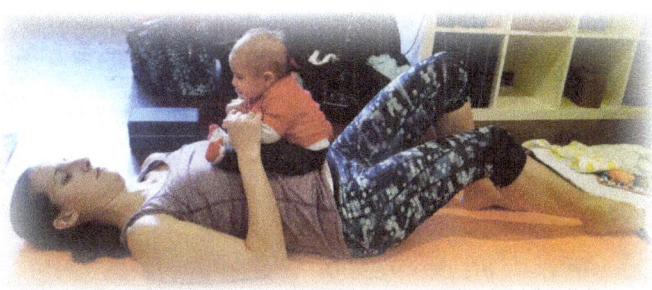

Having extended the hip, on the exhale, slide the heel back against the ground, resisting the movement either internally or by

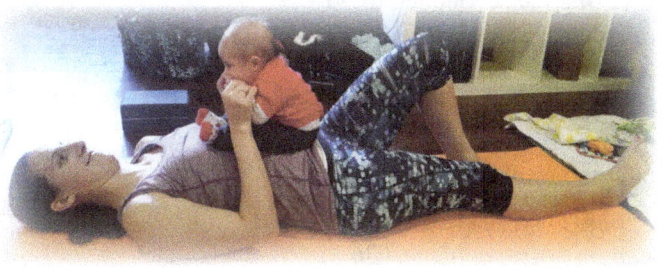

placing a hand or yoga block against the moving thigh. The aim is to create some resistance while maintaining the existing pelvic stability throughout the whole movement. As the heel draws towards the sitz bone, imagine the pelvic floor is drawing the foot in and up. Once the heel is so close it cannot move further, raise the leg back to the 90 degree bend.

Through the whole movement the pelvis remains stable and the abdominal wall continues to lift in and up with the ribs remaining quiet. Repeat the heel slide five times on the right side before switching to the left leg, and make sure you continue breathing. If the abdominals begin to "tent" or the pelvis wobbles during the movement, the body may not yet be ready for this level of challenge.

After completing five repetitions on each leg, return to constructive rest and allow the core to release on an inhale. Pause to feel the impact on the body before moving on.

Double knee lifts

This progression would be appropriate when the single leg lift can be performed with ease for several repetitions and the heel slide can be done with stability.

Beginning in constructive rest, begin engaged TA breathing. On an exhale, raise one leg to the 90 degree bend. Inhale and hold the foot in the air.

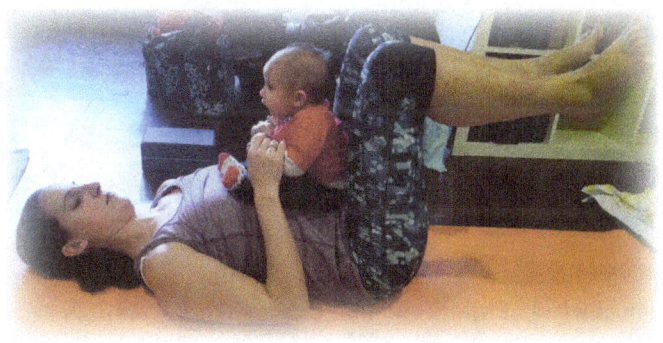

On the NEXT exhale draw the pelvic floor in more strongly and raise the second leg off the floor, bringing it alongside the first leg. The second raise will load the lower abdominals and pelvic floor further. The pelvis should not wobble, the ribs should remain quiet, and the navel should continue to draw in and up towards the heart (no tenting).

If lifting both legs feels manageable, then on the next exhale, slowly lower both feet back to the mat, maintaining the core engagement. Then repeat, lifting the opposite leg first.

Double knee lift progression

If lifting the second leg to 90 degrees feels steady and supported, a further progression of this exercise is to make the lifted leg position the starting position and tap the toes from there.

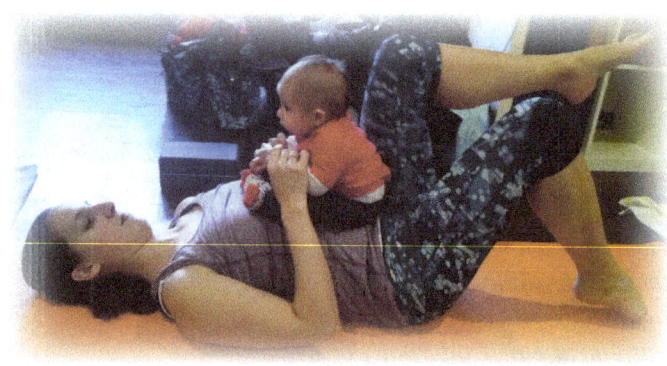

Exhale to lift the first leg. Inhale to pause, then exhale to lift the second leg to come into the new starting position. From this legs-up position, inhale to tap one toe to the floor, and immediately lift it back into the air on the exhale. Then repeat the same movement with the second leg. The result is a marching movement, but instead of starting from the floor, the legs hover in the air.

The real challenge of this movement isn't lifting the leg but switching from side to side. The obliques have to adjust their support to stabilize the other leg in the center. Since you are using the leg lift to activate the core, there is some engagement of the hip flexors. But if the hip flexors begin to burn or struggle, it may either mean that this muscle group is trying to do work intended for the abdominals or that the hip flexors are themselves weak and in need of attention. Either way, take a break, possibly stretching out the hips before continuing.

Beginning yoga Bicycle

From the lifted leg toe-tap variation, we finally progress into a common core exercise in general population yoga classes: the yoga Bicycle. I have seen more than a fair share of yoga Bicycles practiced without

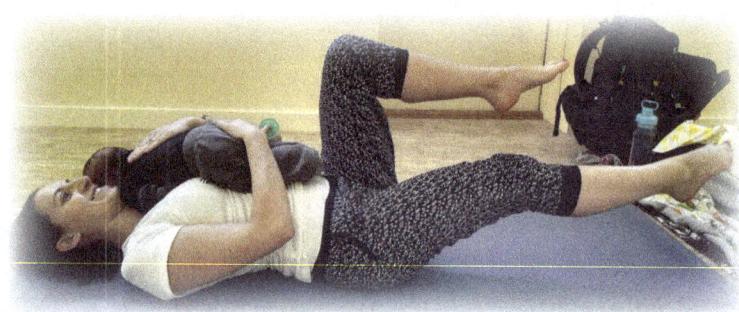

awareness of the deep core and with significant front wall tenting or lower back instability. In this progression, however, you have built up enough internal strength and awareness that you can safely and mindfully load the abdominal wall. Note that you are still not lifting the head here.

Having exhaled and lifted both feet off the floor, hold the knees at 90 degrees to the hips. On an inhale, maintaining the TA engagement, extend the right leg out in front until the knee is straight. The height of the extended leg will depend on where the core can remain integrated and supportive. Lower will be more challenging, higher will be less of a muscle load. Find the height where the TA and pelvic floor can maintain stability.

On the exhale, switch which leg is extended, moving both legs simultaneously. The front abdominals should remain supportive and not tent throughout the whole exercise, and the breath should still be deep and full. Inhale and exhale smoothly, switching extended legs 10 times. Then pause with the legs lifted at 90 degrees and check your stability. If all is well, continue for another set. If you lose support from the front wall at any point, return to a less intense version of this exercise.

These exercises are intended to be done progressively. If you overload the core at any point during this progression of exercises, the body will find ways to cheat. That's why it's always better to drop down to the previous level than strain or struggle at a "higher" stage. Moving slowly builds your foundation, and a strong foundation then supports the wider practice.

Head-lift core exercise/crunches

I hate crunches! They hurt my neck, wreck my back, and make me feel completely incapable of lifting up off the floor. The good news is that in my years of teaching I have found these exercises are not the best focus for gaining abdominal strength. In fact, they're usually done with so little awareness that I encourage students to stop doing them altogether! Yes, you read that right: STOP DOING CRUNCHES!

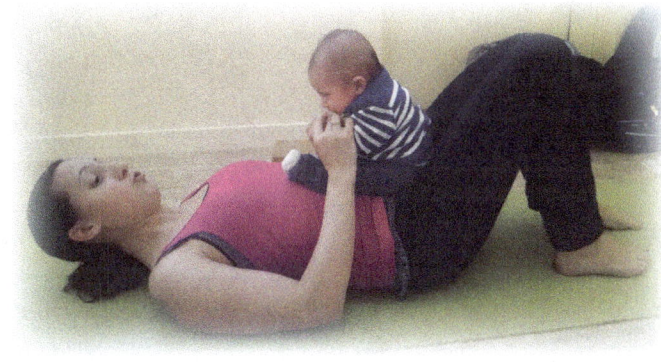

But that doesn't mean you are never going to do head-lift core exercises again. As you've probably figured out by now, the focus for front core work is always on whether the deep abs are stabilizing appropriately. If these muscles are online, you can begin introducing head lifts, provided you take precautions around diastasis recti and focus on building stamina, not speed.

Start lying on your back, knees bent and hip distance apart. Bring both hands to your lower thighs with the arms extended. Inhale deeply. As you exhale, engage the pelvic floor and TA muscles, and draw your ribs towards your hips so that the deep core engages. Start to roll your upper body off the mat while reaching fingertips towards your knees. See how far you can reach the hands, aiming to cup the palms over the knees. DO NOT let the abdominals pop out or tent. If they do lose the connection, you have gone too high and should lower until you can keep the engagement throughout the whole range of motion.

Inhale, and slowly lower while maintaining core engagement. If the neck begins to hurt during this exercise, place one hand behind the head to support it—keeping the elbow out to the side so the arm doesn't pull on the head. You'll be able to gradually reduce the support as the rectus abdominis gains enough strength to support the weight of the head as well as the upper body. Repeat 5-10 times.

Plank progression

Plank is one of those postures which gets so much focus in the fitness world and a bad rap in the perinatal exercise world. The truth is Plank can be more complicated than it seems. A proper expression requires deep core support to be intact. Because of the gravitational pressure on the front abdominal wall (the weight is falling into the front of the body after all) and the possibility of recruiting the back and shoulders to do the work instead of the core, I find that Plank needs to be rebuilt from the ground up. You may still be in the early stages of a Plank progression at six weeks postpartum.

Activated Table

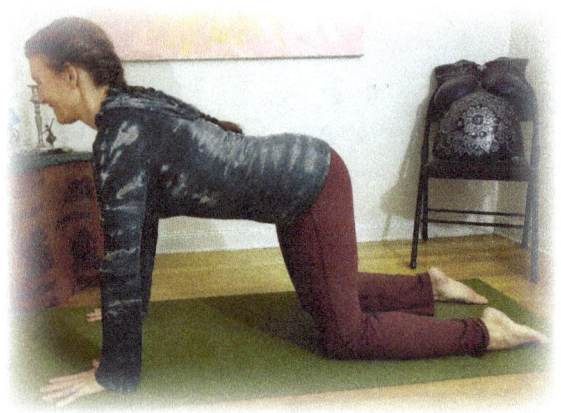

A healthy Plank progression begins in Table. Start on hands and knees. Take a moment to bring the spine into the arch of Cow pose, then reverse to pull the pubis towards the sternum to come into Cat pose. Having felt each extreme, return to the middle and lift the front chest and collar bones as though moving into Cow, but at the same time, gather the hip points together, lengthening the tail as though coming into Cat. Basically, practice Cow from the waist up and Cat from the waist down. The result will be an activated version of Table with the spine stabilized in its neutral curvature.

Remember the pelvic floor is strongest with the pelvis in neutral position, so for moving further, supporting this position will be key. Inhale, holding the abs in and up, then exhale and draw the pelvic floor strongly inward (swimming the jellyfish towards your head). Continue breathing fully, feeling the pelvic floor and deep core respond in support. This Table could be practiced as early as 3-4 weeks postpartum, but make sure lochia bleeding has stopped before attempting something that actively compresses the lower pelvis.

To activate the deep core further, take one hand and place it on your abdomen. Relax the muscles and feel how the abdomen is able to drop into your hand. Now, on an exhale, draw the pelvic floor muscles in and see if you can move the abdomen up away from your hand and slightly forward, as though drawing the navel towards the back of the heart. Don't move your hand with the abdominal muscles or you won't feel the movement. This is the same movement created through engaged TA breathing. If your internal support collapses and can't be recovered, the body is not yet ready for this movement.

Beginning Bird Dog

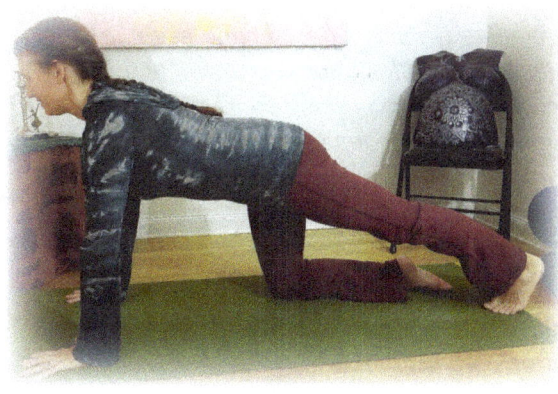

From an activated Table pose, tuck the right toes and extend them back, straightening the knee. Be sure to maintain the deep core control as the leg extends and watch for sinking in the lower back or dropping the front abdominal wall. Holding the leg extended, imagine lifting the second knee off the floor—don't actually do it yet! Feel the deep core organize further. Then inhale to return to Table and exhale to change sides.

Repeat five times on each side or as often as the core can stabilize the action.

As with heel slides and single leg taps, the greatest challenge in this exercise is maintaining pelvic stability when switching from one side to the other. Watch for the abdomen falling or the pelvis shifting during the switch. A simple way to ensure you maintain a stationary pelvis is to place a yoga block on your lower back while practicing. If the block falls off, you know you shifted the pelvis instead of stabilizing from the deep center.

Table hover

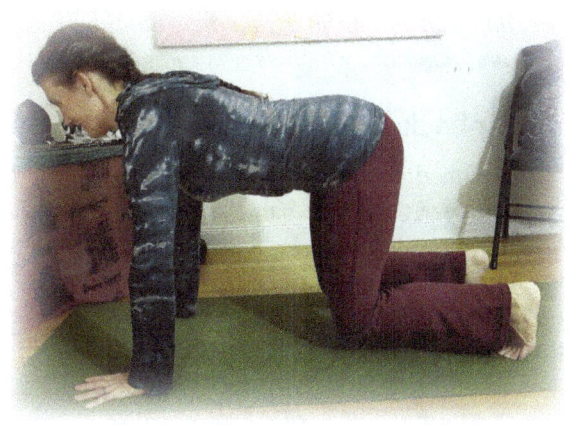

From activated Table, place a block between the upper thighs. Inhale to tuck the toes, and then on an exhale draw in the pelvic floor and deep core as you float the knees one inch off the floor. Feel as though you are lifting from deep in your "guts" rather than using your thighs or arms excessively.

Squeeze the block with the thighs, maintaining the abdominal lift and containment. Hold for 2-3 breaths (and keep breathing!), then release the knees back to the floor. The point is to maintain a neutral spine through the whole exercise, neither rounding nor arching in the mid-back.

Downward Dog into Plank

Once you can stabilize the Bird Dog variation and hold a sustained float of the knees off the floor, you're ready to approach full Plank pose. You want to start this progression in such a way that losing core support won't lead to abdominal separation or other injuries. For this reason, I have students begin in a Downward Dog once they can solidly practice all of the previous exercises.

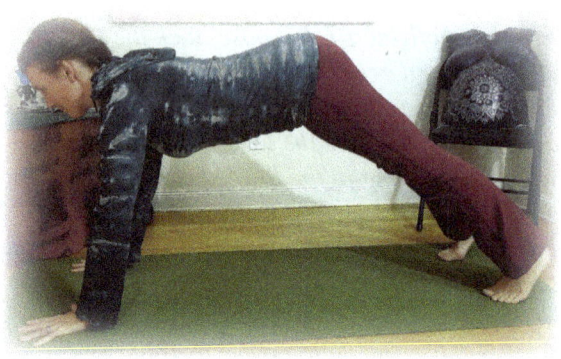

From Downward Dog, take an exhale to gather the pelvic floor in and begin to move the shoulders forward as though the pelvic floor was pushing the rest of the body toward the top of the mat. The spine moves towards neutral curvature, with the chest opening and the pubis and tail merging towards one another.

As the shoulders shift forward, watch the front abdominal wall. When you feel the deep core beginning to work, or you can see the abdomen beginning to drop, pause and see if you can lift the core again by drawing the front hip points together and bringing the navel up towards the center of the chest. This is more than just sucking the abs in. The movement starts at the base and comes up the front body. If you can't regain the lift, back up an inch and try there. Wherever you can maintain a stable center is your Plank for the moment. For most students this means Plank is not a straight line or even parallel to the floor when they begin.

Try this exercise alongside a mirror, as it is extremely easy to lose control and not know it (as I humbly found out myself nine months postpartum). Often it can take months before this coordination comes back together, but the gradual progression builds much deeper awareness and function, which serves in numerous other postures.

Upper back and shoulders

In the immediate days and weeks postpartum it may seem almost as though mom's body wants to re-envelop the baby into itself. Parents curl forward around their children, hunching forward to nurse, or slump into couches from fatigue or lack of back strength. Cue "new parent posture!" I often find that postures which passively shorten the muscles are more beneficial initially. You can progress into active engagement and strengthening *asanas* once the muscles have had a chance to release their built-up tension. Additionally, strengthening the back muscles helps in overall toning of the core body, since the paraspinals and multifidus muscles form the back of the core wall.

There are myriad yoga movements that target the upper back. As I mentioned on pg 172, my absolute favorite is the Upper Back Bolster exercise, lying back over a rolled blanket, towel, yoga block, or foam roller. When working on spinal movement and stability I nearly always begin with some bolster work. Then, having freed some of the chronic tension, I have students turn to more targeted strengthening and stretching.

Other good postures for the upper back include:

Sphinx

You probably are familiar with Sphinx pose as a precursor to prone backbends such as Cobra or Downward Dog. If you are ready to move on from the Slouchy Sphinx variation (page 294), you can take the classic posture, which strengthens the upper back by lifting the head and activating the arms and mid-back.

From Slouchy Sphinx, begin drawing the pelvic floor in and up on an exhale. Then, on the inhale, lift the head from the middle of the back, initiating the action from between the shoulder blades. Press the forearms down into the floor and slightly drag them back against the mat to pull the sternum forward. The action should begin to focus into the upper back between the shoulder blades.

Actively press the knees into the floor and feel the pubis lift subtly, further engaging the pelvic floor. DO NOT grip the glutes! As the neck and head lift, imagine pinwheels on the outsides of the shoulders, softly spinning towards the back. The head lifts as the very last movement, almost as if someone were pulling you up from the tips of your ears. Stay here for a few breaths, then release back to the floor and rest. If the lower back is tender after this pose, engage the glutes and tuck the tail to relieve the excess tension. It might also be worth doing a psoas release and then trying the pose again.

Shalabhasana progression

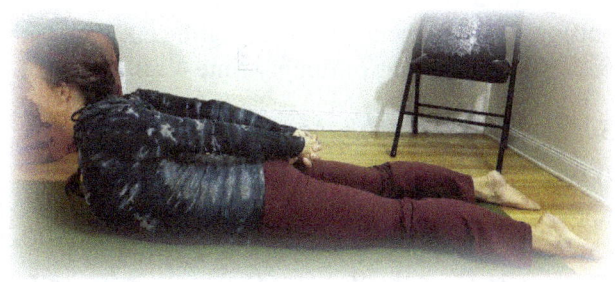

From Sphinx, the next step in strengthening the upper back and posterior core is to remove the support of the arms and let the back muscles bear more weight. As with the supine core progression, be conscious of how much the abdomen presses into the floor when practicing these exercises. The same deep core engagement is required here as you focus on the back side of the abdominal "soda can."

Begin lying on your stomach with the head down and the hands along your side. If possible, clasp the fingers behind your back (or hold a strap if the shoulders are too tight). On an exhale, draw up the pelvic floor and engage the TA. On the inhale, reach the hands back towards the feet, raising the shoulders and chest as much as the body allows. Exhale here.

You might simply repeat this step a few times, moving with the breath. Or, if your body allows, you can try raising the legs (straight knees) on the next exhale, lifting as much as possible off the floor. Remember to lift from the back muscles rather than pushing the belly into the floor to rise. Hold the lift for one more inhale, then release to the ground. Clasping the hands makes it slightly easier to lift the upper back.

Note: It's not uncommon to have one glute that is more responsive than the other. As you lift the legs, notice if one side of the bum engages more readily. This is your strong side, and it impacts the tone of the pelvic floor. Try actively engaging the sleepy side before lifting so both sides work equally, which helps the pelvic floor take a break.

Shalabhasana/Locust

From the clasped hands beginning variation, we can progress to what most of us recognize as the more classic pose of Shalabhasana (Locust Pose).

Begin lying prone with the arms alongside the body. Exhale to engage the deep core and TA. On the inhale, raise both the arms and legs off the floor simultaneously. The focus is on lifting as much from the ground as possible, maintaining good deep core engagement during the full movement.

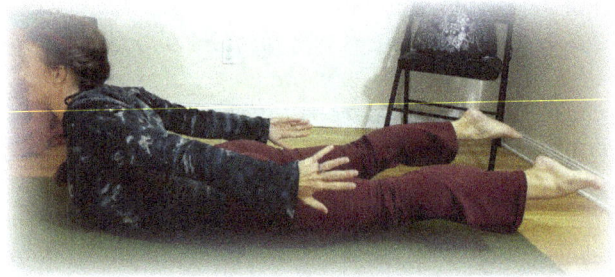

Hold for a couple rounds of breath, then release on the exhale. Squeeze the glutes to tuck the tail if the lower back aches. Repeat several times.

I often find this pose is a great way to commiserate with your baby, who is also doing lots of tummy time to strengthen these same muscles. Try getting down on the floor and doing the exercise with them. You may realize why some babies aren't big fans of tummy time—it's hard!

Super-person Shalabhasana

If you're comfortable lifting both the upper body and legs, you can further challenge your body by raising the arms out in front of you instead of keeping them by your side. Moving the arms forward increases the load the back muscles are asked to support.

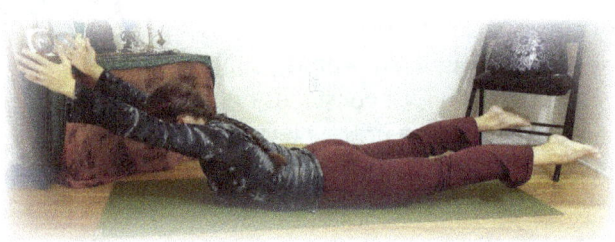

Beginning as for classic Shalabhasana, exhale to engage, then inhale to raise both the arms and legs off the floor. Once up, exhale as you sweep the arms out to the side and then forward towards the front of the mat. Roll the collar bones up, remembering the pinwheels from Sphinx pose. Make sure the breath keeps moving and that the deep core stays connected.

Lift for two more breaths, and on the third gracefully flop onto the floor and release your lower back. You can repeat this action with the arms by the side again or raise the whole pose straight up from the floor where it is. This variation will engage the whole back line, from the shoulders down to the glutes, hamstrings, and even calves. When finished, push back to Child's Pose or take a Downward Dog to stretch.

Bathtub scuba-person

Remember those wind-up scuba people you might have had as bath toys? This final variation mimics that movement, which begins incorporating a twist to recruit the obliques on the front body.

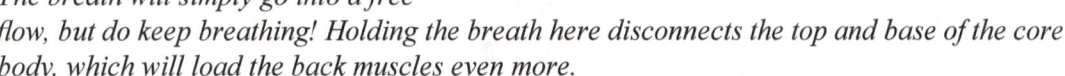

From the super-person variation, with the arms stretched out in front, begin alternately kicking the legs and pulsing the arms up and down, as though swimming in a bathtub. The breath will simply go into a free flow, but do keep breathing! Holding the breath here disconnects the top and base of the core body, which will load the back muscles even more.

Kick up and down for 10 seconds (maintaining deep core connection the whole time), then relax (or gracefully flop) on the floor and take a break. Repeat several times, then push back to Child's Pose.

Shoulder releasing

There are numerous yoga postures for releasing the back and shoulder muscles: Garudasana, Gomukhasana, and even simply standing at a door frame with the arms up in a cactus shape leaning through the door while holding the frame.

It can be helpful to combine several shoulder and upper back movements into a gentle *vinyasa* to work around the whole shoulder girdle in one sequence (because let's face it: we are busy people and sometimes postpartum you only have two minutes!). It can also be fun to involve baby in this sequence!

Garudasana vinyasa sequence

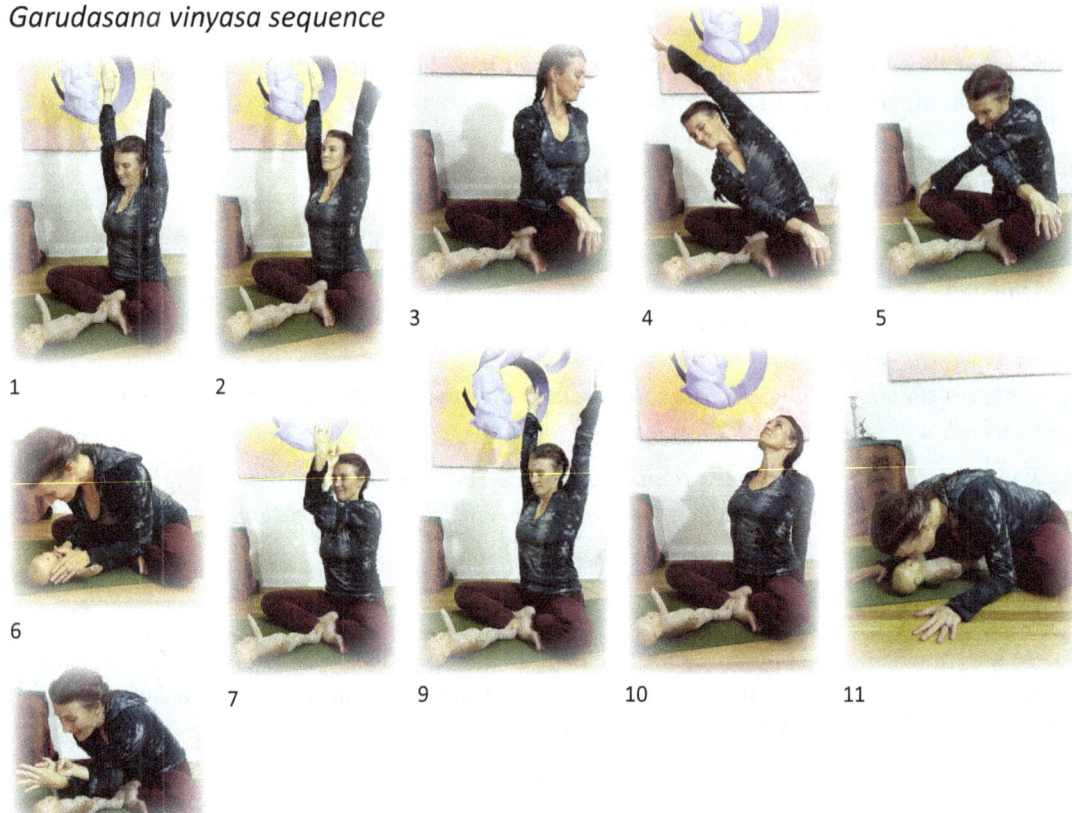

Sit up and switch the cross of the legs. Repeat on the second side.

Hips

Hip stretching

The pelvis continues to need attention postpartum. Just as the psoas can become shortened and tense with prolonged sitting, so too can the gluteal muscles become tense from the hours of holding, soothing, and feeding. Regaining balanced strength in the pelvic bowl can help with overall body movement and enhance recovery because the pelvic joints are better supported as the body readjusts to the postpartum shifts of weight and the center of gravity.

While the internal and external hip rotators do need to be stretched, they also need strength and tone. Otherwise, the body will compensate by recruiting other muscles for support and stability. Compensation leads to unnecessary tension, including lower back pain, pelvic floor dysfunction, and other aches and pains. Yoga offers many options for stretching and strengthening the hips. Here are a few of my favorites:

Figure 4

You can practice this pose seated or supine, but the focus remains the same: increasing flexion at the hip socket to stretch the outer glutes and piriformis.

Begin either seated on a chair, with the weight on the front of the sitz bones, or lying on your back with the knees bent. Cross one ankle over the opposite knee and allow the lifted knee to drop, creating a "4" with your thighs. If seated, work to keep the weight on the front of the sitz bones; avoid letting the pelvis rock backwards. There is no need to lean forward. Simply anchor the inner thighs and ground and stretch up through the spine.

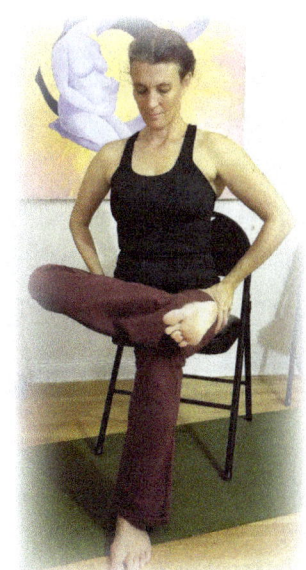

If lying supine, see if you can reach through your legs to hold your thigh, drawing the "4" towards your chest. Don't let the lower back press into the floor. Instead, send the inner groins and tailbone down to the floor. If holding the thigh is not feasible, place the supporting foot against a chair or the wall, and ground the inner thighs towards the floor.

Breathe deeply, bringing the breath into the pelvic floor if possible. Stay here for maybe 30 seconds, then return to the starting position and switch legs.

Ankle to Knee (with baby)

Make sure it is actually the ankle (not the toes or side of the foot) on the knee, and actively flex the crossed ankle so the inner border of the ankle stretches out. The foot should not sickle or twist towards the ceiling. If anything, the outer edge of the foot should reach towards the floor. Activating the foot in this way creates muscular support for the base of the knee, which is where the body will try to borrow the movement from if the hips are tight.

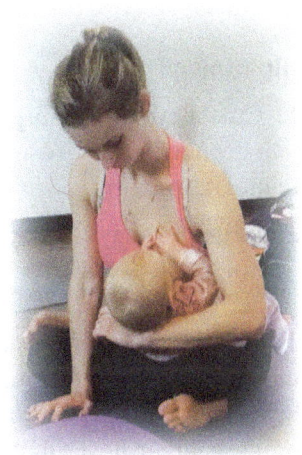

Additionally, the pelvis may try to rock backwards to borrow movement from the lower back, so either press the hands into the floor to tilt the pelvis forward or sit up on a yoga block or blanket. If there is any pressure in the knees, place a block beneath the knee(s) for support, or simply come out of the pose and try the gentler version in a chair or on the floor.

A fun addition is to sit your baby at the top of the crossed thigh and use their weight to anchor the leg down. Fair warning: this will almost certainly increase the sensation. But as a bonus, the bigger baby gets bigger, the more they help you stretch!

Come out by straightening the legs in front and shaking the thighs to unwind any holding. Then repeat on the second side.

Baddha Konasana (with baby)

We did it during pregnancy, but Baddha Konasana (Bound Angle Pose) is also a wonderful hip and pelvic floor release postpartum. It's also a great pose for involving baby!

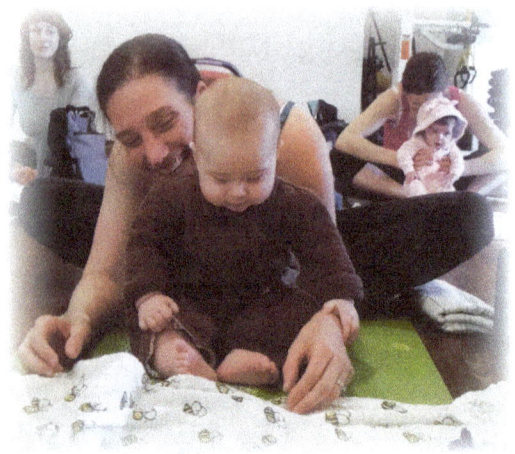

Begin seated with an upright pelvis (weight on the front sitz bones). Bring the soles of the feet together, with the heels close enough to offer a gentle stretch to the inner thighs but also far enough away that the pelvis does not tip backwards. Inhale, stretch up through the spine, and exhale to gently lean forwards, initiating the movement from the hip joint and maintaining a long spine.

If incorporating baby, you may be able to rest them in your lap, with their head cradled by the arches of your feet and their legs draped over or pushing on your inner thighs. Inhale to stretch up, and on the exhale lean forward, making funny faces as you come closer to your child. Some babies enjoy having their parents chant sounds associated with the different chakras, such as "OM," "RAM," "HAM," "LAM," and so on. Sing on the way down, then inhale to roll up. If your baby does not like lying on their back, this is not the time to practice this variation. You can always try again later or practice on your own.

Hip toning

Just about every standing yoga posture uses the glutes for stability. But jumping right back into deep lunges and Warriors is asking for a lot of coordination from muscles that are still reintegrating.

Some gentler ways to begin strengthening the hips and lower back muscles might be:

Utkatasana (with a strap or block)

This exercise was also used for prenatal pelvic floor strengthening. What was good then is still good now. Reintroduce this pose by using a chair to ensure pelvic support and alignment, then progress to the hovering squat once the legs feel strong enough.

Utkatasana for adductor engagement

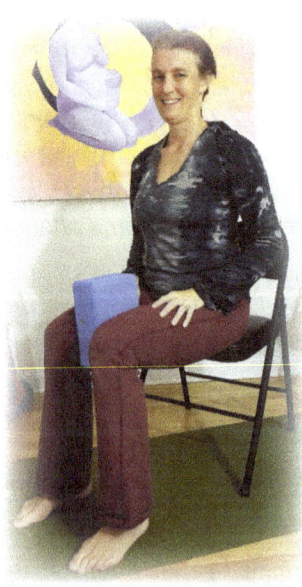

Sit on a firm chair or yoga ball, with the knees at or below the level of the pelvis and the feet planted firmly on the floor. Place the weight on the front of the sitting bones so the pelvic bowl comes into neutral and stretch the spine gently upwards. With the pelvis balanced, place a yoga block between the inner thighs. In your own time, lightly pulse the knees against the yoga block, activating the adductor muscles of the inner thighs. The goal is to pulse for about 60 seconds to begin, then give the legs a break.

Keep the toes relaxed on the floor. Relax and inhale, allowing the pelvic floor to drop, then exhale and engage upwards as though lifting something with the walls of the vagina or like a jellyfish swimming upwards (whichever image works better for you). What sort of response do you get? Repeat this exercise two or three times.

Abductor engagement

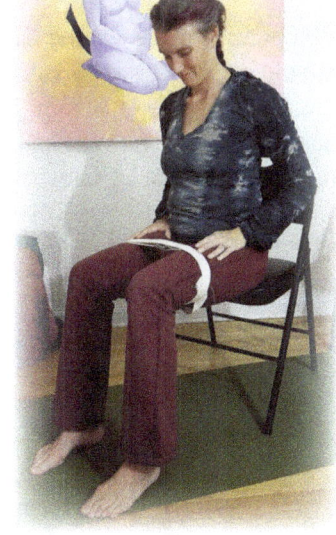

To tone the glutes, sit once again on the chair with the weight forward on the sitting bones. Take a yoga strap (or a scarf or belt if you lack an actual strap), and buckle it into a circle around the mid thighs so it provides some resistance to the outside of the leg. It's important not to place the belt too high or too close to the knees. Gently stretching the spine upright and relaxing the toes, begin to pulse the thighs outwards into the strap. Focus on moving the upper thigh bones apart, as though trying to fit a yoga block back between the legs, rather than simply pushing the knees apart against the strap. It may also feel as though the sitz bones are trying to spread apart. Pulse out with about 50% of the effort you think you could, then relax and repeat. Pulse for 60 seconds, then rest.

Clamshells

Clamshells, while not technically a yoga *asana*, are a great way to directly target the outer glutes and strengthen the pelvic floor. And they can be done lying down—a bonus for tired parents!

Start lying on one side, with knees bent and the legs resting together. The angle of the thighs will depend on what gives you the most access to your glutes (and is therefore appropriately challenging). You can line up the feet with the sitz bones, creating a 45 degree angle in the thighs, or swing the knees forward, making a 90 degree angle with the hips. In either variation, keep the feet together throughout the whole movement. The 90 degree variation will incorporate the smaller glute muscles, while the 45 degree variation will focus more on the gluteus maximus.

Exhale and begin lifting the top knee upwards, keeping the feet together. Lift only as much as is possible without moving the sacrum. The key to practicing Clamshells is to keep the sacrum stable and vertical. This means no rocking back on the pelvis when lifting the top

leg! It may be helpful to place a yoga block behind the hips or, better yet, slide the back up against a wall. If the yoga block falls over, or if you feel the hips trying to press the wall, you're moving the pelvis, not the thigh.

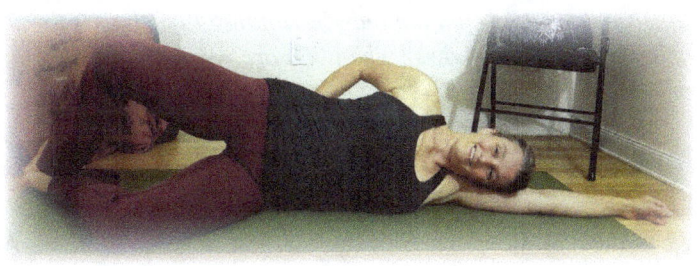

On the inhale, lower the knees back together and repeat. Lift 10 times or until the outer glutes fatigue and it is challenging to keep the pelvis stable. Then drop the top knee over to the floor to stretch the outer hip line before rolling over to practice the second side. Repeat as needed. This is also a great single-sided exercise if you have one glute that is stronger than the other.

I'll confess I always hated Clamshells because this was my weak area (and because it reminded me of ballet class, when I struggled with my relative lack of turnout). When I was practicing these exercises postpartum, I often could not lift my knee more than a few inches before my pelvis wanted to move—and it felt like lifting cement! But that very lack of hip rotation taught me how to practice Clamshells properly rather than cheating through excess flexibility.

Bridge (with baby)

After working the inner and outer hip stabilizers, you can progress to full back-chain activation with Bridge. This pose is also a fun one for involving baby.

Beginning in constructive rest, exhale and press your feet into the floor, opening space

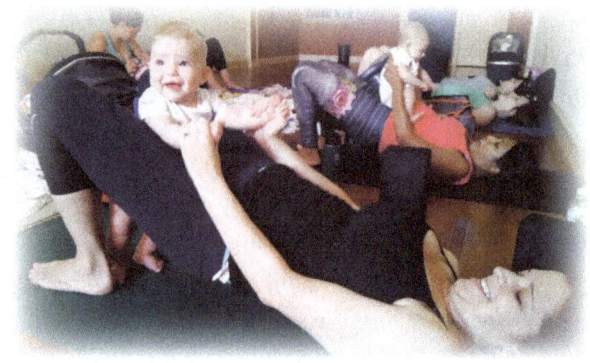

behind the knees. This will raise the hips and shift the weight backwards towards the shoulders. DO NOT FOCUS ON TUCKING THE TAIL! Rather, allow the glutes to engage and float the whole pelvic bowl up towards the ceiling. Allow the back to bend and gently stretch the hip flexors and abdominals. If the lower back feels compressed, pull with the heels as though dragging yourself across the floor to lengthen your spine.

Exhale and hiss through your teeth, pulling your navel and pelvic floor inward as you roll down to the floor. Repeat a few times.

If practicing with your baby, start with them sitting on your abdomen, with your hands stabilizing their core and head. Lift up into Bridge, then pulse the glutes to bounce your hips farther up in the air to give baby a ride. If your baby has good head control, you could instead place them lying between your legs on your stomach. Then, holding their hands, press the feet into the floor and lift them up into a "standing" position between your thighs (Do not squeeze your thighs on the baby!). Holding their hands for stability, add the glute pulses to help them "jump." Lower when you are ready, and hug baby and your knees into your chest and rock side to side.

Involving baby

Let's be honest. If you're only practicing yoga when you have someone to watch the baby or when they are sleeping, your time will be severely limited. After years of teaching postnatal classes, I've found that the true practice of yoga in early parenthood almost always involves bringing the baby into practice rather than trying to keep them out.

It's wonderful to practice alone when possible, but just as the yoga practice eventually bleeds off the mat and into the rest of our lives, so too does postpartum life bleed back onto the yoga mat. In some cases, that means letting go of the posture or *vinyasa* you thought you were going to do and instead being fully present with what is feasible in the moment. But it can also mean physically incorporating baby into the practice. I've included several ways to incorporate baby in the previous exercises. Here are a few other ideas:

- Place them on a blanket near you while you stretch.
- Do mini push-ups from Table while blowing kisses at them.
- Come into Pigeon or Upavistha Konasana, then offer a breast for a long yoga breast-feeding session.

The options are endless once you drop the picture of what you thought postpartum practice would be and instead lean into what it is.

Given that you're effectively engaging in partner yoga, the focus won't solely be on the physical asana but also on your interactions with baby. As many of my own teachers have pointed out, yoga isn't about having the most perfect Downward Dog or Headstand. It is about being a good person and loving ourselves and those around us.

When you share your yoga practice with your baby, you become present to the moment by moment shifts that occur as you and your child grow. That practice is ultimately what transforms you into the conscious parent you hope to be.

Sun Salutations with Baby

Repeat as able (your baby may influence how long you can continue)

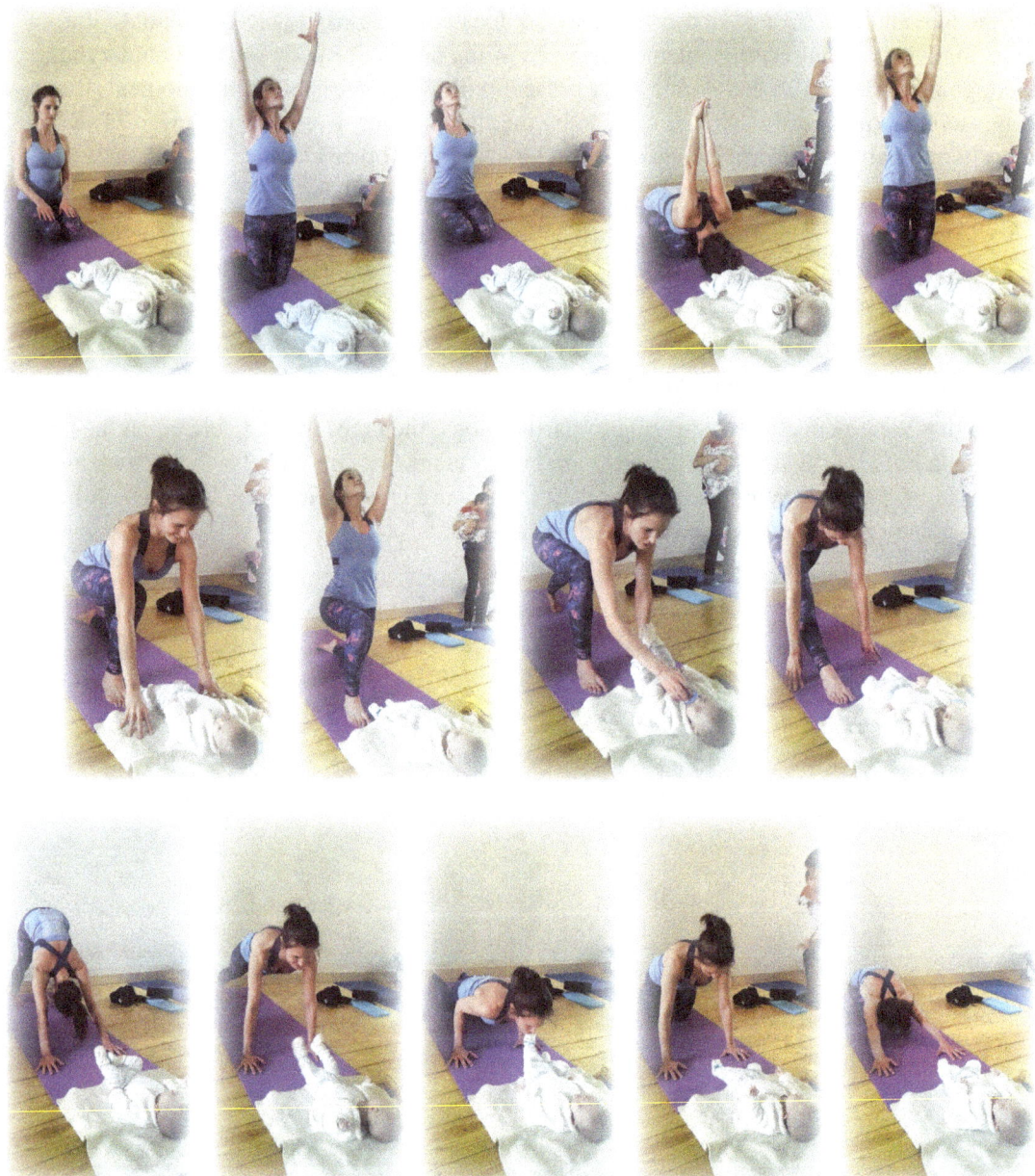

There are numerous ways to involve baby in your yoga practice. We simply need to think beyond the formal *asana* shape.

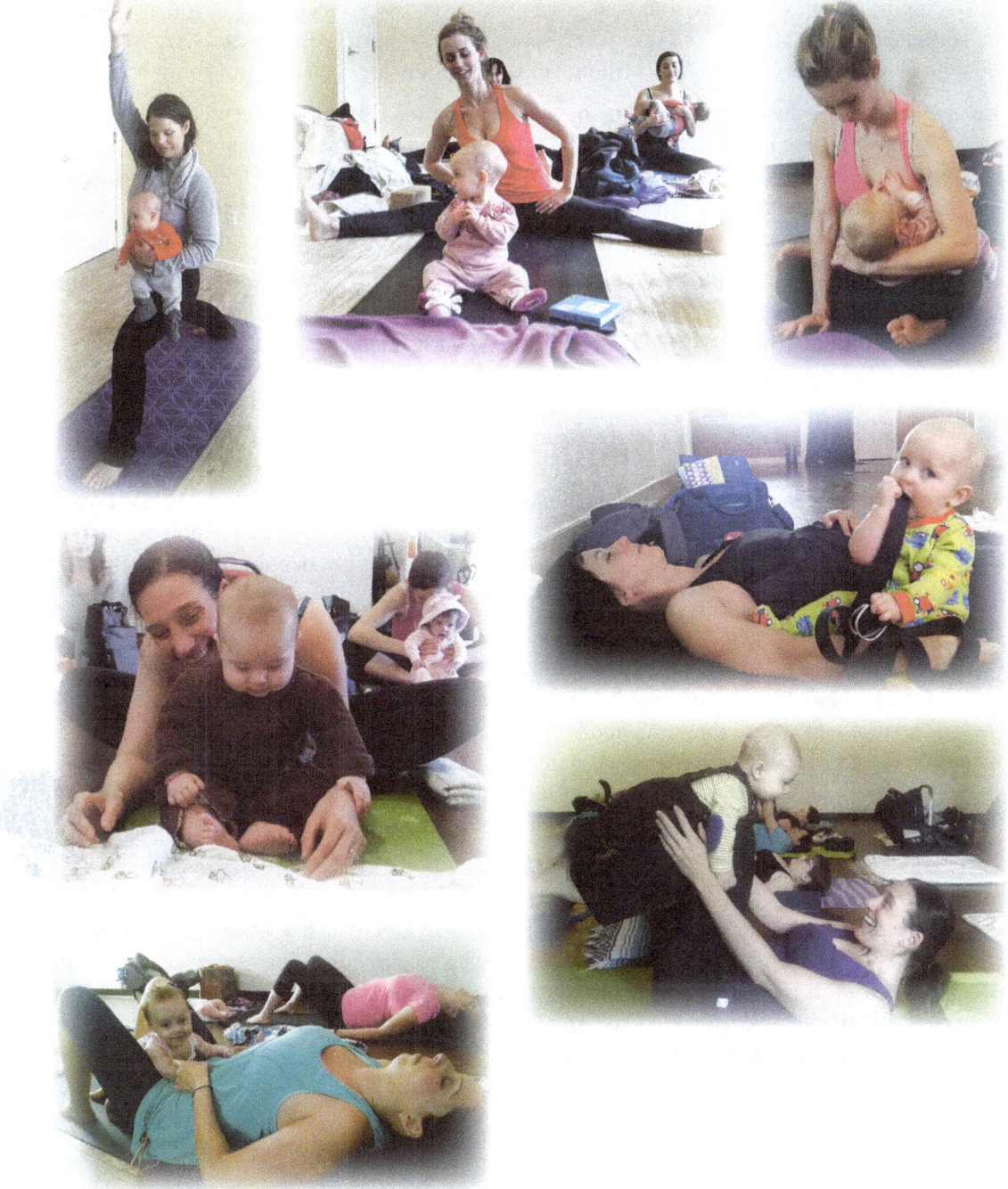

There is more to postpartum yoga than the practices listed in this book. But these exercises are a starting place. Pregnancy can massively shift how you see your body and yourself, and that transformation doesn't disappear when the baby is placed in your arms. That moment is the beginning of a new journey, and your yoga practice can be a touchstone as you navigate the landscape of parenthood. The way you respond to the experiences you encounter shapes the type of parent you become. You will move on, but ultimately you are not "going back."

I remember leaving the hospital with my newborn son in his carseat, my partner at the wheel. As we began the drive home, I voiced the thought that many new parents share: "Honey! They let us leave with a baby!" In that moment, I felt the gravity of what I had gone through and the enormity of what was before me. I was keenly aware of how much had changed, that I was not quite the same person who had conceived this baby nine months earlier. And yet, at the same time, I was.

As the days and weeks progressed, I lost myself in the fog of early parenting and sleep deprivation. But I also had flashes of clarity about who I wanted to be as a parent. There were ways that I both met and fell short of the expectations I had set for myself pre-baby (my expectations were way too high). I expected to be practicing yoga with my baby daily, to meditate during every breastfeeding session. In reality, I mostly forgot about my yoga practice for the first few weeks while I strove to be present during the daily, mundane tasks. Pre-baby, I had been a dancer, a triathlete, a meditator, a size 8, and half a dozen other things. Now I found myself just trying to be present enough to take in my son's face, knowing that in a few days, it would be different (I took many, many pictures of my sleeping baby to help me remember).

The process of matrescence is long and gradual. In many ways, we don't see it happening. I was happy to take on the title of "mom," but I discovered I didn't know who exactly that person was. I've had friends describe it as putting on a pair of shoes that are a bit too big and having to wait to grow into them. I found it to be like discovering which parts of myself were always there and which parts were never really me. Like shedding outfits that had clothed a deeper self, I gradually arrived at a sense of self that was unchanging. The awareness came and went, but it was there—and still is. I sometimes mention this in yoga classes. Deep beneath all the changes and shifts, there is a part of me, of you, that is still here. And maybe that was always your true self.

Beyond the physical balancing, preparation, coping skills, and recovery, our yoga practice offers us the tools to remain curious and present in who we are becoming as parents, and as people, through this process of pregnancy, birth, and parenthood. We can take these moments to step into who we truly are and work with the events surrounding us. May your yoga practice help you walk more fully in the moments of your life. May you welcome your baby with love and joy. And may you find your own way to work with whatever circumstances you encounter on your journey through parenthood.

Appendix: Your Baby Is a Raisin

"We come to know the world through our senses—seeing, touching, hearing, smelling, tasting—and through the knowing faculty of the mind"

—Nancy Bardacke

One common form of mindfulness meditation engages the senses: sight, sound, smell, touch and taste. The classic mechanism for doing this is to use a raisin as an object of meditation, employing the sensory experiences of the raisin to develop and strengthen the ability to be mindful and present. For some parents, engaging the senses can be more stabilizing than trying to focus on something as slippery as the breath in meditation.

While the raisin exercise can be extremely grounding and beneficial in developing awareness, when I have thrown the idea out to new parents coping with the ever changing circumstances a new baby presents, the idea of slowly and mindfully consuming a single raisin seems completely out of reach. For many parents, eating slowly doesn't feel possible when you are grabbing bites of food between feeding sessions or diaper changes. And the baby in your arms presents a constant distraction that seems to interfere with the mindfulness practice.

As with all meditation practice, it is not the object of meditation that matters but the awareness cultivated through that object. Developing this awareness can be a key component in gathering clarity in the midst of the fog of parenthood. Being able to step out of the rambling chatter of the thinking mind offers an opportunity to drop back into the present moment, which in turn offers a chance to see more clearly what is actually going on and whether you are responding in the way you would like.

With all that in mind, there is a way to adapt the raisin meditation to use an object that is very accessible to new parents: the baby! This simple mindfulness exercise helps cut through the stress responses ingrained within our biological instincts as parents. It has been shown via MRI that it's physically painful for mothers to hear their own babies cry. While this response has value, we want the ability to override it in certain instances. Babies will cry, and being in a constant state of stress (i.e., fight/flight/freeze) doesn't benefit you or your child. The way to drop in and be present is by cultivating awareness and, eventually, acceptance of the way things are. We can learn to relax in imperfect circumstances rather than needing everything to be calm and still before we can rest. As I often remind parents during Shavasana practice, "If you are waiting for the baby (or the world) to calm down before you let yourself relax, you are going to be waiting a very long time."

Your baby as the raisin:[69]
(Recorded practice available at: www.ombirths.com/ombirthsbook/your-baby-is-a-raisin)

Sitting, lying, or standing exactly as you are, bring your attention to your body. Feel where you are in contact with the ground. Notice if you wish to shift your posture to be more comfortable, and go ahead and do so if you wish. Do not worry about taking a better or different posture if you are not able to. Simply become aware of the fact that you have a body and that your body is in a posture right now.

Assuming you are holding your baby, bring your focus to the feeling of your baby touching your body. (If you are not holding your baby, simply continue feeling your own body.). Feel your baby's weight against you. The temperature of their body. Any movements they might be making. If your baby is fussy, you might feel their muscle tension or the way their body arches and twists. If they are resting, maybe you can feel their breathing or the little motions of their arms and legs as they shift. Notice if your own body is responding to their movements. How do you shift to continue balancing them as they move? Do you feel any muscle tension of your own?

From feeling (or more likely along with it), shift the attention to looking at your baby. You might already be doing this, but for this moment, truly look and see your baby. What is their facial expression? Again, if they are fussy, this can be challenging, and there is no problem with noticing your own emotional reactions to them being upset. But for this moment, see if you can bring your attention back to simply seeing them.

How is their expression changing? What does their hair look like? Do they have hair? What is their skin tone? What color is the outfit they are wearing (and your mind might remember how many other outfits they have worn today)? Do you have feelings about this outfit? Do you notice any baby acne or cradle cap, and are there accompanying thoughts with those observations? For the moment, try and simply stay with the seeing, and don't solve whatever issues you might be wondering about. Just see this person you are holding or standing near.

Now shift the focus to hearing. What sounds are they making? Crying? Cooing? Do you wish these sounds would cease? Or continue? What responses arise in your own mind? Especially during times when our babies are fussy, it is normal to want to find ways to stop those sounds. Perhaps notice your own desire to make them stop, or perhaps note your own exhaustion. Can you expand your awareness into the sounds in the world around you and your baby? For the moment can you simply hear them as sound? What is the postmodern symphony that provides the soundtrack to your life?

Now, if it is possible, I invite you to bring your nose close to your baby and to breathe in. What does baby smell like? Are you inclined or disinclined towards this smell? Notice if additional thoughts begin to arise, such as, "Do I need to give baby a bath?" or "Is that a

---

[69] This practice is adapted from one originally developed by Nancy Bardacke and used as part of the Mindfulness Based Childbirth Program. Bardacke, N., & Bardacke, N. (2012). The World in a Raisin. *In Mindful birthing: Training the mind, body, and heart for childbirth and beyond* (pp. 31–41), HarperOne.

dirty diaper? When did I last change them?" Take note of these thoughts without necessarily immediately reacting to them. See if you can come back to the simple experience of taking in your baby's smell, just as it is, without judgment.

The final sense of the raisin meditation, taste, is probably not appropriate when focusing on your baby. But if you feel inclined, you could possibly lightly lick your baby's cheek. This is not part of the usual meditation, but you can take a moment to simply notice your reaction to the idea of licking your baby. Animals lick their children quite often; are we so different? Perhaps you feel you are, and that is fine.

To finish, let your awareness spread out to take in the whole dyad of you and your child. You might acknowledge any insights you gathered while practicing mindfulness or just feel the simple feeling of being here with another person. Maybe your mind begins to call up thoughts of how this baby has changed since you have known them. Indeed, how they have changed since they were conceived. From one sperm and egg combining into a single cell, they have grown into this amazing, complex being, just as you also grew from a single cell within your own mother, and she grew from hers, and on and on.

When engaging each sense in this exercise, the others will also come along. Like picking up beads on a string, each sense is entwined with the others in the dance of awareness. You may hear your baby start to fuss and simultaneously feel their body tense and shift as their breathing begins to quicken. You may also notice your own body tensing as you try to stave off what you perceive to be the impending cry. Are you seeing clearly and responding as you intend? Or has your anticipation in fact created a self-fulfilling prophecy in the feedback loop of anticipation and avoidance? You can only know if you are able to sit in the present moment long enough to see clearly.

Acknowledgements

This book was the compilation of over 25 years of teaching experience as well as 5 years of hard work to bring it all together. I want to express my immense gratitude to everyone who supported me through this process to my teachers, all my prenatal students, and all the many Om Births Teacher Trainees who have come through our program over the years. A deep bow to you all for all you have taught me.

Thank to Cyndi Lee for your inspiration and encouragement in starting on this yoga path so many years ago, and helping me see how to be playful alongside mindfulness.

Thanks to Barbara Benagh for the many years of teaching and guidance and showing me how to slow down and truly explore my own internal world more and more.

Thanks to Janice Clarfield for getting me started on the road to prenatal yoga.

Thanks to Judith Lasater for clearing the fog and showing me the true power of the female body in yoga and birth.

Thanks to Leslie Howard for your wisdom, humor, and insight into the world of the pelvis.

Thanks also to David Nichtern for the years of mindfulness instruction, and for the nudge to trust my own instincts.

Thanks also to all my teachers and colleagues in the birth world. To Gail Tully and Lorenza Holt for your wisdom in the birth process. To Kerry Hinds and Sarah Kearns for all the hours of discussion and support with this project and the program.

A huge thank you to Kristen Sweeney and Every Little Word for the editing help, and to Jenny Putnam for holding my hand through the final steps of birthing this "baby."

Thank you to Natalie Nigito for the amazing photos and Dave Stubbart for the cover photo, and to Laura, Kate, Meera, Shilpi, Rebecca, and Kristen for being such awesome models.

Thank you to Lauren Levine for such awesome illustrations and for your never failing friendship all these years.

Thank you to my husband Ryan and my son Sawyer who helped keep me grounded and focused in tough moments.

Thanks to Kim Leuders and Beth Hardiman for making Sawyer's birth the most amazing and enlightening experience it could be.

Thanks to my parents and my sister for their unfailing confidence in my work, and of course. Thank you to my mother Roberta Dew Conant, for everything.

Glossary: Yoga and Prenatal anatomical terminology

Abhinivesha: Sanskrit term for the fear of death (one of the kleshas-obstacles)

Amniotic fluid: The fluid in which the baby floats while gestating

Anal sphincter: The muscular opening at the end of the colon that regulates defecation

Adho Mukha Vrksasana: Yoga Pose. Often translated as Handstand Pose (Literally downward facing tree pose)

Agnistambhasana: Yoga pose. Often translated as Fire Logs, Double Pigeon, or Ankle to Knee

Ananda Balasana: Yoga pose. Often translated as Happy Baby Pose

Anjaneyasana: Yoga pose. Often translated as Lunge, both high and low variations

Annamaya Kosha: The "food" body, the physical sheath of the yogic body view

Anterior pelvic tilt: An orientation of the pelvis which tilts the top of the pelvic bowl towards the front of the body – also called nutation

Anterior superior iliac spine: The bony protuberance at the top of the pelvic bowl in the front, often referred to as the "Hip points" or "headlights". Abbreviated as ASIS

Apana Vayu: The downward energy current of the energy body governing the area from the navel to the perineum

Ardha Chandrasana: Yoga pose. Often translated as Half Moon Pose

Ardha Matsyendrasana: Yoga pose. Often translated as Half seated spinal twist pose (literally translated as Half Lord of the Fishes pose)

Asanas: Yoga Postures, the 3rd limb of yoga practice

Ashtanga: The 8 limb system of organizing the yoga practice and also the name of one of the primary schools of yoga instruction founded by Pattabhi Jois.

Ashwini Mudra: The upward engagement of the anal sphincter brought about either through active contraction, or as a reflexive action after expanding the anal sphincter as in defecation or childbirth.

Asmita: Egoism (one of the kleshas-obstacles)

Asynclitic presentation: When a baby's head enters the pelvis with the neck tilted to the right or the left presenting the side rather than the back of the head to the internal pelvic dimensions.

Atman: The eternal self which does not change throughout our life (or lives)

Anandamaya Kosha: The Bliss body. The deepest sheath of the yogic view of the body.

Avidya: Sanskrit term for ignorance (one of the kleshas-obstacles)

Ayurveda: The holistic health profession associated with yoga

Baddha Konasana: Yoga pose. Commonly translated as Butterfly Pose, literally translated as Bound Angle. Balasana: Yoga pose. Commonly translated as Child's pose

Bandhas: Muscular and energetic actions said to lock energy in the body at certain points. The 3 main bandhas are Mula Bhanda, Udiyana Bandha, and Jalandara Bandha

Bhastrika: A fast paced pranayama, also called Breath of fire.

Bhramari: Bees Breath. A pranayama involving humming

Bhujangasana: Yoga pose. Commonly translated as Cobra Pose

Bodhichitta: The Buddhist principle of the awakened heart

Bradley Method: A method of Childbirth education created by Robert A. Bradley, M.D also sometimes called husband coached childbirth

Breech: When a baby is positioned head up rather than head down in it's mother

Bulbocavernosus: A muscle of the first layer of the pelvic floor

Cervical Spine: The group of 7 vertebrae that compose the neck at the top of the spinal column. These are notated as C1-C7

Cervix: The muscular opening at the bottom section of the uterus that opens during the birth process

Chakra: The wheels of energy said to reside at 7 locations within the body where the main 3 energy channels cross

Chakravakasana: Yoga pose. Commonly translated as rocking child's pose (as though moving back and forth on a wheel)

Chaturanga: Yoga pose. Commonly translated as 4 limbed staff pose, also called low push-up

Colostrum: The precursor to breast milk produced in the breasts in the second and third trimester of pregnancy and what the baby feeds on for the first few days of life.

Constructive rest: Yoga position on the back with the knees bent- no sanskrit name

Corpus luteum: The structure left after an egg breaks out of the developing follicle in the ovary which produces the hormone progesterone to support the pregnancy until the placenta is mature enough to take over.

Dandasana: Yoga Pose. Commonly translated as Staff pose

De Quervain's Syndrome: An inflammation of a nerve bundle in the wrist causing pain to shoot from the thumb and medical side of the wrist joint. Common amongst new mothers and elderly populations

Deep six: A shorthand reference to the 6 primary pelvic stabilizing muscles- Piriformis. Gemellus superior. Obturatur internus. Gemellus inferior. Obturatur externus. Quadratus femoris

Dhanurasana: Yoga pose. Often translated as Bow pose- usually contraindicated for pregnancy

Diastasis recti: A separation along the central fascial sheath of the rectus abdominis muscle (linea alba) of the abdomen. Often discovered postpartum, it can impede core recovery.

Dvesha: Sanskrit term for aversion. (one of the kleshas-obstacles)

Eka Pada Rajakapotasana: Yoga pose. Commonly translated as King Pigeon Pose, or Pigeon pose

Fascia: Connective tissue web running throughout the body interweaving around and between different structures.

Garudasana: Yoga pose. Commonly translated as Eagle Pose

Golgi Tendon Reflex: Also called inverse stretch reflex or autogenic inhibition. An inhibitory effect on the muscle resulting from the muscle tension stimulating Golgi tendon organs (GTO) of the muscle. The result is the muscle fibers relax under pressure.

Gomukhasana: Yoga pose. Commonly translated as Cow-Face-Pose

HELLP syndrome: A life threatening condition during pregnancy consisting of liver dysfunction and red blood cell breakdown. The Acronym stands for Hemolysis, Elevated Liver enzymes, Low Platelets

Hypermobile: Excessive mobility in a joint

HypnoBirthing: A childbirth education technique developed by Marie Mongan utilizing self hypnosis.

Ida nadi: One primary energy channel winding through the body terminating in the left nostril. Said to correspond to the lunar/female/quieting side of the nervous system

Iliacus: Muscle of the hip originating on the interior of the Ilia bone

Ilipsoas: Combination of the Psoas and Iliacus muscle forming a deep hip flexor and spinal stabilizer

Ilium/Ilia: Curving wing bone on each side of the upper pelvis

Innominate/Os-inominata: Latin name for the side pelvic bones composed of the Ilium, Ischium, and Pubis

Interdigitation: Interweaving of muscle fibers

Ischial tuberosities: The sitting bones at the base of the pelvis

Ischiocavernosus: A muscle of the first layer pelvic floor

Ischium: The lower segment of the side bones of the pelvic bowl

Isometric: A muscle contraction that neither shortens or lengthens the muscle

Iyengar: One of the primary schools of yoga instruction founded by BKS Iyengar and known for use of props to facilitate postures

Jaiasana: Yoga pose. Commonly translated as Goddess Pose or wide squat

Janu Sitsasana: Yoga pose. Commonly translated as Head to knee pose

Kapalabhati: Yoga pranayama- involving fast abdominal pulsing. Usually contraindicated in pregnancy

Kapotasana: Yoga pose. Commonly translated as Full Pigeon (not to be confused with Eka Raja Kapotasana)

Kegels: Exercises for the pelvic floor developed by Dr Arnold Kegel, M.D.

Kleshas: Sanskrit term for the characteristics said to cause all human suffering

Koshas: Sanskrit term for the 5 subtle layers of the body

Kumbhaka: Sanskrit term for breath retention

Kundalini: A school of yoga instruction founded by Yogi Bhajan focused on energy work and cleansing practices

Kurmasana: Yoga pose. Commonly translated as tortoise pose

Lamaze: A method of childbirth education founded by Ferdinand Lamaze, especially known for labor breathing practices

Levator ani: A muscle of the third layer of the pelvic floor

Linea alba: The line of fascia connecting the two halves of the rectus abdominis muscle on the front of the body

Lumbar spine: The lower 5 vertebrae of the spine

Malasana: Yoga pose. Commonly translated as garland pose, more commonly known as the squat

Marichyasana: Yoga pose. Commonly translated as Pose of the sage Marichi. Twisting seated posture

Matrescence: Term to describe the period of transformation in becoming a mother. Coined by Aurelie Athan, Ph.D.

Mudras: Symbolic or ritual hand gesture, also said to create seals of energy within the body.

Mula Bandha: The energy lock at the base of the spine said to direct the flow of energy within the body, often associated with a strong engagement of the pelvic floor

Muladhara Chakra: The energy center at the base of the spine

Multifidus: Muscle of the back along the spine

Myofascia: The combined system of muscles and fascia that move and support the body

Nadi Shodhanam: Yoga pranayama breathing practice of alternate nostril breathing

Nadis: Channels of energy within the body like little rivers. Said to number 72,000

Natarajasana: Yoga pose. Commonly translated as Dancer pose

Niyamas: Observances- practices for good living. The second limb of yoga practice

Occiput: Back of the head or skull

Om: Sanskrit seed syllable said to encompass all other sounds within it

Osteopath: Medical profession focused on interconnectedness within the body. Practice includes manual manipulation along with conventional medical practice

Pranamaya Kosha: The energy layer of the body

Paraspinals: A group of muscles on the back of the body

Parasympathetic nervous system: The relaxation response side of the nervous system

Parighasana: Yoga pose. Commonly translated as Gate pose

Parivritta Janu Sirsasana: Yoga Pose. Commonly translated as Rotated head to knee pose

Parivrtta Prasarita Padottanasana: Yoga pose. Commonly translated as Rotated wide legged forward fold

Parivrtta Trikonasana: Yoga pose. Commonly translated as rotated triangle pose

Parsva Virabhadrasana: Yoga pose. Commonly translated as Side/Reverse Warrior Pose

Parsvakonasana: Yoga pose. Commonly translated as Side Angle pose

Parsvottanasana: Yoga pose. Commonly translated as Intense side stretch, also translated as half intense forward fold

Paschimottoanasana: Yoga pose. Commonly translated as Stretch of the west, also called seated forward fold

Pelvic floor: Muscles in the floor of the pelvic bowl responsible for bladder and bowel function as well as deep core support

Perineum: The space between the vagina and anus where the first and second layers of the pelvic floor interweave

Pincha Mayurasana: Yoga pose. Commonly translated as Forearm stand pose

Pingala nadi: One primary energy channel winding through the body terminating in the right nostril. Said to correspond to the solar/male/active side of the nervous system

Placenta previa: A condition in pregnancy when the placenta fully or partially covers the cervix

Posterior chain: The muscles located on the back of the body. Involved in almost all bodily movement

Posterior superior iliac spine: The bony protuberance on the back of the pelvic wing bones

Posterior pelvic tilt: A position of the pelvis rocking the top of the pelvic bowl towards the back of the body. Also called counternutation.

Prana Vayu: The upward energy current in the body running from the navel to the throat

Pranayama: Yogic breath practices

Prasarita Padottanasana: Yoga pose. Commonly translated as Wide legged forward fold pose

Progesterone: A hormone secreted during menstrual cycle and pregnancy that sustains the uterine lining

Prolapse: A condition where an organ slides downward from its normal position in the body and often pushes into another organ or body structure

Proprioception: The internal sense of the body's placement in space

Psoas: The muscle running from the front of the spine beginning at T12, and ending on the lesser trochanter of the inner femur. Primary hip flexor in the body

Pubic symphysis: The joint between the two pubic bones at the front of the pelvis

Raga: Sanskrit term, attachment. (one of the kleshas-obstacles)

Rebozo: Traditional Mayan and Mexican shawl woven for work in labor and birth

Rectus abdominis: The surface abdominal muscle composed of 2 bands of muscle connecting the lower ribcage to the pubis. Also known as the "six pack" muscle

Relaxin: A hormone released during pregnancy which relaxes connective tissue throughout the body

Round ligament: A uterine ligament running from the upper uterine segment over the pubic bone and attaching into the outer labia

Sacroiliac joint: A joint in the back of the pelvis between the sacrum and the ilium

Sacrum: The triangular bone making up the back of the pelvic bowl

Sahajoli Mudra: An engagement of the front of the pelvic floor.

Samana Vayu: The sideways moving current of energy between the navel and lower ribs

Samma Vritti: Yoga pranayama practice with even inhalation and exhalation

Sarvagasana: Yoga pose. Commonly translated as Shoulderstand

Sciatica: A condition involving compression of the sciatic nerve, usually characterized by shooting nerve pain from the glutes to the outside of the knee

Setu Bandha: Yoga pose. Commonly translated as Bridge pose

Shakti: The feminine energy in the body said to rise through the central channel along the spine; also a Hindu Goddess.

Shavasana: Yoga Pose. Commonly translated as Corpse pose or the relaxation at the end of an *asana* practice.

Sirasana: Yoga pose. Commonly translated as Headstand

Sitali: Yoga pranayama practice said to be cooling to the body

Skandasana: Yoga pose. Commonly translated as Side Lunge

Soma: The physical expression of matter (as opposed to energy)

Spinning Babies®: A childbirth education program developed by Gail Tully focused on myofascial balance and making space for the baby within the body

Sthira: Sanskrit term meaning steady

Sukha: Sanskrit term meaning easy or sweet

Sukhasana: Yoga pose. Commonly translated as easy pose or simple crossed legged pose

Supine hypotension: A condition of low blood pressure brought on from reclining or lying supine. Commonly of concern after 20 weeks of pregnancy

Supta Baddha Konasana: Yoga pose. Commonly translated as Reclining Bound Angle Pose

Supta Virasana: Yoga Pose. Commonly translated as Reclining Hero's pose

Sushumna nadi: The primary energy channel running through the center of the body along the spine

Tadasana: Yoga pose. Commonly translated as Mountain pose

Tantric yoga: A style of yoga involving various ritual practices along with *asana*. Often associated with sexuality in the west.

Tensile strength: The ability to resist movement or bear a physical load

Thoracic: The middle section of the spine consisting of 12 vertebrae from the base of the neck to the top of the lower back. Numbered T1-T12)

Titibhasana: Yoga pose commonly translated as Firefly pose

Transverse abdominis: The deepest muscle layer of the abdominal wall

Trikonasana: Yoga pose commonly translated as Triangle pose

Trochanter: A bony protrusion from the femur

Udana Vayu: The energy current said to inhabit the arms and legs

Uddiyana Bandha: The energy lock in the abdomen. Usually involves a strong upward engagement of the abdominal wall and diaphragm. Generally contraindicated during pregnancy

Ujjayi: Yoga pranayama practice that involves creating a soft audible sound from the back of the throat

Upavista Konasana: Yoga pose. Commonly translated as the straddle split or seated wide legged forward fold

Urdhva Dhanurasana: Yoga pose. Commonly translated as Wheel pose

Ustrasana: Yoga pose: Commonly translated as Camel pose

Utero-sacral ligaments: A set of ligaments extending from the sacrum to the lower segment of the uterus and cervix.

Utkatasana: Yoga pose. Commonly translated as Chair pose

Utthita Hasta Padangustasana: Yoga pose. Commonly translated as Extended hand to big toe pose

Vairagya: Sanskrit term meaning detachment or letting go

Vajrasana: Yoga pose. Commonly translated as Thunderbolt pose or kneeling pose

Vayus: The subtle energy currents within the sheath of the energy body

Vena cava: The primary vein returning blood from the lower to the upper body which runs slightly to the right side of the spine in the back of the pelvis.

Vertebra: The bones of the spine

Vertex: Term referring to a baby being positioned head down in its mother's pelvis

Vijnanamaya Kosha: The subtle layer of the body associated with instinct and wisdom

Viloma pranayama: Pranayama breathing practice involving consecutive inhalations with out an exhale between

Viniyoga: One of the 3 primary school of yoga founded by TKS Desikachar which focuses on adapting the practice individually to each student.

Viparita Karani: Yoga posture. Commonly translated as Legs up the wall, or Deep lake pose

Virabhadrasana: Yoga pose. Commonly translated as Warrior. Several different variations

Virasana: Yoga pose. Commonly translated as Hero's pose

Vishnu Mudra: Hand gesture involving folding the first and second finger into the palm

Vrksasana: Yoga pose. Commonly translated as Tree pose

Vyana Vayu: The energy current running throughout the body said to enliven the tissue

Yamas: Practices of restraint for good living. The first limb of yoga practice.

Bibliography

Americanpregnancy.org/healthy-pregnancy/pregnancy-complications/hellp-syndrome

Anatomytrains.com

B, B., and Marelli, F. "Emotions in Motion: Myofascial Interoception. *Complementary Medicine Research*. March 10, 2017. https://pubmed.ncbi.nlm.nih.gov/28278494/

Bardacke, Nancy. *Mindful Birthing: Training the Mind, Body, and Heart for Childbirth and Beyond*. HarperOne, 2012.

Bardacke, Nancy. *Mindfulness-Based Childbirth and Parent Education*. Mindful Birthing, 2005.

Birth Day. Film Australia, Sydney. 2001.

Boddy, A.M., Fortunato, A., Sayres, M.W., & Aktipis, A. "Fetal Microchimerism and Maternal Health." Bio Essays. August 28, 2016. https://onlinelibrary.wiley.com/doi/full/10.1002/bies.201500059.

Broad, Matthew. *The Science of Yoga*. 1st ed. Simon & Schuster, 2012.

Cassidy, Tina *Birth: The Surprising History of How We are Born*. Reprint. Grove Press, 2007.

Centers for Disease Control and Prevention. "Products - Health e Stats - Maternal Mortality Rates in the United States, 2019. Centers for Disease Control and Prevention. March 23, 2021. www.cdc.gov/nchs/products/hestats.htm

Chan, W.F.N., Gurnot, C., Montine, T.J., Sonnen, J.A., Guthrie, K.A., and Nelson, J.L. "Male Microchimerism In the Human Female Brain." *PLOS ONE*. September, 26, 2012. https:/journals.plos.org/plosone/article?id=10.1371%2Fjournal.pone.0045592

Coventry, P.A., Brown, J.V.E., Pervin, J., Brabyn, S., Pateman, R., Breedvelt, J., Gilbody, S., et al. "Nature-Based Outdoor Activities for Mental and Physical Health: Systematic Review and Meta-Analysis." *SSM - Population Health*. October 1, 2021. https://www.sciencedirect.com/science/article/pii/S2352827321002093?via%3Dihub

Davis, Elizabeth, and Debra Pascali-Bonaro. *Orgasmic Birth: Your Guide to a Safe, Satisfying, and Pleasurable Birth Experience*. Rodale Press, 2010.

England, Pam. *Birthing From Within: An Extra-Ordinary Guide to Childbirth Preparation*. Partera Press, 1998.

Floyd-Davis, Robbie. *Birth as an American Rite of Passage.* 2nd ed. University of California Press, 2004.

Gaskin, I. M. *Ina May's Guide to Childbirth.* Bantam Books, 2003.

Gray, Henry. *Anatomy of the Human Body.* 20th ed. Lea & Febiger, 1918.

Hall, S.J., "Equilibrium and Humman Movement." In Basic Biomechanics, edited by S.J. Hall, New York, NY: McGraw-Hill; https://accessphysiotherapy.mhmedical.com/content.aspx?bookid=2433&sectionid=191511590

Heazell, A., Li, M., Budd, J., Thompson, J., Stacey, T., Cronin, R.S., Martin, B., et al. "Association Between Maternal Sleep Practices and Late Stillbirth - Findings from a Stillbirth Case-Control Study." *BJOG: An International Journal of Obstetrics and Gynaecology.* November 20, 2017. https://pubmed.ncbi.nlm.nih.gov/29152887/

Hinde, N. "Nearly Half of Women Can't Identify the Vagina, So How Can They Spot Cancer?" *HuffPost UK.* September 12, 2022. https://huffingtonpost.co.uk/entry/half-of-women-cannot-identify-vagina-eve-appeal-survey_uk_57c6e0f7e4b085cf1ecccea5.

Hjarttardóttir, S., Nilsson, J., Petersen, C., Lingman, G. "The Female Pelvic Floor: A Dome not a Basin." *Acta Obstetrica Et Gynecologica Scandinavica.* July, 1997. https://pubmed.ncbi.nlm.nih.gov/9246965/

Howard, Leslie. *Pelvic Liberation: Using Yoga, Self-Inquiry, and Breath Awareness for Pelvic Health.* Leslie Howard Yoga, 2017.

Jansen, L., Gibson, M., Bowles, B.C., Leach, J. "First Do No Harm: Interventions During Childbirth." *The Journal of Perinatal Education.* 2013. www.ncbi.nlm.nih.gov/pmc/articles/PMC3647734/

July, Miranda. *The First Bad Man: A Novel.* Canongate Books, 2015.

Kinsella, M.T. and Monk, C. "Impact of Maternal Stress, Depression and Anxiety on Fetal Neurobehavioral Development." *Clinical Obstetrics and Gynecology.* September, 2009. https://wwwncbi.nlm.nih.gov/pmc/articles/PMC3710585/

Matressence.com

Medical Dictionary. "Walcher Position." https://medical-dictionary.thefreedictionary.com/Walcher+position.

Medscape. "How Are the Cardinal Movements of Labor Characterized?" www.medscape.com/answers/260036-172113/how-are-the-cardinal-movements-of-labor-characterized.

Milunksy, A., Ulcickas, M., Rothman, K.J., Willett, W., Jick, S.S., and Jick, H. "Maternal Heat Exposure and Neural Tube Defects." *JAMA.* August 19, 1992. https://www.ncbi.nlm.nih.gov/pubmed/1640616

Moore, Keith, and T.V.N. Persaud. *The Developing Human.* 11th ed. Saunders, 2019.

Nutritiousmovement.com

Osterman, M.J.K, Hamilton, B.E., Martin, J.A., Driscoll, A.K., & Valenzuela, C.P. "National Vital Statistics Reports - Centers for Disease Control and ..." National Vital Statistics Reports. February 7, 2022. https://www.cdc.gov/nchs/data/nvsr70/nvsr70-02-508.pdf.

Peart, K.N. "The Science of Baby-Making Still a Mystery for Many Women." *YaleNews.* January 28, 2014. https://news.yale.edu/2014/01/27/science-baby-making-still-mystery-many-women.

Plant, R. "What is Relaxin?" Verywell Family. June 14, 2021. https://www.verywellfamily.com/what-is-relaxin-5180381.

Silver, R.M., Hunter, S., Reddy, U.M., Facco, F., Gibbins, K.J., Grobman, W.A., Mercer, B.M., et al. "Prospective Evaluation of Maternal Sleep Positions Through 30 Weeks of Gestation and Adverse Pregnancy Outcomes." *Obstetrics and Gynecology.* October, 2019. https://pubmed.ncbi.nlm.nih.gov/31503146/

Shah, N. "The Rise of C-Section – and What it Means." *U.S. News and World Report.* September 25, 2019. https://www.usnews.com/news/healthiest-communities/articles/2019-09-25/the-rise-of-c-sections-and-what-it-means.

Sperstad, J.B., Tennfjord, M.K., Hilde, G., Ellström-Engh, M., Bø, K. "Diastasis Recti Abdominis During Pregnancy and 12 Months After Childbirth: Prevalence, Risk Factors and Report of Lumbopelvic Pain." *British Journal of Sports Medicine.* September, 2016. https://www.ncbi.nlm.nih.gov/pmc/articles/PMC5013086/

Soet, J.E., Brack, G.A., and Dilorio, C. "Prevalence and Predictors of Women's Experience of Psychological Trauma During Childbirth." *Birth.* Berkeley, California. March, 2003. https://pubmed.ncbi.nlm.nih.gov/12581038/

Spinning Babies. https://spinningbabies.com/pregnancy-birth/techniques/other-techniques/rebozo-manteada-4.

Stacey, T., Thompson, J.M.D., Mitchell, E.A., Ekeroma, A.J., Zuccollo, J.M., McCowan, L.M.E. "Association Between Maternal Sleep Practices and Risk of Late Stillbirth: A Case-Control Study." *The BMJ.* June 14, 2011. https://www.bmj.com/content/342/bmj.d3403

Stahl, J.E., Dossett, M.L., LaJoie, A.S., Denninger, J.W., Mehta, D.H., Goldman, R., Fricchione, G.L., et al. "Relaxation Response and Resiliency Training and Its Effect on Healthcare Resource Utilization." *PLOS ONE.* March 13, 2015. https://journals.plos.org/plosone/article?id=10.1371%2Fjournal.pone.0140212

The Complete Guide to The Alexander Technique. https://alexandertechnique.com

Tozzi, P. "Does Fascia Hold Memories?" *Journal of Bodywork and Movement Therapies.* 2014. 18(2), 259-265. https://doi.org/10.1016/j.jbmt.2008.09.001

Trueba, G., Contreras, C., Velazco, M.T., Lara, E.G., Martinez, H.B. "Alternative Strategy to Decrease Cesarean Section: Support by Doulas During Labor." *The Journal of Perinatal Education.* 2000. https://wwwncbi.nlm.nih.gov/pmc/articles/PMC1595013/

Verny, T. R., and J. Kelly. *The Secret Life of the Unborn Child.* Dell Pub. Co., 1988.

Visco, C. "Promoting the Health of Mother and Baby During Pregnancy Using Ayurveda." *California College of Ayurveda.* April 9, 2014. https://www.ayurvedacollege.com/blog/pregnancy.

Index